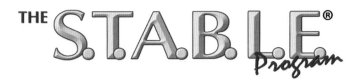

Post-resuscitation/Pre-transport Stabilization Care of Sick Infants — 7th EDITION

Guidelines for Neonatal Caregivers

Kristine A. Karlsen

Learner Manual

This educational program provides general guidelines for assessing and stabilizing sick infants in the post-resuscitation / pre-transport stabilization period. Because of rapid advances in nursing and medicine, independent verification of diagnoses, stabilization recommendations, and drug utilization and doses should always be made by the healthcare professional. Medical decisions should not be made based solely upon the content herein. Changes in nursing and medicine may impact the patient care recommendations in this book. It is the reader's responsibility to verify their care practices are current with any new evidence that arises. To the fullest extent of the law, no responsibility is assumed by, and no damages may be assessed against the authors, the content reviewers, the publisher, or S.T.A.B.L.E., Inc. for any injury and/or damage to persons as a matter of negligence, or otherwise, or from any use of the instructions, guidelines, or recommendations contained in the content herein. While caring for infants, healthcare professionals may encounter situations, conditions, and illnesses not described in this book. It is strongly recommended that additional nursing and medical education materials and consultation with neonatal and other subspecialists are utilized when necessary. Use of this book implies your acceptance of this notice and disclaimer. Prior to implementing these program guidelines, the content of this manual should be reviewed and approved for use by appropriate policy committees at your institution or facility.

A very special thank you to the families and staff at Children's Minnesota Minneapolis and St. Paul campuses, Northfield Hospital in Northfield, MN; Lakeview Hospital in Stillwater, MN; Rush University Medical Center in Chicago, IL; and University of Utah Hospital, Salt Lake City, UT for allowing our photography team to take photos and videos of their patients and staff for this 7th edition.

ISBN: 978-1-937967-20-8

Address communications to:

Kristine A. Karlsen, PhD, NNP-BC, FAAN
The S.T.A.B.L.E.® Program
P.O. Box 980023
Park City, Utah 84098 USA
Phone 1-435-655-8171
Email: stable@stableprogram.org
www.stableprogram.org

Copy Editor
Nichole DelValley, WriteRN

Graphic Designer
Kristin Bernhisel-Osborn, MFA

Medical Illustrator
John Gibb, MA

Photographers
Jill A. Bauer, MAN, RNC
Susan Sieg, MSN, NNP-BC

PowerPoint Designer
Mary Puchalski, DNP, CNS, NNP-BC

This book is dedicated to my twin grandchildren—Lilianna Grace and Stella Willow. Taking you home from the hospital and watching you grow and develop has been a constant reminder of the power of this education. And to my family, Torbjorn, Annika, and Solveig, you have been with me every step of the way, and without your love and support, there would be no S.T.A.B.L.E. Program. And to the many incredible and dedicated neonatal health caregivers I have had the privilege to meet, your expertise and knowledge impact so many and help to improve the lives of babies and their families.

Content Reviewers

Specialty Reviewers

Sugar Module

Camilia R. Martin, MD, MS
Division Chief of Neonatology
Weill Cornell Medicine
New York, New York

Michael Narvey, MD, FRCPC, FAAP
Associate Professor
Section Head, Neonatology
Medical Director - Child Health
Transport Team
Winnipeg, Manitoba
Canada

Paul J. Rozance, MD
The Frederick C. Battaglia Chair in
Neonatology Research
Children's Hospital Colorado
Professor of Pediatrics, Neonatal
Medicine
University of Colorado School of
Medicine
Perinatal Research Center
Aurora, Colorado

**Elizabeth Sharpe, DNP, APRN,
NNP-BC, FAANP, FAAN**
Associate Clinical Professor, College
of Nursing
The Ohio State University
Columbus, Ohio

Paul S. Thornton, MD
Medical Director of Diabetes and
Endocrinology
Director of the Congenital
Hyperinsulinism Center
Cook Children's Medical Center
Fort Worth, Texas

Temperature Module
Appendix 2.1 HIE

Tara L. DuPont, MD, FAAP
Neonatologist
Associate Professor of Pediatrics
University of Utah
Salt Lake City, Utah

Sonia L Bonifacio, MD
Neonatologist
Director NeuroNICU
Clinical Professor, Pediatrics
Neonatal and Developmental
Medicine
Stanford University School of
Medicine
Palo Alto, California

**Kathi Salley Randall, MSN, CNS,
NNP-BC**
Neonatal Nurse Practitioner
International NeuroNICU Consultant
Synapse Care Solutions
Las Vegas, Nevada

Airway Module

Kimberly S. Firestone, MSc, RRT
Director of Respiratory Care and
Clinical Outreach Services
Akron Children's Hospital
Akron, Ohio

Donald M Null, MD
Emeritus Professor of Pediatrics,
Division of Neonatology
University of Utah School of Medicine
Salt Lake City, Utah

Howard Stein, MD
Medical Director, NICU, ProMedica,
Ebeid Children's Hospital.
Section Head, Neonatology
Professor of Pediatrics, University of
Toledo College of Medicine and Life
Sciences
Toledo, Ohio

Bradley A. Yoder, MD
Professor of Pediatrics, Division of
Neonatology
University of Utah School of Medicine
Salt Lake City, Utah
Airway and Lab Work modules

Blood Pressure Module

**Collin G. Cowley, MD, FAAP, FACC,
FAHA**
Professor of Pediatrics
Division of Pediatric Cardiology
University of Utah
Salt Lake City, Utah

Lab Work Module

Robert D. Christensen, MD
Professor of Pediatrics
University of Utah Health, and
Director, Neonatology Research
Intermountain Health
Salt Lake City, Utah

Michael Kuzniewicz, MD, MPH
Neonatologist/Research Scientist II
Director, Perinatal Research Unit
Kaiser Permanente Northern California
Oakland, California

Robin Ohls, MD
Division Chief, Neonatology
University of Utah School of Medicine
and Primary Children's Hospital
Neonatal Intensive Care Unit
Salt Lake City, Utah

Quality Improvement

Taylor Sawyer, DO, MBA, MEd
Division Head & William Alan Hodson
Endowed Chair of Neonatology
Medical Director, Seattle Children's
Simulation Program
Professor of Pediatrics
Division of Neonatology
Seattle Children's Hospital
Seattle, Washington

Neonatologists
Neonatal ICU Nurses
NICU Nurse Practitioners

Jill Bauer, MAN-Ed, RNC
NICU nurse and former Neonatal
Outreach Educator (MN, Western WI)
S.T.A.B.L.E. Program Lead Instructor
Children's Minnesota
St Paul/Minneapolis, Minnesota

**Adelaide B. Caprio, MSN, APRN,
ACCNS-N, RNC-NIC**
Neonatal Clinical Nurse Specialist
Rush University Medical Center, Rush
Children's Hospital
Owner, Hatch & Bloom Consulting
Chicago, Illinois
Temperature and Emotional Support

**Prof. Bill Chan, MBBS, FHKCP,
FHKAM, FRCPCH, FRCP**
Clinical Professional Consultant
Professor of Practice in Paediatrics
The Chinese University of Hong Kong
Hong Kong
Sugar Module

Bridget Cross, DNP, APRN, NNP-BC
Neonatal Nurse Practitioner
Texas Children's Hospital
Assistant Professor, Baylor College
of Medicine
Houston, Texas

**Alice Eames, RN BSc (Child Branch),
Grad Cert (Neonate Crit Care)**
Neonatal Clinical Nurse Educator
Fiona Stanley Hospital
Perth, Western Australia
Sugar Module

Brigitte A. Grissom, MSN, NNP-BC
Neonatal Nurse Practitioner
S.T.A.B.L.E. Program Coordinator
for Landstuhl Regional
Medical Center (LRMC)
Germany
Sugar and Temperature modules

**Elaine R. Hamilton, MS, MBA, CPNP,
NNP-BC**
Neonatal Nurse Practitioner
Camp Pendleton
Camp Pendleton, California

Tracy Karp, MS, NNP-BC
Advance Practice Practitioner (APP)
Neonatology (Emeritus)
Primary Children's Hospital
Salt Lake City, Utah

**Anil Kumar N. Lakkundi, MBBS,
MRCPCH, FRACP**
Consultant Neonatologist
John Hunter Children's Hospital
Newcastle, NSW
Australia
Sugar Module

**Pong Kwai Meng, FRCPCH,
FRCP, CHSE**
Consultant Neonatologist
Certified Healthcare Simulation
Educator
Penang Adventist Hospital
Penang, Malaysia
Sugar Module, HIE Appendix

**Sally Overington, RGN/RSCN NNP
MSc**
Neonatal Nurse Practitioner
NICU Waikato Hospital
Hamilton, New Zealand
Airway and Blood Pressure Modules

**Webra Price-Douglas, PhD, CRNP,
IBCLC**
Former Coordinator Maryland
Regional Neonatal Transport Program
University of Maryland Medical Center
and Johns Hopkins Hospital
Baltimore, Maryland
S.T.A.B.L.E. National Faculty

**Mary Puchalski, DNP, APRN, CNS,
NNP-BC**
Ann & Robert H. Lurie Children's
Hospital of Chicago
Clinical Assistant Professor, University
of Illinois at Chicago
Chicago, Illinois

**Dr Kirsten Ramadas, FRACP, DCH,
MBChB**
Consultant Neonatologist
Fiona Stanley Hospital
Perth, Western Australia

**Patricia A. Scott, DNP, APRN,
NNP-BC, C-NPT**
Coordinator of Neonatal
Transport Services
Centennial Medical Center
Assistant Professor
Vanderbilt University
School of Nursing
Nashville, Tennessee
S.T.A.B.L.E. National Faculty

Catherine Smith, MSN, RN
Clinical Nurse Educator, NICU
S.T.A.B.L.E. Program Director for
Walter Reed National Military
Medical Center
Bethesda, Maryland

**Dr. Rory Trawber, FRACP, MBBS,
BSc**
Director Medical Education
Neonatologist
Fiona Stanley Fremantle Hospitals
Perth, Western Australia

**Mary Youngblood, RN, BSN,
RNC-NIC**
Neonatal Intensive Care Nurse
S.T.A.B.L.E. Lead Instructor
Johns Hopkins All Children's Hospital
St. Petersburg, Florida

Neonatal Pharmacist

Danielle M. Scott, PharmD, BCPPS
Advanced Clinical Pharmacist
Neonatal Intensive Care Unit
Intermountain Medical Center
Murray, Utah

Obstetrics

Michael W. Varner, MD
Professor Emeritus, Obstetrics and
Gynecology
Maternal-Fetal Medicine Division
University of Utah
Health Sciences Center
Salt Lake City, Utah

Ross McQuivey, MD
Adjunct Clinical Instructor
Stanford University School of
Medicine
Department of Obstetrics &
Gynecology
Stanford, California

Pediatric Surgery

Earl C. (Joe) Downey, MD
Clinical Professor of Pediatric Surgery
Formerly, University of Utah
Salt Lake City, Utah

Table of Contents

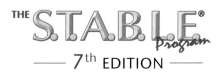

Introduction

Program Philosophy

All hospitals or birthing centers must be prepared for the resuscitation, stabilization, and transport or transfer of sick and/or preterm infants. Hospitals without delivery services should also prepare for the unexpected arrival of sick infants in the emergency department. A uniform, standardized process of care and a comprehensive team approach can improve the infant's overall stability, safety, and outcome.[1-4]

Program Goals

The S.T.A.B.L.E. Program is designed to provide essential information about neonatal stabilization for maternal/infant caregivers in all settings—from first responders, rural hospitals, and birth centers to emergency departments and more complex hospital environments.

Goal 1: Improve patient safety for infants by:

   (a) Standardizing processes and approach to care,

   (b) Encouraging teamwork,

   (c) Identifying areas where medical errors can and do occur, and

   (d) Reducing and eliminating preventable adverse events and errors.

Goal 2: Organize this information using a mnemonic to assist with the retention and recall of essential stabilization activities necessary for the post-resuscitation/pre-transport care of sick infants.

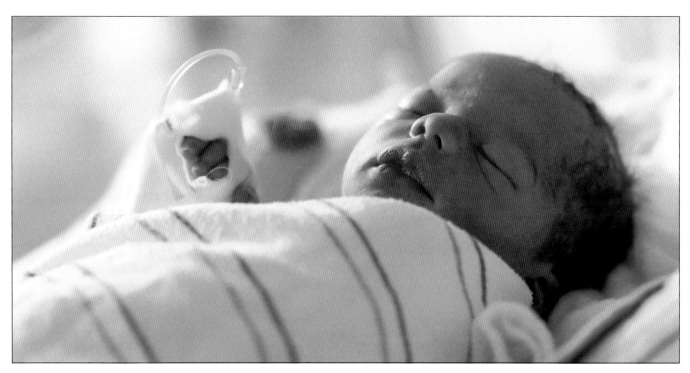

The S.T.A.B.L.E. Mnemonic

Healthy infants far outnumber those who are sick. Therefore, in some settings, caregivers may have difficulty remembering what to do for the sick infant. The mnemonic "S.T.A.B.L.E." was created to assist with the recall and retention of information and to standardize and organize care in the post-resuscitation/pre-transport stabilization period.[5-7]

S stands for SUGAR

The Sugar module contains care recommendations that outline actions to take when an infant is sick and cannot tolerate enteral feedings. The initial intravenous (IV) therapy and how to monitor for and treat hypoglycemia are explained in detail. Infants at-risk for hypoglycemia but who are healthy enough to tolerate enteral feedings are also discussed. Additionally, this module reviews indications for and safe use of umbilical catheters.

T stands for TEMPERATURE

This module reviews the special thermal needs of infants, including those at increased risk for hypothermia, how body heat is lost and how to reduce heat loss, the consequences of hypothermia, and precautions about how to rewarm hypothermic infants.

A stands for AIRWAY

This module reviews the evaluation of respiratory distress, common neonatal respiratory diseases, airway challenges, detection and treatment of a pneumothorax, blood gas interpretation, signs of respiratory failure, and when to initiate and/or increase the level of respiratory support.

B stands for BLOOD PRESSURE

This module reviews the four major causes of shock in infants: hypovolemic, obstructive, cardiogenic, and septic shock, and how to assess and treat shock.

L stands for LAB WORK

This module focuses primarily on neonatal infection: maternal and neonatal risk factors, clinical signs, laboratory tests to obtain, and the initial antibiotic treatment for suspected infection.

E stands for EMOTIONAL SUPPORT

This module reviews the emotional crisis surrounding the birth of a sick infant and how to support families when their infant needs intensive care.

A 7th module, Quality Improvement, completes the course to discuss methods to improve patient safety and the importance of effective communication and teamwork. Providing safe, quality care and eliminating preventable errors is a top priority of The S.T.A.B.L.E. Program curriculum.

 This caution symbol is used throughout the program to draw attention to safety concerns and precautions so that extra care and attention may be taken.

The ABCs . . .

When faced with an unexpectedly sick newborn, caregivers often ask, "Where should I start?" In any critical care situation, rapidly assess the infant and first devote attention to immediate resuscitation needs. As we progress through the mnemonic of **S.T.A.B.L.E.**, remember that the ABCs of resuscitation—Airway, Breathing, and Circulation—are the first priority. Although the algorithm for cardiac resuscitation care prioritizes high-quality cardiopulmonary resuscitation for children and adults, the priority for neonates remains **Airway** first.[8,9] Therefore, this program mnemonic is based upon:

$$A \ B \ C \ \rightarrow \ S.T.A.B.L.E.$$

Although a resuscitation course is not a prerequisite for the S.T.A.B.L.E. curriculum, it is strongly recommended that participants also complete the Neonatal Resuscitation Program (NRP; aap.org),[10] the American Red Cross Neonatal Advanced Life Support (NALS) program (redcross.org), or an equivalent newborn resuscitation course.

Note:
Throughout this manual, the word "infant" will be used to describe babies from birth through the twenty-eighth day of life (the neonatal period).

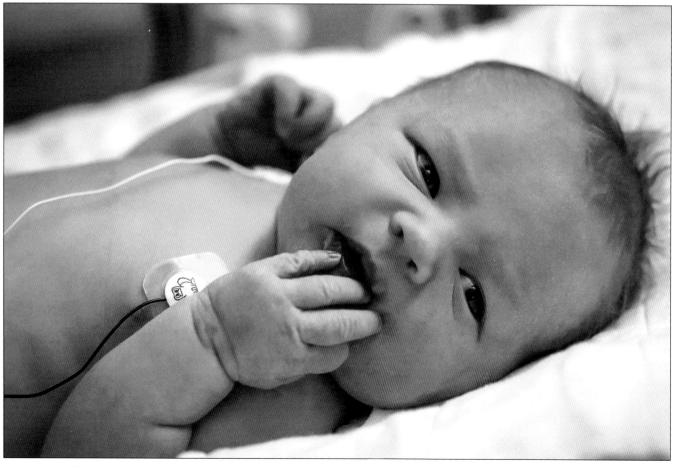

Safe, Evidence-Based Patient Care

Every year, tens of thousands of infants are transported or transferred to neonatal intensive care units (NICUs) to receive specialized care for various reasons: prematurity, problems related to delivery, infection, cardiac or surgical problems, genetic, and complex medical conditions.[11] Preparing maternal/child providers for the unexpectedly sick or preterm infant includes resuscitation and stabilization education, skill acquisition, ensuring proper equipment and supplies are available, and simulation training.[12-14] The benefit of simulation in neonatal education is well established in developed nations and increasingly in limited resource settings. Simulation training aims to help establish safe, reliable, and high-quality systems and provide opportunities to practice the technical, cognitive, and behavioral aspects of time-pressured emergencies.[4,8,11,14-16]

The public expects safe, quality care every time they interact with healthcare providers and health systems. Standardized care processes use guidelines and protocols to improve the effectiveness of patient care and patient safety and to avoid reliance on memory. Vulnerable infants require more technology, medications, treatments, and procedures—all of which increase the potential for making errors. Actions taken in the first minutes, hours, and days after birth may affect short- and long-term outcomes. Accurate diagnosis, monitoring, and clear, unambiguous communication contribute to patient safety and improved outcomes. **Module 7, Quality Improvement,** further explores methods to improve communication and reduce errors and adverse events and discusses the value of simulation-based training for healthcare teams.

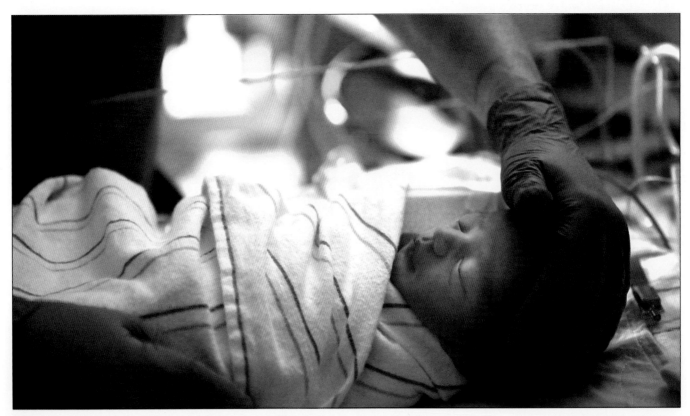

Sugar, Temperature, Airway, Blood Pressure, Lab Work, Emotional Support

Neonatal Transport

Ideally, patients with identified high-risk pregnancies should deliver in a facility with maternal and infant specialists capable of caring for both the mother and baby.[13] However, many infants who require neonatal intensive care do not present until the late intrapartum or early neonatal period, thus precluding safe maternal transport prior to delivery.[17-22] Therefore, it is vitally important that birth hospital providers are prepared to resuscitate and stabilize unexpectedly sick and/or preterm infants. Adequate preparation includes education and training in resuscitation and stabilization and immediate access to necessary supplies and equipment.[14,17,20] Combined with an accurate neonatal assessment and appropriate actions, such preparations will contribute to optimizing stabilization efforts before the transport team arrives or the infant is transferred to a NICU.[13,23]

Referring Hospital Responsibilities

The goal of all neonatal transport teams is to transport a well-stabilized infant. This goal is best achieved when care is provided in a timely, organized, comprehensive manner by all members of the healthcare team.[4,20] Referring hospital responsibilities include the following:

- Knowing how to activate a neonatal or maternal transport
- Discussing patient questions and the stabilization care with the medical control transport physician
- Knowing how to assess and monitor the infant's condition
- Beginning the necessary actions needed to stabilize the infant
- Providing detailed medical records and imaging
- Keeping the family updated and involved as much as possible

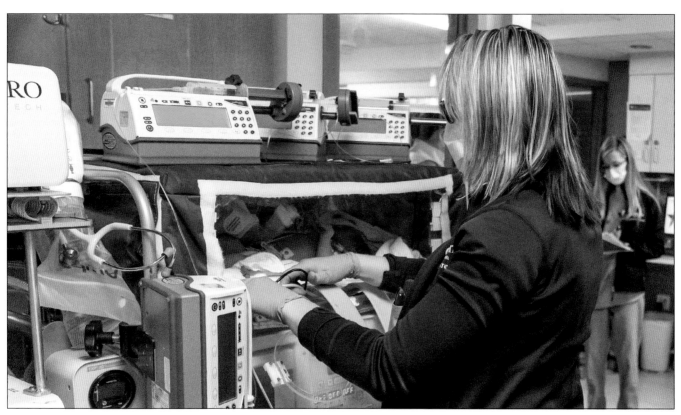

Transport Team Responsibilities

The transport (retrieval) team is responsible for assessing the maternal and infant history, current condition, diagnosis, and stabilization care that was completed. This information is used to decide the next steps in stabilization, including any necessary changes in the IV fluid and/or rate, the need for additional venous and/or arterial access, changes in respiratory support, or medications. The team responds to the changing clinical situation, utilizing protocols to guide their care and assessing clinical data to decide how to optimally prepare and stabilize the infant before departing in a transport vehicle.[4] Referring hospital staff should not be alarmed or discouraged by changes made by the transport team.

Developing a close relationship between referring hospitals and their respective retrieval or transport teams can help improve mortality and morbidity outcomes of sick infants who require transport to a tertiary center.[24] One way to enhance this relationship is to incorporate post-event (post-transport) debriefings and involve as many of the patient caregivers as possible. Debriefing can help improve future patient care, identify knowledge and/or equipment deficits, and identify any procedural changes that can improve care in similar situations.[25,26] The Pre-Transport Stabilization Self-Assessment Tool (PSSAT) found on page 270 is designed to guide a review of the stabilization care provided and to help identify questions that can be discussed with the receiving NICU after transport. Concerns specific to the transported infant's case can be recorded on the PSSAT form and addressed during a post-event debrief, case review, or patient simulation.

Inclusivity Statement from The S.T.A.B.L.E. Program

S.T.A.B.L.E. recognizes the existence of diverse gender identities and family structures and supports affirming all the ways in which people differ, identify, and create their families. In healthcare settings, we encourage you to be actively respectful and inclusive by keeping up to date with affirming care practices as they continue to evolve. By embracing gender-affirming care, medical professionals create a welcoming and safe environment for all patients, fostering trust and promoting better healthcare outcomes for all.

A Note on Language Found in The S.T.A.B.L.E. Program

The S.T.A.B.L.E. content sometimes includes gender-specific terms, such as "mother", "maternal", "father", and "paternal". Feel free to substitute alternative gender-specific terms when reading or teaching this content, such as gender-neutral terms like "laboring patient", "birthing patient", "pregnant patient", or "partner". When pronouns such as "she/her", "he/him", or "they/them" are used, it can be assumed the patient identified pronouns for them and their child.

Anticipate problems that may occur, **recognize** problems when they do occur, and **act** on problems quickly to restore stability. **Reassess** the infant at regular intervals to assess the effectiveness of previous interventions and changes in patient status that can occur.

· ·

Let's apply ARAR to a case of a patient with gestational diabetes who presents in labor at 38 weeks with an estimated fetal weight of 4,400 grams. What risk factors would you anticipate for the mother, birth, and infant? *Shoulder dystocia, birth injury, neonatal resuscitation, neonatal hypoglycemia.*

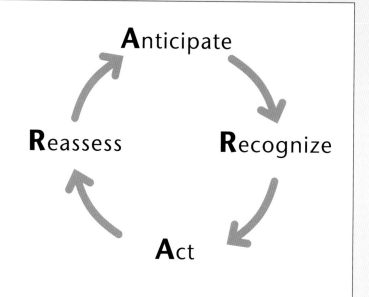

Anticipate

Be prepared to activate emergency notifications applicable to your setting (anesthesia, neonatal care team, other personnel as indicated).

- Verification of fetal position
- Footstool ready to assist with suprapubic pressure (for shoulder dystocia)
- Vacuum and forceps available
- Monitor for fetal distress
- Resuscitation warmer and supplies prepared prior to delivery
- Operating room available and set-up
- Blood glucose monitoring per protocol

Recognize

- Need for cesarean or assisted delivery: Prolonged second stage of labor (pushing) or arrest of descent in the second stage
- Shoulder dystocia: Delivery of head with no further movement or no shoulder delivered
- Newborn injury: Evaluate for brachial plexus palsy, facial nerve injury, arm or clavicle fracture, organ laceration, scalp injury
- Resuscitation needed: Nonvigorous infant in distress
- Signs of hypoglycemia

Act

- Activate emergency notifications if cesarean delivery required or other complications arise (shoulder dystocia)
- Shoulder dystocia maneuvers
- Newborn resuscitation as indicated
- Closely monitor infant's blood sugar / provide appropriate therapy

Reassess

- Maternal injury (cervical/perineal tear), uncontrolled bleeding/postpartum hemorrhage, pain, post-operative management if cesarean delivery
- Care of diabetes in pregnancy as applicable
- Neonatal response to resuscitation and stabilization care

Sugar Module

Sugar

Temperature

Airway

Blood Pressure

Lab Work

Emotional Support

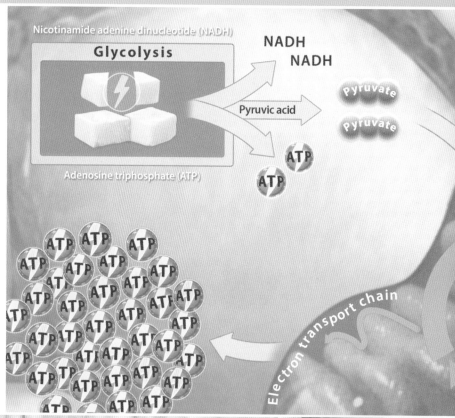

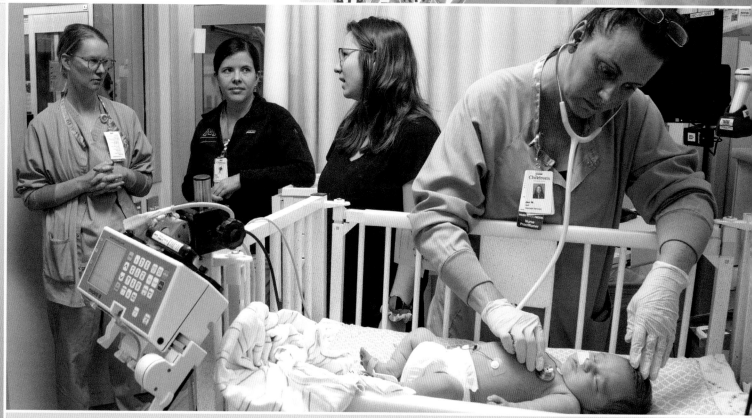

Sugar—Module Objectives

Upon completion of this module, participants will gain an increased understanding of:

1. Why it is important to withhold feedings and establish intravenous (IV) access when infants are sick.

2. The initial intravenous (IV) fluid therapy to provide to sick infants.

3. Preparation for extrauterine life and infants at increased risk for developing hypoglycemia, including preterm and small for gestational age infants, infants of diabetic mothers, and sick, stressed infants.

4. The impact of late preterm birth on increased morbidity and mortality.

5. Signs of hypoglycemia and how to monitor the blood glucose.

6. IV glucose treatment of hypoglycemia and post-treatment reassessment.

7. Infants at-risk for hypoglycemia and treatment with enteral feedings and dextrose gel.

8. Indications for and safe use of umbilical catheters.

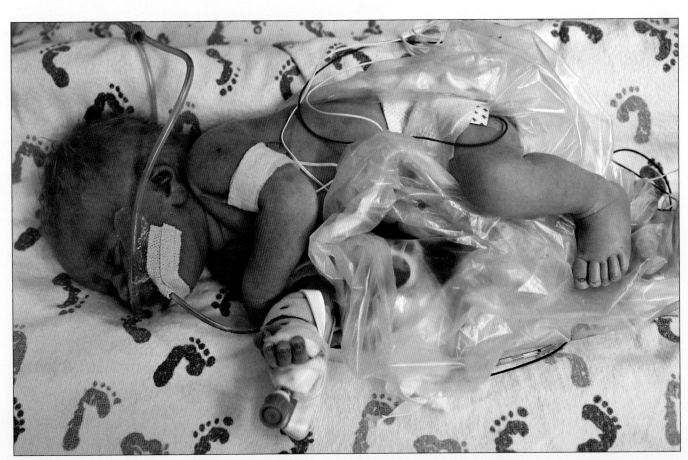

One-hour-old, 36-week gestation infant with gastroschisis (bowel is herniated through a hole in the abdominal wall adjacent to the umbilicus) who delivered unexpectedly after spontaneous labor.

S

Sugar

Guideline 1

If the Infant Is Sick, Especially If Unstable, Do Not Give Enteral (Oral or Gavage) Feedings

Care Recommendation 1

In the initial stabilization period, enteral feedings may not be tolerated and can increase the risk for aspiration. Once the infant stabilizes and the medical diagnoses are known, the introduction of enteral feedings can be considered.

When an infant is sick, there are good reasons to withhold breast, bottle, and gavage feedings. Offering nothing by mouth is called "NPO" after the Latin term "nil per os," or in some nations, NBM for "nil by mouth."

> **NPO**
> Nothing by Mouth
> *nil per os*

Rationale for Making the Baby NPO

- Infants with respiratory distress and increased work of breathing have poor suck, swallow, and breathing coordination, which places them at increased risk for choking episodes and aspiration of stomach contents into the lungs.[27-29]

- Some illnesses, including infection or the effects of hypoxia secondary to a stressful birth or clinical deterioration, may result in delayed gastric emptying because of intestinal ileus.[30,31]

- If the infant's blood pressure was low (hypotensive) before, during, or after birth, intestinal blood flow and oxygenation may be reduced, making the intestine susceptible to ischemic injury.[32,33] It is important to allow the bowel time to recover from injury that may have occurred.[3]

- If the infant has a bowel obstruction, secretions collect in the stomach and increase the risk for aspiration. Intermittent gastric decompression, set to a suction level of 30 to 40 mmHg, should be initiated to prevent aspiration pneumonia. If this suction equipment is not available, insert an 8 French gastric tube into the stomach and secure it well. Every 5 or 10 minutes, use a syringe to aspirate and discard the secretions. For more information about bowel obstruction, see Appendix 1.1 on pages 67 to 71.

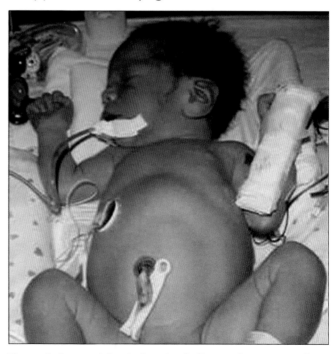

Term infant with abdominal distension secondary to imperforate anus (a bowel obstruction).

Rationale for Making the Baby NPO *(Continued)*

○ If esophageal atresia is suspected, use a double-lumen tube to remove secretions from the esophageal pouch. One lumen of the tube suctions secretions while the other lumen vents the tube to air to keep it from adhering to adjacent tissue.[4,35] Low intermittent suction set to 30 to 40 mmHg is usually adequate to clear secretions.

○ Although bilious (green-colored) emesis can be seen in infants with or without a bowel obstruction, it is a common clinical presentation of a potentially catastrophic surgical condition called *midgut volvulus*.[30,35] For more information, see *Let's Learn More: Malrotation with midgut volvulus* on page 14.

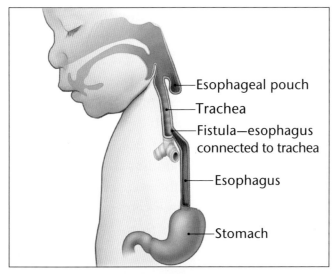

86% of cases of tracheoesophageal fistula/ esophageal atresia (TEF/EA) are Type C.

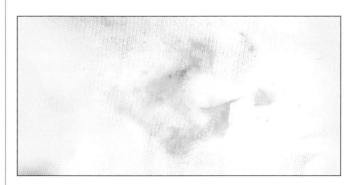

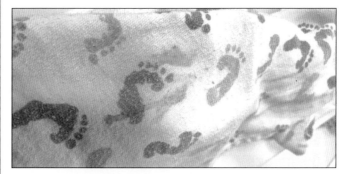

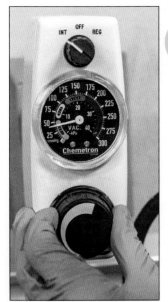

 Bilious (green-colored) emesis should be reported promptly to the infant's medical team as a potential sign of bowel obstruction, the most serious being a surgical emergency called midgut volvulus.

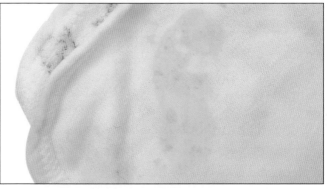

Bile colored emesis from three infants with malrotation and midgut volvulus.

Nutritional Support of the Preterm Infant

Although early protein intake and initiation of enteral feedings, preferably with human milk, are important to support the nutritional needs of preterm infants, these infants are often critically ill.[36] Early initiation of intravenous protein has proven beneficial for preterm infants and is a standard of care in the neonatal intensive care unit (NICU).[36,37] The decision to offer enteral feedings to preterm and other sick infants is made following careful evaluation of the infant's history, diagnosis, exam findings, and laboratory data. Some preterm infants may be healthy enough to tolerate the introduction of enteral feedings on the same day they are born. The goal of the care team is to decide when it is safest to proceed with offering small-volume milk feedings and how these feeds should be incrementally increased.[36]

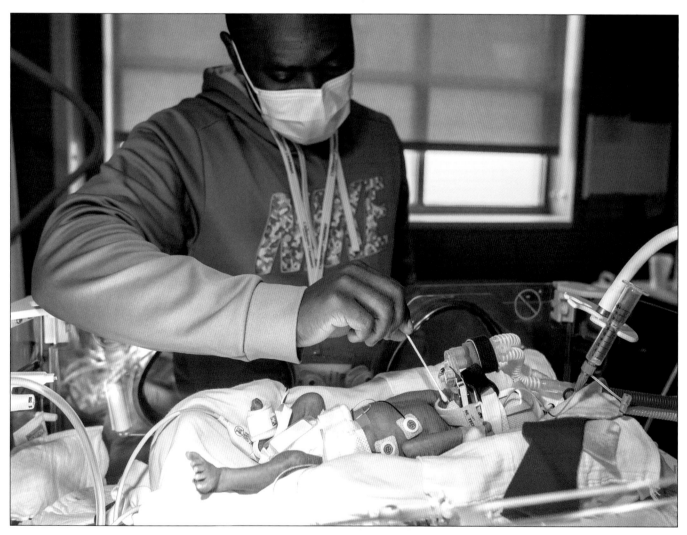

Breast milk swabs being given by the infant's father. This 24-hour-old, 30-week gestation infant is on nasal continuous positive airway pressure (CPAP) for treatment of respiratory distress syndrome.

Let's Learn More... **Malrotation with midgut volvulus**[30,32,38-42]

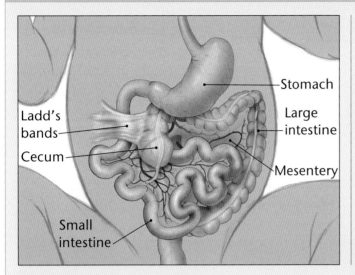

Malrotation without volvulus.

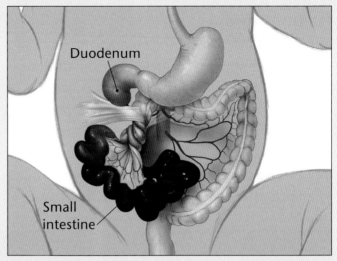

Intestinal malrotation with midgut volvulus (twisting of the bowel).

A review of fetal embryology helps to better understand how malrotation occurs.

In the 6th week of gestation, the intestine is herniated into the umbilical cord. Between 8 and 10 weeks of gestation, the intestinal tube dynamically grows and elongates and begins a process of rotation that ends with the intestine entering the abdominal cavity. If all proceeds normally, the duodenal-jejunal junction will be located in the left upper quadrant of the abdomen, and the cecum, which is the beginning part of the large intestine, will be located in the right lower quadrant of the abdomen. The small and large intestines become anchored or fixed to the retroperitoneum by a specific tissue called the

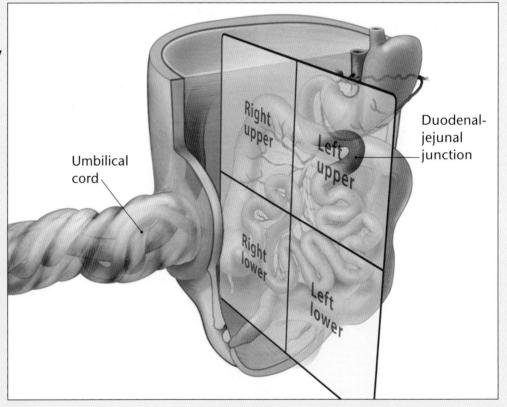

mesentery. In addition to securely holding the intestine in position, the mesentery provides a conduit for blood vessels that perfuse the intestine, as well as a conduit for lymph nodes, lymphatic vessels, and nerves.

Let's Learn More... *Malrotation with midgut volvulus*

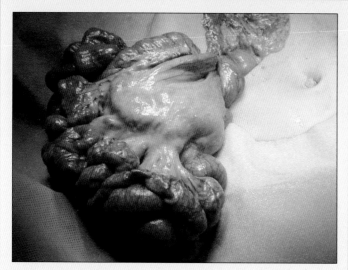

Surgical finding of malrotation with midgut volvulus in a two-week-old infant.

With malrotation, the intestine fails to properly rotate and fixate to the retroperitoneum. Instead of the intestine being securely "fixed" or "anchored" by the mesentery, the stalk-like mesentery is vulnerable to twisting at any time. The term 'midgut volvulus' describes twisting of the bowel that affects the midgut regions of the intestine: structures distal to the second portion of the duodenum, including the jejunum, ileum, and proximal two-thirds of the transverse colon. When volvulus occurs, the blood supply to the intestine is cut off, leading to ischemic injury. Immediate surgery is necessary to untwist the bowel to restore blood flow and remove any nonviable necrotic bowel.

Often, the only clinical indicator of malrotation with midgut volvulus is the presence of green bilious vomit. There is no known correlation between the number of bilious vomits or amount of bilious vomit to the severity of intestinal injury. Thus, one bilious vomit must be treated as malrotation and volvulus until proven otherwise.

An infant with malrotation may initially look healthy with no abdominal distension, a soft and non-tender abdomen on palpation, and a normal-appearing abdominal X-ray. However, when volvulus occurs, there will be a deterioration of physical exam findings, and the patient will be in significant pain, with abdominal distension, tenderness, guarding, and signs of shock.

Physical examination and a diagnostic workup should be initiated as quickly as possible. Radiographic tests may include an upper gastrointestinal study (UGI), abdominal x-ray, and in some centers, other imaging such as an abdominal ultrasound. The UGI study is best performed at a hospital with pediatric surgical services and radiologists experienced in pediatric evaluation, as well as radiology staff who are prepared to monitor the infant and protect the infant from aspiration and hypothermia during the study.

The incidence of malrotation is 1 in 2,500 to 1 in 6,000 live births, and depending on the case series reported, between 45 and 65% of cases of malrotation result in volvulus. Interestingly, about half of the cases of midgut volvulus occur in the first month of life, another 25% within the first year of life, and the remaining 25% at any other time in life.

Occurrence of Midgut Volvulus

50%
1st month of life

25%
1st year

25% Any other time of life

Incidence of malrotation is 1 in 6,000 live births; 45 and 65% of cases of malrotation result in volvulus.

Guideline 2

Provide Glucose via Intravenous (IV) Fluids

Care Recommendation 2

If the infant is not well enough to tolerate enteral feedings, establish IV access and infuse a glucose-containing solution.

Supporting the energy needs of sick infants with IV fluids containing glucose is an important component of stabilization. As shown in Figure 1.1., the brain requires a steady supply of glucose to function normally. Unlike the liver, kidneys, skeletal muscle, and cardiac muscle, the brain stores minimal amounts of glucose in the form of glycogen.[33,43,44] Almost all of the circulating glucose is used by the brain, and when the glucose concentration (blood sugar)* is low, permanent brain damage can occur.[45-49]

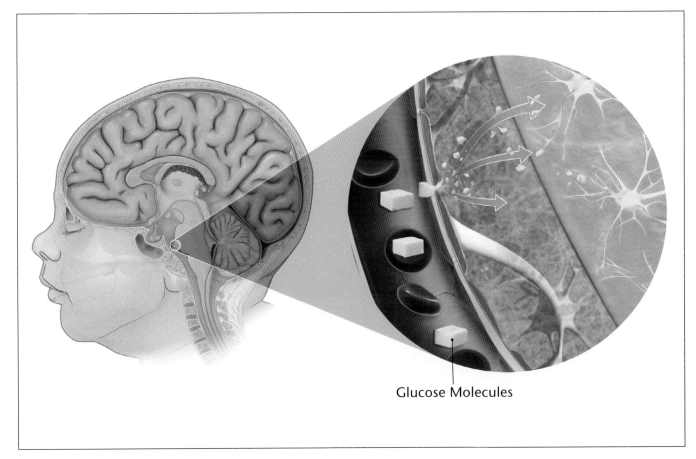

Glucose Molecules

Figure 1.1. The brain requires a steady supply of glucose to function normally.

Note:
*The term *glucose concentration* is used interchangeably with *blood sugar* and *blood glucose*.

Establishing IV access allows for

- Infusion of a glucose-containing solution, such as $D_{10}W$, to help stabilize the blood sugar

- A route for medications needed in the treatment of sick infants

- Venous access if needed in an emergency

 It is also important to remain alert to the infant identified as "at risk" for feeding intolerance or hypoglycemia (e.g., infants who are late preterm, small for gestational age, large for gestational age, and infants of diabetic mothers), as these infants may also need an IV glucose infusion and/or feeding support while oral feedings are being established.

*For infants, the best peripheral IV insertion sites are in the hand, foot, ankle, forearm, or scalp veins.[50] See Figure 1.2 on page 18 and the **Clinical Tip** on page 25 for helpful information about inserting and securing IVs.*

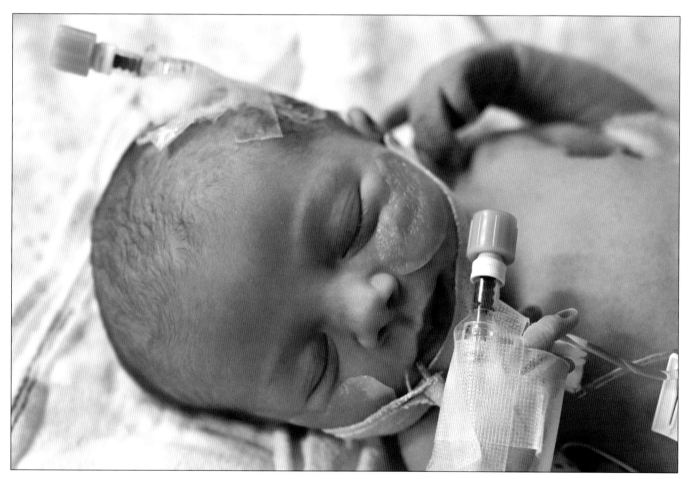

Scalp and peripheral IV lines placed in a 39-week gestation infant who was distressed at birth and required resuscitation.

Figure 1.2. Setting up for and securing a peripheral IV.[50-53]

Peripheral IV Catheter Size

For most infants, an appropriate size is a 24-gauge IV catheter or, if not available, a 23 or 25-gauge butterfly needle (with ¾ inch needle length).

 Use a needle or catheter with a safety device to reduce the risk of a needle stick injury and exposure to bloodborne pathogens. When finished with the procedure, promptly and properly dispose of the shielded needle in a regulation sharps container.

Preparing to Insert a Peripheral IV

- Observe evidence-based guidelines for hand hygiene before and after patient contact. Before beginning, wash and dry hands or apply an antiseptic solution to hands.
- Plan for infant comfort interventions to reduce pain: swaddling, offering a pacifier, sucrose, and facilitated tucking.
- Assemble all of the equipment that will be necessary for the procedure.
- Prepare the tape and semipermeable transparent sterile dressing so that it is ready to use after the needle is inserted.
- Apply gloves. Note that sterile gloves are used in some situations.
- Disinfect the skin prior to IV insertion. Alcohol is acceptable for a simple IV start, but if this site will also be used for a blood culture draw, ensure that you use an appropriate antiseptic solution to sterilize the skin. Some facilities prohibit drawing a blood culture from a newly inserted IV because of the risk of contaminating the blood culture sample and/or losing the line. Follow your hospital's protocol.
- Optional: A non-latex material tourniquet may be placed on the extremity above the needle insertion site. Loosen or remove the tourniquet before flushing the IV. In very small infants, a 2 X 2 gauze sponge under the tourniquet may help protect the skin.

Step 1

- A transillumination light (cold light) or a bright pen light held beneath the hand or foot helps the veins become visible. In some centers, ultrasound-guided IV placement may be available.

 Ensure the light source does not transmit heat, which could burn the skin.

- Select a vein in the hand, foot, ankle, forearm, or scalp. Cleanse the area with antiseptic solution. Begin more distally in case additional attempts are required. Avoid inserting a scalp IV in any areas below the hairline in case the IV extravasates, which could leave long-term visible damage or scarring

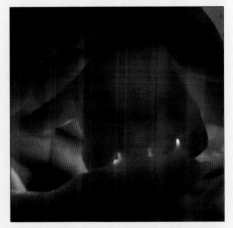
Transillumination of the hand.

- Blood return may be very slow in a baby who is hypotensive or otherwise compromised. Once you see a flashback of blood, remove the tourniquet (if used), lower your angle, and advance a small amount to ensure the needle and catheter sheath are in the vein. Then, gently slide the IV catheter off the needle to advance into the vein.

Step 2

- Place a ½ inch (1.3 cm) piece of tape over the hub. Apply additional tape to secure the IV catheter and tubing. Note that some prefer to apply the clear dressing in step 3 before applying the tape. To allow

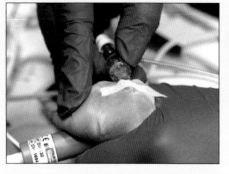
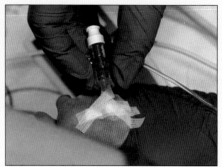

observation, don't tape over the needle insertion area that will be secured by the transparent dressing.

- While taping, periodically ensure patency by flushing the IV with a small amount of sterile normal saline (NS).

Step 3

- Secure the catheter by placing a small piece of transparent dressing from the hub down to below the insertion site to allow observation for redness or swelling.

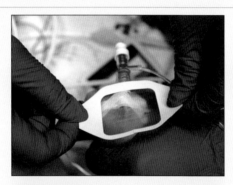
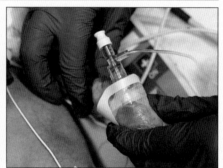

- If a transparent dressing is not available, secure the hub with a piece of ½ inch (1.3 cm) clear tape. If using a butterfly needle, place the tape such that it also covers the butterfly wings.

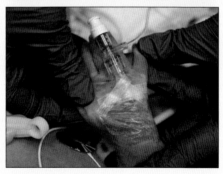

Step 4

- If the IV is over a joint, use a padded "board" to prevent flexion of the elbow, wrist, or ankle. Gently support the extremity in the most neutral and natural position. Prevent pressure injuries from any IV tubing by protecting the skin with a cotton ball or gauze sponge.

- To help prevent accidental dislodgment of the IV tubing pulling on the catheter, secure the tubing with a ½ inch (1.3 cm) piece of tape such that the tape does not touch the hub or wings of the IV needle.

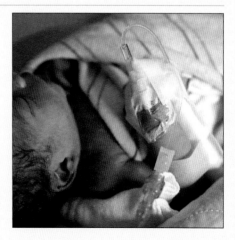

Continued on next page

Figure 1.2. Setting up for and securing a peripheral IV.[50-53] *(Continued)*

Document the following:

- Where the IV was placed

- The size and device used

- The number of attempts

- Any bruising or other notable skin finding in the area of insertion

- If an extremity was avoided because of concerns for poor perfusion or plans for a future central or arterial line placement

- Document hourly the appearance of the IV and the amount of fluid that was infused in the prior hour

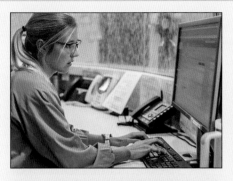
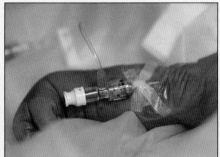
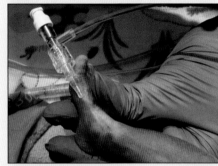
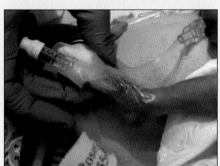
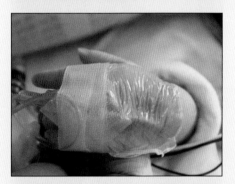

Monitoring

Once an IV is inserted, inspect the IV site at least hourly so that any swelling or redness can be detected. Swelling may indicate the IV infiltrated and needs to be removed. Some medications and IV fluids can be very irritating to the skin and can damage the skin if they leak into the surrounding tissues (extravasation injury).

Protect the IV from dislodgment when the infant is moved.

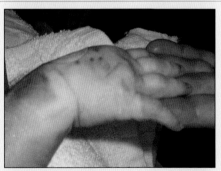
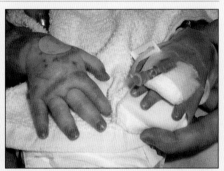
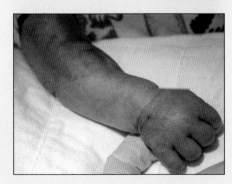

 Extravasation injury following unintended leakage of IV fluids or medications can occur and require prompt assessment and treatment.[54-56]

Vascular Access in the NICU

Midline Catheter[57,58]

An extended dwell peripheral intravenous (abbreviated EDPIV or EPIV) catheter is an option for infants with difficult vascular access. These 4 to 8-centimeter-long catheters are placed by NICU nurses skilled in vascular access. The advantages of the EPIV over the PIV are longer dwell times, fewer placement attempts required, and fewer complications.

Peripherally Inserted Central Catheter (PICC)[59-66]

For long-term nutrition of NICU patients, a PICC may be placed in the upper or lower extremities.

An upper extremity PICC is in a central location when the tip is located in the superior vena cava (SVC) but not deeper than the junction of the SVC and right atrium (RA). After initial insertion, periodic X-ray or imaging surveillance is important to monitor for tip migration to an undesirable location.

A lower extremity PICC is in a central location when the tip is located in the inferior vena cava (IVC) below the RA. The ideal tip location is at the level of the diaphragm. Complication rates increase when the tip is located at or below the common iliac vein (iliac bifurcation), so this location should be avoided. Please consult additional evidence-based materials for guidelines on optimal tip location. When the PICC is initially placed in the IVC, both anterior-posterior and lateral abdominal X-rays are recommended to ensure the catheter tip is located in the IVC and not in unintended locations, such as lumbar, epigastric, spermatic, kidney, or liver vessels. Periodic abdominal X-ray or imaging surveillance should also occur to monitor for tip migration to an undesirable location.

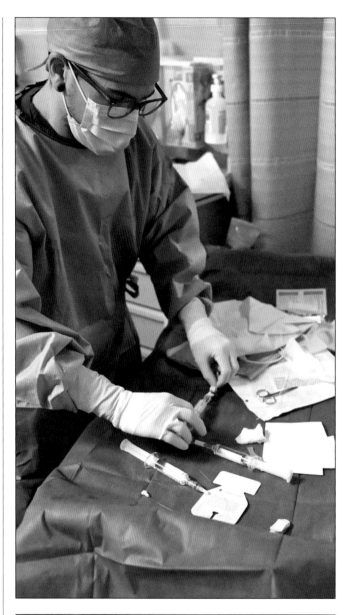

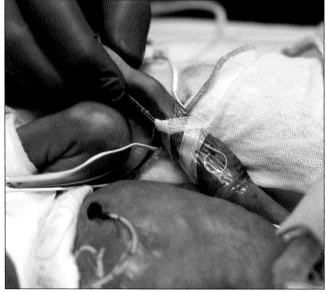

Guideline 3

Initial IV Fluid and Glucose Infusion Rate (GIR)

Care Recommendation 3

After inserting an IV, infuse a 10% dextrose solution ($D_{10}W$) at a rate of 80 mL per kilogram per day (80 mL/kg/day).

Infusion of $D_{10}W$ at 80 mL/kg/day will provide a GIR of 5.5 mg/kg/minute. This GIR is similar to the liver glucose production rate in healthy, term newborns—4 to 6 mg/kg/minute.[67-70] In the absence of conditions related to hyperinsulinemia or other pathologic forms of hypoglycemia, a GIR of 5.5 mg/kg/minute is usually sufficient to maintain the blood glucose above 50 mg/dL (2.8 mmol/L). Table 1.1 shows the GIR with different fluid infusion rates and dextrose concentrations. Figures 1.3 and 1.4 summarize how to calculate the hourly infusion rate and GIR.

Initial IV Fluid Management for the Sick Infant
$D_{10}W$ (without sodium or potassium)*
80 mL per kilogram per 24 hours (80 mL/kg/day)
Infuse via an infusion pump
*If the infant is older than 24 to 48 hours, it may be necessary to add electrolytes to the IV solution.[70,71]

If the blood glucose is persistently elevated or the electrolytes (sodium and potassium) become deranged, consult the tertiary center physician for guidance regarding fluid and electrolyte management.

Care in the NICU—Special Circumstances

Infants who experience birth stress, including those who require cardiopulmonary resuscitation or who have significant respiratory distress, are at increased risk for poor kidney function. A lower IV infusion rate of 60 mL/kg/day is not uncommon while awaiting kidney recovery. Initially, infants who require resuscitation may have stress-induced hyperglycemia that may be followed by hypoglycemia. While fluids are restricted, closely monitor the blood glucose and be prepared to increase the dextrose concentration to increase the GIR as necessary.

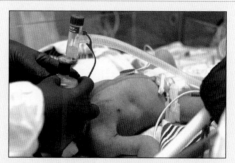

37-week gestation infant delivered emergently for fetal distress.

Preterm infants often require a higher volume of fluid than term infants because of increased water losses through their thinner, less developed skin. Increased insensible water loss (IWL) occurs because of skin immaturity, providing care under a radiant warmer, and the use of phototherapy to treat hyperbilirubinemia.[37,72]

Appendix 1.4 on pages 74 and 75 provides dextrose preparation charts should the IV dextrose concentration need to be adjusted down or up.

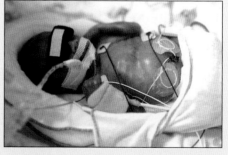

25-week gestation, 1-day-old infant.

Infusion Volume in mL/kg per 24 hours (mL/kg/day)	IV Infusion Rate in mL/Hour *Multiply this number by the infant's weight in kilograms to provide the correct hourly infusion rate*	Dextrose Concentration					
		D_5W	$D_{7.5}W$	$D_{10}W$	$D_{12.5}W$	$D_{15}W$	$D_{20}W$
		Glucose Infusion Rate (mg/kg/minute)					
60	2.5	2.1	3.1	4.2	5.2	6.3	8.4
70	2.9	2.4	3.6	4.8	6	7.3	9.7
80 Usual starting rate	3.3 Usual starting rate	2.8	4.1	5.5 Usual starting dose	6.9	8.3	11
90	3.8	3.2	4.8	6.3	7.9	9.5	12.7
100	4.2	3.5	5.3	7	8.8	10.5	14
110	4.6	3.8	5.8	7.7	9.6	11.5	15.4
120	5	4.2	6.3	8.4	10.4	12.5	16.7
130	5.4	4.5	6.8	9	11.3	13.5	18
140	5.8	4.8	7.3	9.7	12.1	14.5	19.4
150	6.3	5.3	7.9	10.5	13.2	15.8	21

Table 1.1. Effect of different dextrose concentrations (horizontal peach-colored row) and infusion rates (purple and blue vertical columns) on the glucose infusion rate (GIR; yellow box area). For example, if the desired fluid rate is 80 mL/kg/day, multiply 3.3 by the infant's weight in kilograms. If the infant weighs 2.5 kg, then 3.3 multiplied by 2.5 is 8.25. Round up to 8.3 and infuse the IV fluid at that rate on an IV pump.

Figure 1.3. How to calculate the hourly fluid infusion rate to provide 80 mL/kg/day.

Step 1. Multiply the body weight in kilograms by 80 (mL): kg x 80

Step 2. To find the hourly rate, divide this number by 24 (hours): (kg x 80) ÷ 24 = fluid rate in mL per hour to infuse the IV fluid

Example 1: Body weight 4,200 grams or 4.2 kg

Step 1. 4.2 (kg) X 80 = 336 (mL)

Step 2. 336 (mL) divided by 24 (hours) = 14 (mL per hour)

Step 3. Infuse the IV fluid on an infusion pump at 14 mL per hour

Example 2: Body weight 1,800 grams or 1.8 kg

Step 1. 1.8 (kg) X 80 = 144 (mL)

Step 2. 144 (mL) divided by 24 (hours) = 6 (mL per hour)

Step 3. Infuse the IV fluid on an infusion pump at 6 mL per hour

Figure 1.4. How to calculate the glucose infusion rate (GIR) in mg/kg/minute.

To calculate the GIR in mg/kg/minute, the formula is:
(% dextrose in solution **X** IV rate in mL/hour **X** 0.167) divided by weight in kg

Example 1: 4.2 kg infant is receiving $D_{10}W$ at a rate of 14 mL/hour = 80 mL/kg/day

Step 1. (10 X 14 X 0.167) = 23.4

Step 2. Divide by the weight in kg: 23.4 / 4.2 (kg) = 5.6 mg/kg/minute GIR

Example 2: 3.5 kg infant is receiving $D_{12.5}W$ at a rate of 14.6 mL/hour = 100 mL/kg/day

Step 1. (12.5 X 14.6 X 0.167) = 30.5

Step 2. Divide by the weight in kg: 30.5 / 3.5 (kg) = 8.7 mg/kg/minute GIR

Note:
A pounds/ounces to kilograms weight converter may be found on the STABLEize® app (available for Apple and Android phones).

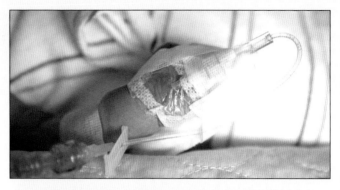 Clinical Tip   *Starting IVs in infants—Tips from NICU nurses*

1. To promote success, consider this a two-person procedure. One should stabilize and comfort the infant while the other person prepares the materials and places the IV. Discuss your plan, including how the other person can best assist you (flushing the IV when asked, applying the tape, etc.).

2. IV insertion is a painful procedure. Sucking on a pacifier can help reduce discomfort. Oral sucrose can help with pain control. If parents choose to be present, they can be coached on how to help comfort their baby.

3. Although practice guidelines vary, many NICUs allow two insertion attempts per person. Multiple IV sticks can be very stressful for the baby and can reduce available IV sites for later attempts. If having difficulty inserting the IV, contact the infant's medical team to discuss alternatives such as an umbilical venous catheter insertion. In critical, life-threatening situations, an intraosseous needle insertion may be necessary.

4. Although rarely used, if the only IV device available is a butterfly needle, enter the skin approximately ¼ inch (0.6 cm) away from where you enter the vein. This technique will improve the stability of the IV needle once it is placed. Once you have a blood return, don't try to cannulate the vein further because the butterfly needle may go through the vein.

Scalp Vein Insertion Pointers

- At times, a scalp vein may be the best option. If hair needs to be removed, try to trim rather than shave the hair. Shaving can cause skin abrasion. Minimize the amount of hair removed and save the baby's hair for the parents. Label the bag, "Your baby's first haircut."

- Apply gentle traction on the skin with the non-dominant hand to prevent the vein from moving. Insert the needle or catheter in

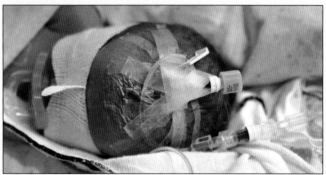

the direction of venous flow, which is toward the heart.

- Swabbing the skin with alcohol immediately before piercing the vein helps to dilate it for easier visualization. Because the alcohol dries quickly, the infant should not feel a sting.

- Veins fill from above, and arteries fill from below. Veins and arteries can be difficult to tell apart, so palpate for arterial pulsation prior to insertion. Once inserted, flush a small amount of sterile saline to check for patency and for any blanching (which represents arterial spasm). If in an artery, remove the catheter or needle and apply pressure to the site for at least 5 minutes to be sure all bleeding has stopped.

- An IV placed in the scalp can be scary for parents to see. Prior to insertion or after one has been placed, try to inform the parents of the IV location before they see it. Also, explain that the IV is in a superficial vein (blood vessel) and not in their baby's brain, which is a fairly common misunderstanding.

Guideline 4

Sick and Preterm Infants Are at Increased Risk for Hypoglycemia

Care Recommendation 4

 Identify infants at risk for hypoglycemia and monitor their blood sugar at an interval that allows for prompt treatment.

Infants at risk for hypoglycemia[73,74] include

- Preterm (<37 weeks gestation)
- Small for gestational age (SGA)
- Intrauterine growth restricted (IUGR)

- Large for gestational age (LGA)
- Infant of a diabetic mother (IDM)
- Sick and stressed, especially if unstable

In addition, some medications given to pregnant patients increase the risk for neonatal hypoglycemia. These medications and their effect on glucose metabolism are described in Table 1.2.

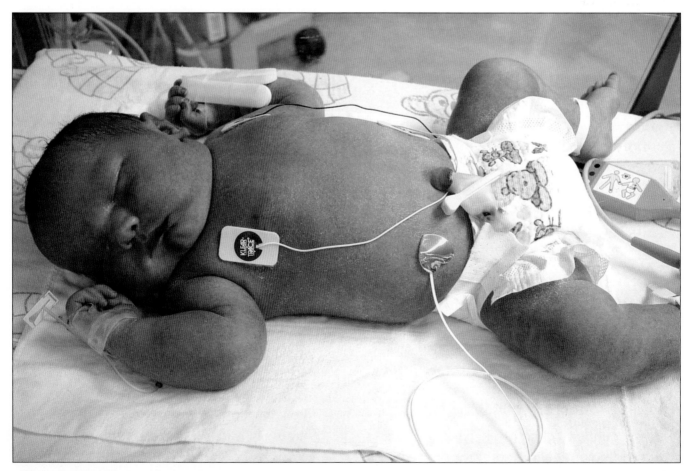

37-week gestation, 5.2 kg, IDM infant. Head circumference 39.5 cm., length 57 cm.

Table 1.2. Maternal medications and how they affect fetal and neonatal glucose metabolism.[44,100]

Medication [a]	Indication	Effect on the Neonate's Glucose Metabolism
Sulfonylureas[75-84] Chlorpropamide [b] Glyburide [c] Glipizide [c]	Type 2 diabetes	Drug crosses the placenta and promotes fetal insulin secretion that can cause hypoglycemia.
Beta-sympathomimetics[85-87] Terbutaline	Preterm labor	Maternal hyperglycemia leads to fetal pancreatic beta cell stimulation and increased fetal insulin secretion. Drug crosses the placenta and breaks down glycogen in the fetus.
Beta Blockers[88-90] Atenolol Carvedilol Labetalol Metoprolol Pindolol Propranolol	Hypertension Migraine headaches Propranolol is also used for thyrotoxicosis	Blocks fetal $ß_2$ adrenergic receptors (adrenocepters), preventing their stimulation of hepatic glycogen breakdown (glycogenolysis) and pancreatic release of glucagon. Drug persists in the neonate after birth and prevents glycogenolysis.
Thiazide Diuretics[91] Chlorothiazide Hydrochlorothiazide Chlorthalidone [d]	Hypertension Edema	Maternal hyperglycemia leads to fetal pancreatic beta cell stimulation and increased insulin secretion.
Tricyclic Antidepressants[92,93] Amitriptyline Desipramine Imipramine Nortriptyline	Depression	Maternal hyperglycemia leads to fetal pancreatic beta cell stimulation and increased insulin secretion.
Corticosteroids[94-98] Betamethasone Dexamethasone	Antenatal corticosteroid for fetal lung maturation with preterm premature rupture of membranes or preterm labor at risk for preterm delivery	Maternal hyperglycemia leads to fetal pancreatic beta cell stimulation and increased insulin secretion.
Maternal IV Dextrose [e] Administration During Labor[99]	Labor hydration	Glucose crosses the placenta and causes increased fetal insulin secretion.

Notes:

a. Not all medications are listed for each class described.

b. First-generation sulfonylurea implicated as a possible teratogen and should not be used in pregnancy.

c. Per the American College of Obstetricians and Gynecologists (ACOG), metformin can be a reasonable alternative to insulin when the pregnant patient declines insulin therapy, or it is not possible to safely administer insulin, or for pregnant patients who cannot afford insulin.[80] Glipizide, metformin, and glyburide cross the placenta to the fetus and have been associated with neonatal hypoglycemia.[81]

d. Chlorthalidone is not recommended in pregnancy because of adverse neonatal effects, including hypoglycemia, hyperbilirubinemia, and thrombocytopenia.[101]

e. IV fluid administration during labor varies based on maternal indication and can include Normal Saline (NS), D_5W, D_5NS, and D_5LR (LR = Lactated Ringers).

Preparation for Extrauterine Life and Factors That Affect Glucose Stability After Birth

In utero, the fetus relies entirely on the placental transfer of glucose, amino acids, and lipids for energy metabolism, protein synthesis, and tissue growth.[37,44,67,68,74] To prepare for extrauterine life, the fetus stores glucose in the form of glycogen in the liver, skeletal and cardiac muscle, lung, kidney, intestine, and in minimal amounts, the brain.[33,43,44] Liver glycogen stores increase slowly during the first and second trimesters, with the majority of glycogen stored starting at 36 weeks and peaking at term gestation.[68,74] The liver is the only organ that can release glycogen for use by other organs.[44] Because little glycogen is stored in the brain, it is essential that a steady supply of glucose is supplied via the bloodstream so the brain can function normally.[102]

Normal Postnatal Decline in Plasma Glucose

As soon as the cord is clamped, the plasma glucose level begins to decline. By 1 to 2 hours after birth, and in some cases by 30 minutes, the lowest point, or nadir, is reached.[74,103] The more preterm the infant, the earlier the nadir occurs.[104] While awaiting a carbohydrate intake from milk or dextrose-containing IV fluid, liver glycogen is broken down into glucose molecules (*glycogenolysis*) that are released into the bloodstream.[105] Liver glycogen stores are depleted by 10 to 12 hours after birth. A process called *gluconeogenesis,* where glucose is formed from non-carbohydrate precursors such as lactate, pyruvate, glycerol, and amino acids, helps to ramp up glucose production again.[68,106,107]

Three Main Factors That Impact Blood Glucose After Birth

Three main factors that can negatively affect an infant's ability to maintain a normal blood glucose (sugar) level after birth include

1 Inadequate glycogen stores and decreased glucose production

2 Hyperinsulinemia, which suppresses glucose production and increases glucose utilization

3 Increased glucose utilization when an infant is sick and has increased energy demands

▲ HIGH-RISK GROUPS: Inadequate Glycogen Stores and Decreased Glucose Production

Preterm Infants—Birth Before 37 Weeks Gestation

In preparation for extrauterine life, glycogen stores progressively increase as the fetus approaches term gestation. Prior to 36 weeks gestation, glycogen stores are minimal, and any available stores are rapidly depleted after birth.[68,108,109]

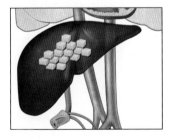
Term liver glycogen stores

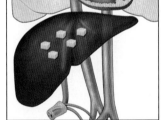
Preterm liver glycogen stores

Worldwide, every year, more than 15 million infants are born preterm, at less than 37 weeks gestation.[109] Preterm infants are metabolically and physiologically immature, and the earlier the gestation, the more pronounced this becomes.

⚠ HIGH-RISK GROUPS: **Inadequate Glycogen Stores and Decreased Glucose Production**
Preterm Infants—Birth Before 37 Weeks Gestation *(Continued)*

Preterm infants have immature liver enzyme systems necessary for gluconeogenesis (making glucose from non-carbohydrate precursors) and glycogenolysis (breaking down glycogen into glucose). Thus, the preterm infant is at high risk for becoming hypoglycemic.

Indications for preterm delivery

There are maternal, fetal, and placental complications that may make preterm delivery necessary.[110-112]

- **Maternal conditions** include hypertensive disorders (chronic hypertension, gestational hypertension, preeclampsia), preterm premature rupture of membranes (PPROM), preterm labor, and other diseases that may jeopardize maternal health. Preterm birth is more common with advanced maternal age and multiple gestation.

- **Fetal conditions** include oligohydramnios with associated maternal complications such as preeclampsia, intrauterine growth restriction, abnormal presentation, fetal heart rate abnormalities, hydrocephalus, or other conditions that may jeopardize fetal health.

- **Placental complications** that can lead to preterm birth include placental abruption or previa and placental implantation abnormalities (e.g., placenta accreta, increta, percreta).

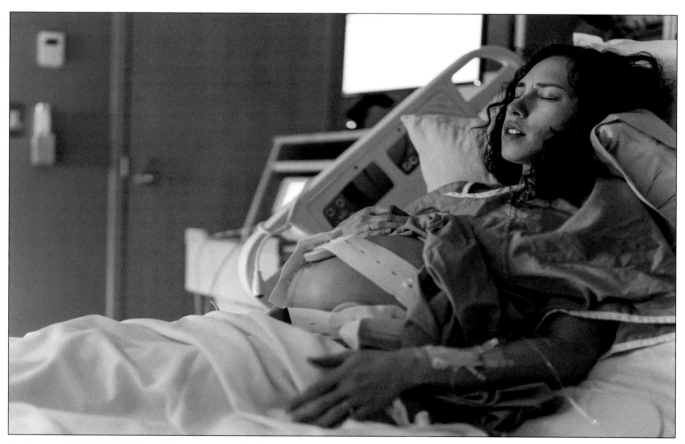

Patient with PPROM and in preterm labor at 32 weeks gestation.

⚠️ HIGH-RISK GROUPS: **Inadequate Glycogen Stores and Decreased Glucose Production**
(Continued)

Late Preterm Infants—Birth Between 34 and 36-6/7 Weeks Gestation

In 2022, 10.4% of all infants born in the U.S. were born preterm, with 70% of those infants born in the late preterm age group. In the U.S., year-to-year, these percentages of preterm birth change minimally.[108,113] Globally, the late preterm birth rate ranges from 3.3% (Finland) to 18% (Southeastern Asia, South Asia, and sub-Saharan Africa).[109,114] In the U.S., late preterm infants have a three-fold higher mortality rate than term infants.[115]

As shown in Figure 1.5, at 34 weeks gestation, the brain weight is approximately 60% that of a term infant's brain,[116] and cortical volume is nearly half, thus making the brain more susceptible to injury and increasing the risk for long-term developmental delays.[109,117] Table 1.3 lists the common clinical complications related to late preterm birth.

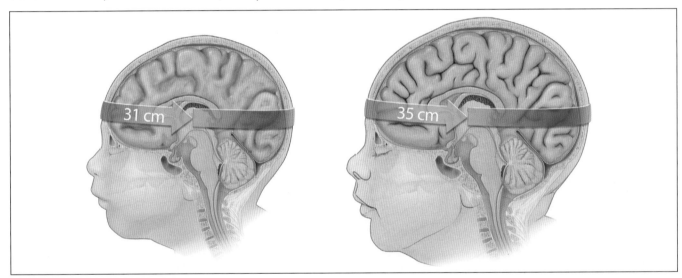

Figure 1.5. Comparison of the brain size and maturation at 34 and 40 weeks gestation. At 34 weeks, the 50th percentile for head circumference is 31 centimeters. By 40 weeks gestation, the head circumference increases to 35 centimeters, representing substantial brain growth and maturation in just 6 weeks. Between 35 and 41 weeks, there is a five-fold increase in brain volume.[116]

- Feeding difficulty (poor feeding, immature suck-swallow coordination, increased sleepiness, immature gut motility, problematic breastfeeding)
- Hypoglycemia
- Temperature instability
- Respiratory problems (respiratory distress syndrome, transient tachypnea of the newborn, pneumonia, apnea/bradycardia, pulmonary hypertension)
- Increased rates of sepsis
- Hyperbilirubinemia
- Higher hospital readmission rates—often because of hyperbilirubinemia and dehydration related to poor feeding

Table 1.3. Clinical complications related to late preterm gestation.[108,109,118,119]

Small for Gestational Age (SGA) and Intrauterine Growth Restriction (IUGR) Infants

SGA infants have a birth weight below the 10th percentile for their gestational age.[120] Other definitions include when the birthweight is more than 2 standard deviations below the mean for gestational age or when the birthweight is below the 3rd percentile.[120-122] When compared with appropriately grown for gestational age (AGA) preterm and term infants, SGA infants have higher complication rates, including death.[120,122-126] Infants with congenital malformations (cardiac or renal structural anomalies, gastroschisis) and multiple anomalies are commonly SGA.[120,125,127]

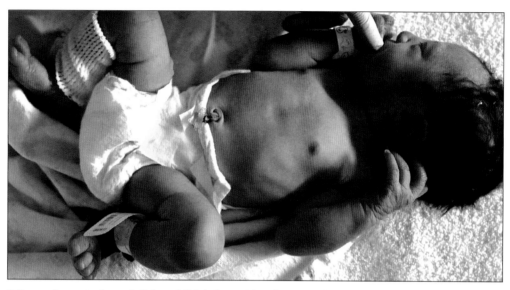

37-week gestation, 2.3 kg, SGA infant. Head circumference 30 cm, length 43 cm.

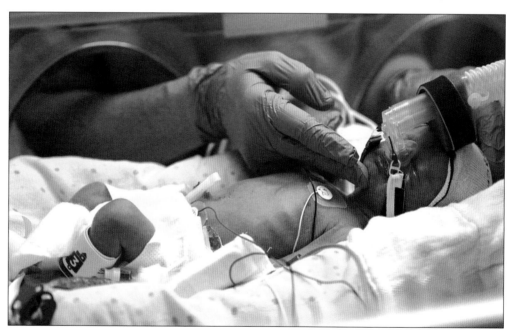

33-week gestation, 1.4 kg, SGA infant. Head circumference 29 cm, length 40 cm.

Symmetric SGA infants have a weight, length, and head circumference that all plot on a growth chart at or below the 10th percentile. Symmetric SGA growth often results from intrauterine viral infection in early gestation, longstanding maternal diseases with placental growth restriction present throughout most of the pregnancy, or chromosomal or genetic causes. Prior to plotting the infant's weight, head circumference, and length on a growth chart, perform an accurate gestational age assessment. See Appendices 1.2 and 1.3 for female and male growth charts.[128]

Intrauterine growth restriction (IUGR) describes when the fetus fails to meet its genetically determined growth potential based on race and gender. The terms IUGR and SGA are often used interchangeably; however, they are not the same. Infants with IUGR have clinical features of compromised in-utero growth and malnutrition.[129] Their birthweight is reduced but may be above the 10th percentile.[126,130] The IUGR infant's weight will be low for their gestational age, followed by some impact on length, but with relatively less restriction in brain growth and head circumference (often referred to as "head sparing").[120,131]

This asymmetric pattern of growth usually results from maternal medical conditions or poor placental function that disrupts oxygen and nutrient delivery to the fetus.

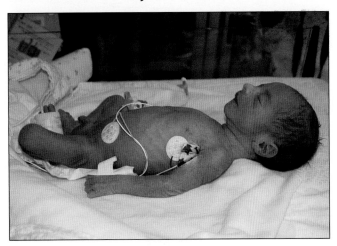

34-week gestation, 1.6 kg, IUGR infant. Head circumference 32 cm, length 47 cm.

SGA and IUGR infants are at increased risk for hypoglycemia

The fetus will make glycogen when fetal glucose uptake exceeds what they need for energy and growth.[74] When the placenta cannot provide enough nutrients and oxygen, the chronically stressed fetus will use most, if not all, of the placentally transferred glucose for growth and survival, thus limiting their ability to make or store glycogen for use after birth.[68,122] Even if glycogen stores are available, SGA infants may have difficulty mobilizing glycogen. In addition, SGA infants have low fat stores and impaired gluconeogenesis.[120,122] In one study of at-risk infants who were ≥35 weeks gestation and well enough to enterally feed, hypoglycemia (defined as a glucose concentration <47 mg/dL or 2.6 mmol/L) occurred in 50% of the SGA infants, with severe hypoglycemia (<36 mg/dL or 2 mmol/L) in 18% of the SGA infants.[132]

Growth in utero is influenced by the ability of the placenta to deliver oxygen and nutrients to the fetus, genetics, and intrauterine growth factors and hormones.[120] Causes of insufficient fetal growth include the following fetal and maternal factors.

Fetal Factors[120,122,129,131,133]

- Chromosomal abnormalities (e.g., trisomy 13, trisomy 18, trisomy 21, monosomy X)
- Genetic abnormalities / syndromes / congenital malformations
- Multiple gestation
- Intrauterine viral infection (cytomegalovirus, rubella, toxoplasmosis, syphilis, varicella, human immunodeficiency virus, parvovirus, and malaria)
- Metabolic disorders

Maternal Factors[120,122,127,129,131,133]

- Nutritional status before and during pregnancy, low maternal prepregnancy weight, low pregnancy weight gain

- Chronic illness / impaired placental function and ability to deliver oxygen and nutrients to the fetus secondary to: hypertension, preeclampsia, diabetes with underlying vascular disease, maternal congenital heart disease, renal disease, chronic anemia, chronic pulmonary illness (asthma, cystic fibrosis)

- Uterine factors: uteroplacental vascular insufficiency, abnormal anatomy, size, multiple gestation, twin-to-twin transfusion, short interpregnancy interval (less than 6 months)

- Chronic psychosocial stress

- Ingestion of substances (not prescribed medications taken as indicated) and toxins: nicotine, heroin, methadone, cocaine, morphine, methamphetamine, alcohol, toluene (glue and paint sniffing)

- Prescription medications used for chemotherapy (methotrexate, aminopterin, busulfan), seizure control (diphenylhydantoin, trimethadione), hypertension (propranolol), anticoagulant therapy (warfarin)

- Genetic and familial factors for small infant size (note that some infants may be "constitutionally small" but otherwise healthy)

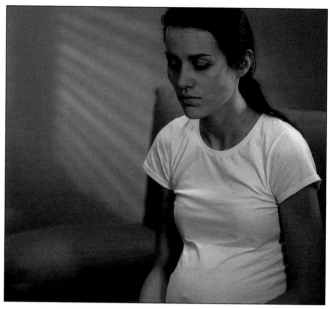

Anorexic patient at a prenatal visit at 34 weeks gestation.

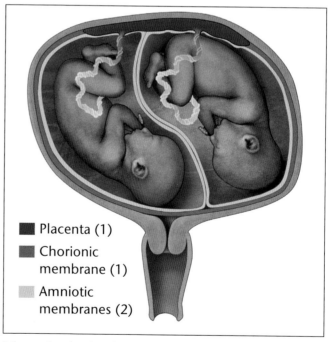

■ Placenta (1)
■ Chorionic membrane (1)
▨ Amniotic membranes (2)

Monochorionic, diamniotic (mono-di) twin pregnancies have a shared placenta and chorion but separate amniotic sacs. There is an increased risk for twin-twin transfusion syndrome (TTTS) where one twin will be the donor and develop hypovolemia and growth restriction, and the other twin will be the recipient and at risk for hypervolemia and congestive heart failure.

▲HIGH-RISK GROUPS: **Hyperinsulinemia**

Infant of a Diabetic Mother (IDM)

Glucose in the mother's bloodstream easily crosses the placenta to the fetus. The fetal blood glucose level is approximately 70% of the mother's glucose level.[68,134] If the mother's glucose is abnormally elevated, as occurs when the mother has uncontrolled diabetes, the fetal blood glucose level will also be elevated. Unlike glucose, **insulin does not cross the placenta.** In response to elevated blood glucose levels, fetal insulin production increases to help lower glucose.

When the umbilical cord is cut, the maternal glucose supply stops abruptly. The infant's insulin secretion can remain elevated for 2 to 4 days or longer as the neonatal pancreas adjusts to the infant's own glucose levels.[135] While awaiting the insulin secretion to down-regulate, IV dextrose (in combination with enteral feedings if the infant is well enough to tolerate feedings) may be required to help maintain the blood glucose at a safe level.[135] Infusing $D_{10}W$ at a lower glucose infusion rate of 3 to 5 mg/kg/minute may help to avoid further stimulating insulin secretion, but this adjustment in GIR is usually decided in the NICU setting.[103,136]

Compared to non-IDM infants, IDM infants may reach their nadir (low point) of blood glucose more quickly, by 60 minutes after birth.[137]

In addition to an increased risk for fetal malformations and preterm birth, IDM infants are at increased risk[134] for

- Respiratory distress syndrome
- Hypertrophic cardiomyopathy
- Polycythemia
- Hyperviscosity
- Renal vein thrombosis
- Hyperbilirubinemia
- Hypoglycemia
- Hypocalcemia
- Hypomagnesemia

Fetal exposure to hyperglycemia secondary to maternal diabetes also has negative health consequences for their offspring, including metabolic syndrome (obesity, hypertension, dyslipidemia, glucose intolerance), childhood obesity, diabetes later in life, and impaired neurodevelopmental outcomes.[135,138]

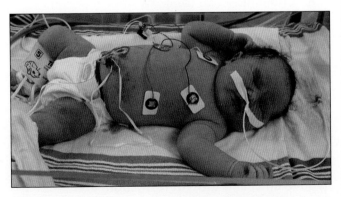

39-week gestation, 5.1 kg, LGA, IDM infant.

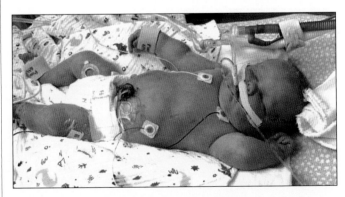

33-week gestation, 4 kg, LGA, IDM infant with complex congenital heart disease.

Large for Gestational Age (LGA) Infants

LGA infants have a birth weight above the 90th percentile for their gestational age.[129,139] Infants may be LGA because of ethnic[120] or genetic factors[140] or a higher percentage of lean body mass.[139] However, infants may also be LGA because of the effects of elevated maternal glucose levels during pregnancy and the subsequent fetal hyperinsulinemia.[121,141] Insulin is very important for fetal growth. Too much insulin causes more fat deposition than would otherwise occur, thus giving the IDM a characteristic overweight (obese) appearance.[74,134,139,141] When trying to determine if an infant is IDM versus constitutionally large without being an IDM, evaluate the infant for increased fat deposition in the face, neck and shoulders, arms, and thighs.[142] If these physical exam findings are present, maternal diabetes is possibly the cause. When an infant is born LGA, investigate the underlying cause, which may include that diabetes was not recognized during pregnancy.[143]

Macrosomia

A fetal weight larger than 4,000 to 4,500 grams is considered macrosomic.[139,142,144] Macrosomia is divided into three categories: 4,000 to 4,499 grams, 4,500 to 4,999 grams, and ≥5,000 grams. Obstetric management and birth planning incorporate this important information since morbidity and mortality, including stillbirth, increase as the fetal weight exceeds 4,500 grams. The most pronounced risk for a negative outcome is when the weight exceeds 5,000 grams.[142]

When macrosomia is produced by maternal glucose intolerance (e.g., in patients with diabetes, including GDM), fat deposition increases in the shoulders and upper extremities.

Birth complications *related to macrosomia include birth injuries (shoulder dystocia, brachial plexus injury, arm and clavicle fractures, and organ injury) and perinatal asphyxia.[138] A smaller head-to-abdominal circumference contributes to a higher incidence of shoulder dystocia.[142] When the fetal weight exceeds 5,000 grams, the risk of stillbirth and neonatal death increases.*

Maternal complications *related to fetal macrosomia include protracted or arrested labor, the need for operative vaginal (vacuum assist/forceps) or cesarean delivery, chorioamnionitis, third- and fourth-degree vaginal lacerations, postpartum hemorrhage, and uterine rupture.[142,144]*

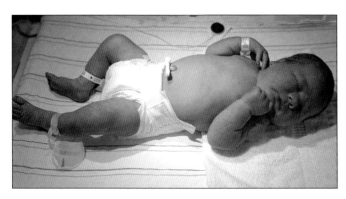

38-week gestation, 4.14 kg, LGA infant (but not an IDM).

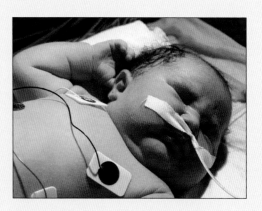

Let's Learn More... Diabetes in pregnancy and what is hemoglobin A1c?

Pregestational type 1 or type 2 diabetes and gestational diabetes mellitus (GDM) affect 7% of pregnancies in the U.S., with 86% of those cases being GDM.[80,138] Glucose intolerance during pregnancy that leads to a diagnosis of GDM is more common in Hispanic, African American, Native American, and Asian or Pacific Islander women.[80,141] In addition to ethnicity, risk factors for developing GDM include obesity, a history of GDM, glycosuria, a history of delivering a macrosomic infant, a maternal family history of type 2 diabetes, and a diagnosis of polycystic ovarian syndrome.[76,134,145-148]

As maternal body mass index (BMI) increases, independent of a diagnosis of diabetes, the risk for fetal death, stillbirth, neonatal death, perinatal death, and infant death also increases.[149] Obesity, defined as a body mass index $\geq$30 in women of childbearing age, is a significant global public health problem.[150] Unless counseled by their care providers, obese pregnant patients may not know they have an increased risk for complications (gestational hypertension, GDM, pre-eclampsia, and cesarean delivery)[151] and neonatal conditions and adverse events (transient tachypnea of the newborn, respiratory distress syndrome, hypoglycemia, and a difficult birth associated with macrosomia).[152]

Worldwide, there is a rise in type 2 diabetes among pregnant patients attributed to increased rates of obesity. Preexisting type 1 and 2 diabetes confers a much greater risk to maternal and fetal health than GDM. Uncontrolled diabetes increases the risk for spontaneous abortion, fetal demise, preeclampsia, fetal anomalies, macrosomia, preterm delivery, neonatal hypoglycemia, and neonatal hyperbilirubinemia.[135,147]

Fetal malformations of the heart, central nervous system, craniofacial area, genitourinary, gastrointestinal, and musculoskeletal systems are attributed primarily to the teratogenic effect of maternal hyperglycemia that impacts weeks 2 to 8 of pregnancy when the organs are first developing.[135,138,153] In women with type 1 and 2 diabetes, pre-pregnancy control of glucose can lower the risk for congenital malformation to levels of nondiabetic women.[135] For women with diabetes who are planning a future pregnancy, it is also very important to ensure pre-pregnancy glucose control is achieved prior to fertilization.[80]

Follow-up of the Pregnant Patient With Gestational Diabetes Mellitus (GDM)

When diagnosed with GDM, there is a 50 to 70% risk of developing type 2 diabetes within 15 to 25 years. Unfortunately, postpartum screening of patients with GDM is low for all racial and ethnic groups.[154] Follow-up evaluation that includes an oral glucose tolerance test should occur 4 to 12 weeks postpartum.[147] If diabetes is not detected in that postpartum follow-up, screening should occur every 1 to 3 years with other risk factors considered, such as prepregnancy body mass index (BMI), family history, and any glucose-lowering medications that were required during pregnancy.[80,147]

What Is Hemoglobin A1c (HbA1c), and How Is This Test Used to Evaluate Average Blood Glucose Levels?

In adults, hemoglobin A is the most abundant type of hemoglobin in the red blood cell (RBC).[155] When RBCs are exposed to glucose in the plasma, some of the hemoglobin becomes 'glycated' or glucose-coated. This glycated hemoglobin A is quantified as hemoglobin A1c (HbA1c). The HbA1c estimates the average

Let's Learn More... **Diabetes in pregnancy and what is hemoglobin A1c?**

blood glucose level over the previous 3 months (the average lifespan of the RBC is 120 days). Individuals with normal blood glucose levels have a baseline HbA1c of about 5%, meaning that 5% of their hemoglobin is glycated. When blood glucose levels are elevated, as can occur with diabetes, more HbA1c is formed.[156] The HbA1c test has become a reliable and valuable indicator of blood glucose control in diabetic patients.[156] HbA1c evaluation is not used in neonatal patients.

Key Points: Hemoglobin A1c

- Formation of HbA1c is an irreversible process, which means until the RBCs die and new RBCs and hemoglobin are formed, HbA1c reflects overall glucose levels for the prior 3 months.[156]

- A non-diabetic HbA1c is <5.7%. Individuals with a HbA1c of 5.7 to 6.4% are considered pre-diabetic. The threshold for diagnosing overt diabetes is when the HbA1c is ≥6.5%.[157]

- Assessment of HbA1c is of limited value in the presence of certain conditions: rapid RBC turnover (e.g., sickle-cell disease), glucose-6-phosphate dehydrogenase deficiency, hemodialysis, recent blood loss or transfusion, erythropoietin therapy, and iron-deficiency anemia.[145,157]

- RBC turnover is also increased in the second and third trimesters of pregnancy, and hemoglobin A1c levels may fall.[157] Therefore, HbA1c levels are not used as a primary measure of glucose control during pregnancy but can assist as a secondary measure for fetal risk assessment in the pregnant diabetic patient.[158,159] In the second and third trimesters, the risk for LGA size was lowest when the HbA1c was <6%.[81] In pregnant patients with type 1 diabetes, a HbA1c between 6 and 6.4% correlated with an increased risk for an LGA infant and between 6.5 to 6.9%, an increased risk for preterm delivery, pre-eclampsia, and need for a neonatal glucose infusion.[160]

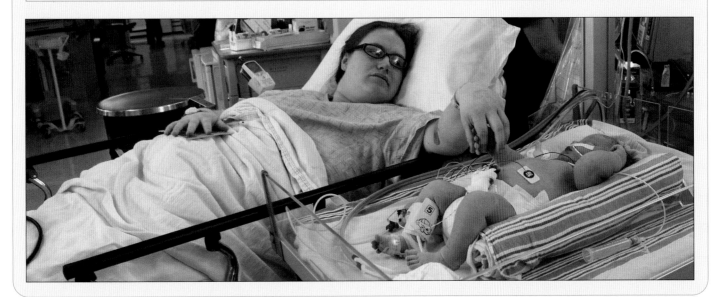

▲ HIGH-RISK GROUPS: Increased Utilization of Glucose

Who Does This Include?

All sick infants, including preterm and small for gestational age infants and those with sepsis, shock, respiratory and/or cardiac disease, hypothermia, or hypoxia.

Under aerobic conditions, when oxygen (O_2) content in the blood is sufficient to satisfy tissue needs, glucose is metabolized into energy.[161] Sick infants have higher energy expenditure than healthy newborns, and they may more rapidly deplete their glycogen stores. Infants who experience birth asphyxia and are hypoxic (O_2 delivery to the tissues is less than what is needed by the cells to function normally) may need to rely on anaerobic glycolysis to produce energy.[44] Anaerobic glycolysis is very inefficient because large quantities of glucose are consumed for a very low yield of energy.[33,162] Lactic acid produced during anaerobic glycolysis causes a decrease in pH and presents as metabolic acidosis.[162-164] In severely hypoxic infants, anaerobic glycolysis can provide enough energy to sustain cellular function for only a short period of time.[162] Figures 1.6 and 1.7 on page 39 illustrate energy production under aerobic and anaerobic conditions.

A significant perinatal event prior to birth can limit brain perfusion and oxygenation and increase the risk of developing a severe clinical problem called hypoxic-ischemic encephalopathy (HIE). Neurodevelopmental outcomes are worse when infants with HIE are hypoglycemic (blood glucose <47 mg/dL or 2.6 mmol/L), hyperglycemic (blood glucose > 150 mg/dL or 8.3 mmol/L), or when they have unstable blood glucose levels.[165-169] The ideal target blood glucose level has not been established, but special attention should be given to tight glycemic control to prevent both hypo- and hyperglycemia.

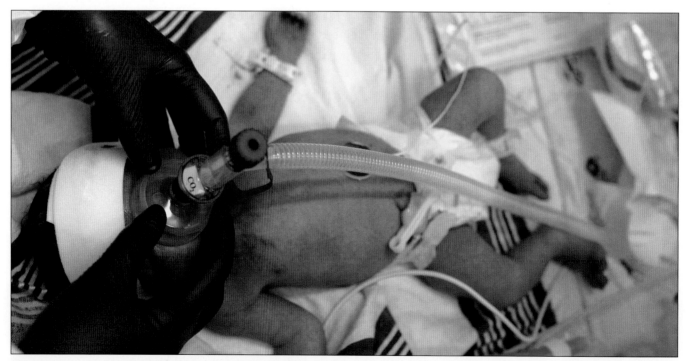

38-week gestation, 2.8 kg infant delivered by emergency cesarean section for fetal distress.

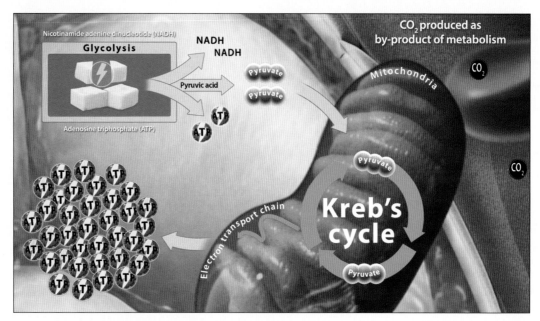

Figure 1.6. Model of aerobic metabolism. Under aerobic conditions, adequate amounts of O_2 are present inside cells to allow for the complete metabolism of glucose into adenosine triphosphate (ATP). For every molecule of glucose that is completely metabolized, 38 molecules of ATP are produced: two molecules from glycolysis of glucose to pyruvic acid and 36 molecules from the metabolism of pyruvic acid to ATP via the Krebs cycle.[162]

NADH = Nicotinamide adenine dinucleotide   ATP = Adenosine triphosphate

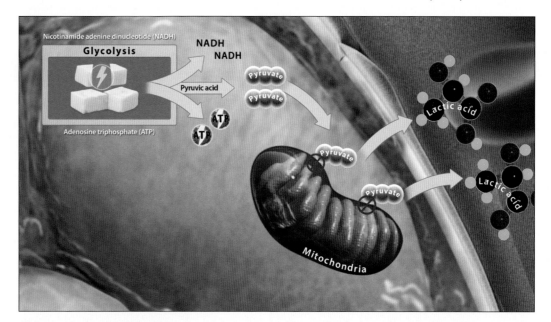

Figure 1.7. Model of anaerobic metabolism. Under anaerobic conditions (when cellular O_2 content is low), incomplete metabolism of glucose occurs. Only two molecules of ATP are produced for every molecule of glucose that is metabolized to pyruvic acid. Pyruvic acid is further metabolized into lactic acid.[162] If O_2 becomes available again, lactic acid is reconverted to pyruvic acid and metabolized as in aerobic metabolism. Evidence of anaerobic glycolysis may be seen as an elevated lactate level and on a blood gas as a low pH, low bicarbonate value, and a worsening base deficit.[163]

Monitoring the Blood Glucose Concentration (Blood Sugar Level)

Carbohydrates, as simple sugars, are the major source of metabolic fuel for the newborn. Glucose is the principal simple sugar: as glucose is transported to organs and tissues in the blood, it is also the principal 'blood sugar.' The gold standard for monitoring the level of blood sugar is the plasma glucose concentration. Either a sample of blood can be sent to the laboratory for analysis (which takes longer and requires more blood), or a bedside glucose oxidase device (e.g., Abbott® iSTAT®)* can be used.[170] Plasma glucose tests sent to the laboratory should be analyzed promptly to prevent red and white blood cells from further metabolizing glucose, which can result in falsely low values.[45]

Bedside "point-of-care" (POC) glucose meters are commonly used to monitor the blood sugar. The advantages of POC glucose devices are ease of use, rapid results, and the small amount of blood required (1 or 2 drops). Whole blood glucose concentrations may be 15% lower than plasma glucose.[45,171,172] Advances have been made in the accuracy of glucometers used in neonatal care to compensate for the difference between whole blood and plasma glucose measurements. One POC device approved by the U.S. Food and Drug Administration (FDA) for neonatal use is the StatStrip® glucometer (Nova Biomedical) because it corrects for the infant's hematocrit, then yields a plasma measurement of glucose.* Using a device with improved accuracy may eliminate the need for confirmatory laboratory testing in many cases.[173]

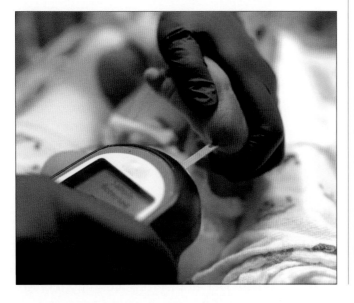
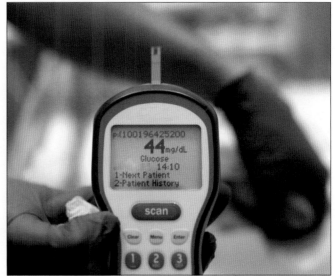

Note:

*There may be other glucometers that are FDA-approved for use in neonates, and this mention does not imply S.T.A.B.L.E.® endorsement of this specific glucometer.

How Often Should the Blood Glucose (Sugar) Be Checked?

The infant's health status and response to therapies will guide the interval for how often and how long to monitor their blood glucose.

For Sick Infants Who Cannot Be Fed

- Check the blood glucose early in the stabilization process and then every 1 to 3 hours until it remains stable ≥50 mg/dL (2.8 mmol/L).

- After 72 hours of age, the target glucose level is raised to ≥60 mg/dL (3.3 mmol/L).[105,174]

- When the blood sugar demonstrates a pattern of stability that is appropriate to the infant's postnatal age, risk factors for hypoglycemia, diagnosis, and clinical status, glucose monitoring can be spaced out, then eventually stopped.[172]

For Infants at Risk for Hypoglycemia (Late Preterm, IDM, LGA, SGA, IUGR) Who Are Well Enough to Feed

A reasonable guideline is to feed the infant within 1 hour of birth, followed by a blood glucose check 30 minutes after the feeding is completed, which will likely be at around 2 hours of age. Depending upon the result obtained at that time, the pre-feeding glucose should be checked at regular intervals until the level remains stable above 47 mg/dL (2.6 mmol/L).[175] After 72 hours of age, the target glucose is raised to ≥60 mg/dL (3.3 mmol/L).[105,174] At-risk infants may require glucose testing for 24 to 72 hours after birth and sometimes even longer. For more information, see Guideline 7: Management of Hypoglycemic Infants Who Are Healthy Enough to Tolerate Enteral Feedings on page 48.

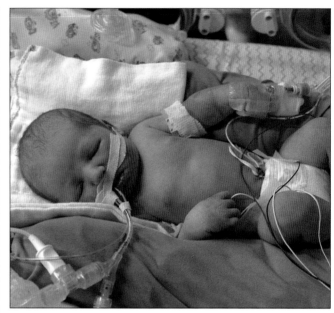

Term infant with pneumonia who was severely hypothermic following an unplanned out-of-hospital birth.

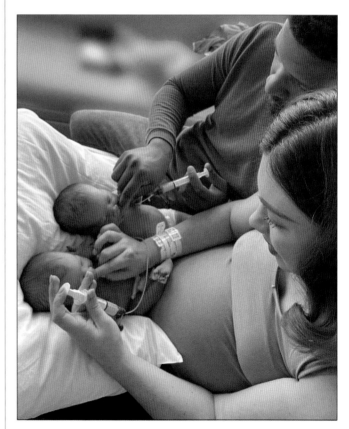

1-day-old, 36-week twins being finger fed by tube and syringe.

Signs of Hypoglycemia

In older children and adults, a low glucose level induces signs and symptoms of impaired cognition and level of consciousness or "neuroglycopenia."[172] In infants, neuroglycopenia can only be assessed by observing tone, feeding ability (suck coordination and strength) or interest in feeding, level of consciousness and response to stimuli, and cardio-respiratory status. Severe signs of neuroglycopenia include coma and seizures. These can often be late signs and indicative of irreversible brain damage.

Many infants who have low blood glucose levels are asymptomatic.[176] Therefore, if the infant is sick or there are risk factors for hypoglycemia, it is important to monitor the blood glucose at regular intervals. Table 1.4 describes the signs that may be observed when the blood glucose is low. Remember that these signs may also be observed because of other clinical problems, such as infection, brain injury, drug withdrawal, metabolic derangements, or respiratory distress. Once the blood glucose is normal again, the clinical signs that were observed should be resolved. If they are still present, then it is likely that the signs were caused by something other than hypoglycemia. Consider other causes, such as sepsis, neonatal abstinence syndrome, and metabolic pathologies.[136,177]

Table 1.4. Signs of hypoglycemia.

Neurogenic Signs (initial response to hypoglycemia related to catecholamine release)	Neuroglycopenic Signs (reflects brain glucose deprivation)	Other Non-Specific Signs
• Jitteriness/tremors • Irritability • Tachypnea • Pallor	• Poor feeding (worse than is expected, complete disinterest in feeding, very poor suck) • Weak or high-pitched cry • Lethargy • Hypotonia that is worse than expected for gestational age • Seizures • Coma	• Hypothermia • Apnea • Bradycardia • Cyanosis

Neurogenic (autonomic nervous system) signs triggered by hypoglycemia are shown in column 1. These signs are usually seen when the blood glucose (sugar) begins to decline below 50 mg/dL (2.8 mmol/L). However, many infants have a blood glucose below this level and do not show any signs. Column 2 lists the signs seen when the blood glucose declines to a level that deprives the brain of enough glucose and, therefore, is insufficient for normal brain function (called neuroglycopenia).[44,45,73,74,172,178,179]

Guideline 5

Recommended Target Blood Glucose Level for Infants Who Require Intensive Care

Care Recommendation 5

Sick and at-risk infants may be more vulnerable to the negative neurological effects of hypoglycemia. Maintain the blood glucose ≥50 mg/dL (2.8 mmol/L). After 72 hours of life, increase the target glucose level to ≥60 mg/dL (3.3 mmol/L).

The S.T.A.B.L.E. Program defines hypoglycemia as "glucose delivery or availability to the brain and organs that is inadequate to meet glucose demand."[105]

Severe and/or prolonged hypoglycemia can cause brain damage.[47,180-190] Furthermore, the impact of asymptomatic and transient hypoglycemia on the brain may not be benign.[189,191-193] If an infant has a low blood glucose level, this does not imply that permanent neurologic damage will occur; however, it means that action should be taken to restore the blood glucose to a safer level.

Sick and especially unstable infants have higher energy expenditure than well infants. Sick infants are often too ill to tolerate enteral feedings, or enteral feedings are contraindicated because of the clinical situation or disease process.

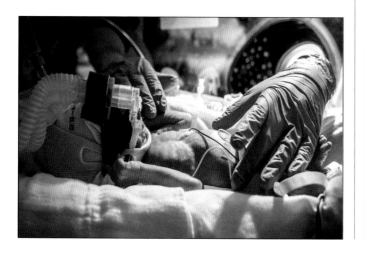

For *SICK* Infants Who Require Intensive Care

To provide a safe and reasonable target and treatment threshold, a whole blood or plasma glucose value <50 mg/dL (2.8 mmol/L) is the value below which The S.T.A.B.L.E. Program recommends corrective intravenous therapy. Ongoing monitoring should continue until the glucose remains ≥50 mg/dL (2.8 mmol/L) on at least two consecutive evaluations.[172]

After 72 hours of age, when **transitional hypoglycemia** in healthy newborns should be resolved, the target glucose level is raised to ≥60 mg/dL (3.3 mmol/L). The rationale for this higher target is that by 72 hours of age, the glucose ranges between 63 and 99 mg/dL (3.5 and 5.5 mmol/L).[105] Infants and children have equivalent ranges of plasma glucose: 70 to 100 mg/dL (3.9 to 5.6 mmol/L).[45,172]

Summary: Target Glucose Level for Sick Infants

Maintain the blood glucose ≥50 mg/dL (2.8 mmol/L).

After 72 hours old: Maintain the blood glucose ≥60 mg/dL (3.3 mmol/L) with an expectation that the normal range of glucose is 70 to 100 mg/dL (3.9 to 5.6 mmol/L).[172,194]

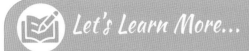

Let's Learn More... Transitional neonatal glucose regulation and pathologic neonatal hypoglycemia[45,68,74,105,172,174,195-199]

Glucose delivery from the mother to the fetus abruptly halts when the umbilical cord is cut and clamped. The newborn's blood glucose concentration declines from the fetal range of 70 to 100 mg/dL (3.9 to 5.6 mmol/L) to a nadir of approximately 55 to 65 mg/dL (3.1 to 3.6 mmol/L) by 1 to 2 hours after birth.[45] The decline in the blood glucose concentration activates a homeostatic response to help restore and maintain the blood glucose in a normal range. This response includes suppressing insulin secretion and releasing hormones: glucagon, adrenalin, cortisol, growth hormone, and thyroid stimulating hormone. Initially, glycogen is broken down in the liver, releasing glucose into the bloodstream at a rate of 4 to 6 mg/kg/minute. Glycogen is formed from non-carbohydrate precursors (*gluconeogenesis*), and fats are broken down (*lipolysis*). Combined with the establishment of breast milk or formula feedings, the blood glucose slowly rises, reaching concentrations above 70 mg/dL (3.7 mmol/L) by 72 to 96 hours after birth. Ninety percent of healthy, term, breastfed infants have a blood glucose concentration >47 mg/dL (2.6 mmol/L) for the first 48 hours after birth, rising to >54 mg/dL (3 mmol/L) by 84 hours and stabilizing at 83 +/- 13 mg/dL (4.6 +/- 0.7 mmol/L) by 4 days of age.[174]

Because the most common time of presentation of pathological hypoglycemic disorders occurs during the first 48 hours after birth, it is essential to distinguish between the normal transition of healthy infants to extrauterine life (transitional glucose regulation) and hypoglycemia caused by pathological, underlying conditions that may be either transient or persistent and capable of causing brain damage.

The common risk factors for pathological transient neonatal hypoglycemia are babies born preterm, small (especially those with IUGR), or large for gestational age, and infants of diabetic mothers. Other at-risk infants include those who are polycythemic or who experienced asphyxia, sepsis, or other illnesses that increase glucose utilization.[45,177] Maternal etiologies that increase the risk for neonatal hypoglycemia include hypertensive disorders, diabetes, obesity, and some medications taken during pregnancy, as outlined in Table 1.2. There is evidence of poorer academic performance[192] and worse neurodevelopmental outcome, executive function, and behavior in at-risk infants who experience hypoglycemia.[191,193] Treatment of transient hypoglycemia includes dextrose gel (if the infant is healthy enough to feed), human milk and/or formula feedings, and IV dextrose as necessary.[136,200]

Persistent, severe hypoglycemic disorders that present in the newborn period can lead to permanent brain injury. Causes include but are not limited to endocrine disorders (e.g., congenital hyperinsulinism, hypopituitarism, adrenal insufficiency), chromosomal or genetic abnormalities (Beckwith-Wiedemann syndrome and others), or inborn errors of metabolism of carbohydrates, fats, or amino acids.[44,45,74,172,201] Treatment often requires prolonged management with IV glucose, medications, and feeding regimens that may include continuous feedings and higher calorie supplementation.[74,194,202]

Let's Learn More...
Transitional neonatal glucose regulation and pathologic neonatal hypoglycemia

Why is this important? From Pediatric Endocrinologist, Dr. Paul Thornton

It is important to understand the physiology of normal glucose regulation in the newborn baby because this explains the common finding of hypoglycemia in the newborn. Up to 30% of otherwise healthy babies will have occasional glucose levels <45 to 50 mg/dL (2.5 to 2.8 mmol/L) in the first 24 hours of life. The difficulty faced by those taking care of newborns is how to differentiate these normal transitional changes in blood glucose from those babies with pathological forms of hypoglycemia, either transient or persistent, and how to prevent the brain damage that occurs in both the transient and persistent forms. The 2015 Pediatric Endocrine Society (PES) recommendations suggest that babies who have symptomatic hypoglycemia, need IV dextrose to treat hypoglycemia, or have **PERSISTENT** glucose values <50 mg/dL (2.8 mmol/L) in the first 48 hours of life or <60 mg/dL (3.3 mmol/L) after 48 hours are those at the greatest risk of pathological forms of hypoglycemia and need to have proof of resolution of hypoglycemia prior to discharge.[172] This evaluation can be done by a simple fasting study of 6–8 hours to demonstrate resolution of hypoglycemia. Those who fail to maintain a blood glucose >60 mg/dL (3.3 mmol/L) during the study will need further evaluation prior to discharge.

What about glucagon?

Administration of glucagon is a safe treatment for persistent or severe hypoglycemia, especially when IV access is a problem, as may be the case with LGA and IDM infants. Glucagon has also been used effectively in IUGR and SGA infants who have problematic and difficult to treat hypoglycemia.[203]

Glucagon is a counterregulatory hormone of insulin that increases hepatic glycogenolysis and gluconeogenesis, causing an increase in blood glucose levels.[69,204] Glucagon may be given intravenous (IV), intramuscular (IM), or subcutaneous (SC). The dose is 0.02 to 0.2 mg/kg/dose up to a maximum dose of 1 mg. While establishing IV access, glucagon may be a very useful medication to help treat hypoglycemia. Check the blood sugar 30 minutes after administration and then every 30 minutes until a glucose treatment regimen has been successfully implemented. In the majority of infants, glucagon administration is effective for 40 to 90 minutes, and the dose can be repeated.[205,206]

If the infant's glucose level is not responding to standard therapy, consult neonatology and pediatric endocrinology experts as quickly as possible since neurologic outcomes may be severely impacted by prolonged and/or persistent hypoglycemia.

Causes of persistent hypoglycemia can include endocrine disorders (e.g., congenital hyperinsulinism, hypopituitarism, hypothyroidism, adrenal insufficiency), chromosomal disorders (Beckwith-Wiedemann syndrome), genetic disorders, or inborn errors of metabolism of carbohydrates, fats, or amino acids.[44,45,74,172]

Guideline 6

IV Treatment of a Blood Glucose <40 mg/dL (2.2 mmol/L)

Care Recommendation 6

Ensure the IV is patent and that a dextrose-containing solution is infusing at an appropriate rate. If the blood glucose is ≥40 mg/dL (2.2 mmol/L) and steadily rising, then continue monitoring it at a regular interval. If the blood glucose <40 mg/dL, a mini-bolus of glucose is recommended.

This information pertains to sick or preterm infants who are too unwell to feed, such as infants with severe respiratory distress, bilious emesis, or tracheoesophageal fistula/esophageal atresia.

- Begin or continue an IV infusion of $D_{10}W$ at 80 mL/kg/day (= 5.5 mg/kg/minute GIR).

- If the blood glucose is **<40 mg/dL (2.2 mmol/L)**, administer a bolus of 2 mL/kg of $D_{10}W$ at a rate of 1 mL per minute.[44] This dose equals 200 mg per kg of glucose.

- If the glucose is ≤30, recheck the glucose 15 minutes after the bolus is completed. If the glucose is >30, recheck the glucose 30 minutes after the bolus is completed.

- If the blood glucose is **still <40 mg/dL (2.2 mmol/L), repeat the bolus** of 2 mL/kg of $D_{10}W$ (at a rate of 1 mL per minute) and increase the IV to 100 mL per kg per day. *(Multiply the infant's weight in kg by 100, then divide by 24 to find the new infusion rate).*

- If the blood glucose **is <40 mg/dL (2.8 mmol/L) after two glucose boluses,** then repeat the glucose bolus and increase the amount of delivered glucose.

To prevent hyperglycemia and rebound hypoglycemia, do not infuse 25% or 50% dextrose solutions. These solutions are also hypertonic and may cause phlebitis or thrombosis.

Two Options for Increasing the GIR

a) Increase the IV infusion to 120 mL/day (a faster option since it just requires increasing the IV rate), or

b) Increase the IV dextrose concentration to $D_{12.5}W$ or $D_{15}W$ if the glucose is very low.

- If the infant is experiencing persistent and severe hypoglycemia, increasing the dextrose concentration to provide a GIR of 12 to 15 mg/kg/minute (or more) may be necessary. Appendix 1.4 on pages 74 and 75 explains how to constitute higher (or lower) dextrose concentrations for IV infusion.

- Monitor the blood glucose every 30 to 60 minutes until it is at least 50 mg/dL (2.8 mmol/L) on at least two consecutive evaluations. Heel stick pokes are painful, so use good judgment to decrease the testing interval if the glucose is trending steadily upward.

- Remain vigilant for signs of hypoglycemia because interstitial blood glucose monitoring has revealed that infants at-risk for hypoglycemia had low glucose concentrations that went undetected after routine monitoring was stopped.[176,191]

Summary: Care Recommendations for the Initial Fluid and Glucose Management of Sick Infants

1 **If the infant is sick, especially if unstable, do not give enteral (oral or gavage) feedings.**

To reduce the risk of aspiration and unnecessary stress on the gastrointestinal tract, withhold enteral feedings, (oral or tube feedings). Once the infant stabilizes and the medical diagnoses are known, the introduction of enteral feedings can be considered.

2 **Provide glucose via intravenous (IV) fluids.**

Establish intravenous (IV) access and provide a glucose-containing solution.

3 **Initial IV fluid and glucose infusion rate (GIR).**

- Infuse $D_{10}W$ at 80 mL/kg/day (equals a GIR of 5.5 mg/kg/minute). If the infant is older than 24 to 48 hours, consider adding electrolytes to the IV fluid.

- If there is a history of significant birth stress, consider starting at a lower infusion rate of 60 mL/kg/day. Anticipate a higher dextrose concentration may be needed.

- Extremely preterm infants may have glucose intolerance and increased insensible water loss. Consider starting at a lower dextrose concentration (but $>D_5W$) and a higher infusion rate.

4 **Sick and preterm infants are at increased risk for hypoglycemia.**

Identify infants at risk for hypoglycemia (SGA, LGA, late preterm, sick) and monitor the blood glucose at an appropriate interval to detect low glucose levels that require treatment.

5 **Recommended target blood glucose level for infants who require intensive care.**

- Sick and at-risk infants may be more vulnerable to the negative neurological effects of hypoglycemia.

- Maintain the blood glucose between 50 and 100 mg/dL (2.8 to 5.6 mmol/L).

- After 72 hours old, the target glucose is raised to ≥60 mg/dL (3.3 mmol/L).

- Heel stick pokes are painful, so once the blood glucose has stabilized, use good judgment to decrease the testing interval.

6 **IV treatment of a blood glucose <40 mg/dL (2.2 mmol/L).**

The brain requires a steady supply of glucose to function. If the glucose is <40 mg/dL (2.2 mmol/L) and especially if not rising:

- Give a 2 mL/kg bolus of $D_{10}W$ (at a rate of 1 mL per minute).

- Evaluate the blood glucose 15 to 30 minutes after completion of the glucose bolus.

- Continue the IV infusion of $D_{10}W$ at 80 mL/kg/day.

- If the blood glucose is not rising following the $D_{10}W$ bolus, be prepared to repeat the bolus and increase the infusion rate and/or dextrose concentration.

 If the blood glucose is persistently >150 mg/dL (8.3 mmol/L) and not decreasing, this may be secondary to glucose intolerance (as may be seen with preterm infants), sepsis, a glucocorticoid (stress) response, or a side effect of methylxanthine medications.[44] Consult the referral center for guidance as needed.

Guideline 7

Management of Hypoglycemic Infants Who Are Healthy Enough to Tolerate Enteral Feedings

Care Recommendation 7

Offer regularly scheduled milk (mother's own milk, donor human milk, infant formula) feedings and consider dextrose gel to maintain the blood glucose ≥47 mg/dL (2.6 mmol/L).

- At-risk infants (late preterm, IDM, LGA, SGA, IUGR) who are well enough to feed should be fed as soon as possible after birth. Check the blood glucose 30 minutes after the feeding, which will likely be around 2 hours of age. Depending on the result obtained, the glucose should be checked at regular intervals and timed with feedings until the glucose level remains stable above 47 mg/dL (2.6 mmol/L).[175,176] After 72 hours old, the target glucose is raised to ≥60 mg/dL (3.3 mmol/L).[105,174]

- Additional strategies to prevent hypoglycemia in at-risk but otherwise healthy infants include skin-to-skin holding as soon as possible after birth to promote successful breastfeeding and avoid cold stress.[103] Sometimes, supplementation with donor human milk or infant formula is needed for a short period of time.

- It is increasingly common to treat hypoglycemia with buccal dextrose gel (40% gel, 0.5 mL/kg/dose = 200 mg/kg/dose) followed by human milk (mother's own milk or donor milk) or formula feedings every 2 to 3 hours.[176] To administer dextrose gel, the buccal area is dried with gauze, and then the dose of gel is massaged into the inner cheek mucosa.[73,207-209] To be effective, human milk or formula *must* be provided with the gel and can be given by syringe or gavage if necessary.

- If the infant's blood glucose is not rising, further declines, or the infant becomes symptomatic after two doses of dextrose gel plus effective feedings, notify the infant's medical staff. If the infant is still healthy enough to tolerate enteral feedings, a third dose of dextrose gel may be given while awaiting medical review. Escalation of therapy may need to include IV dextrose administration.[175,176]

- A useful algorithm for the screening and management of hypoglycemic infants who are well enough to feed uses a treatment threshold of <47 mg/dL (2.6 mmol/L) to administer 40% dextrose gel 0.5 mL/kg, followed by breastfeeding or a measured feeding of 5 mL/kg of mother's expressed milk, donor breast milk, or formula.[175] This algorithm further guides the timing of follow-up glucose evaluation and treatment and when to initiate IV therapy. See Narvey MR, Marks SD. The screening and management of newborns at risk for low blood glucose. *Paediatr Child Health.* 2019;24(8):536-554.

Because of the extra care and vigilance required, it is very important that the nursing assignment allows a mother/infant ratio that permits timely follow-up of the blood glucose levels and time to assist the mother to breastfeed, hand express, or pump their milk.

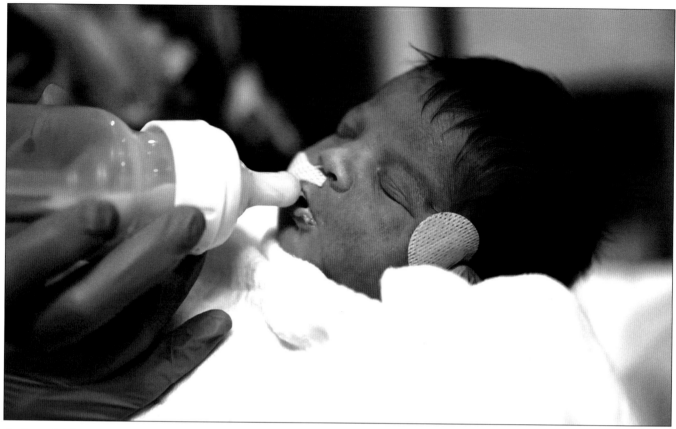

4-day-old former 34-3/7-week gestation infant attempting to bottle feed.

 Let's Learn More... **Dextrose gel study and practice guidelines**

The only evidence-based dextrose gel studies that evaluated long-term neurological outcomes of at-risk neonates 35 weeks gestation and older were done in New Zealand.[176,191] Hypoglycemia was defined as a glucose <47 mg/dL (2.6 mmol/L). Hypoglycemic infants were randomized to receive 40% dextrose gel or a placebo gel, followed by a milk feeding. The dextrose gel clinical practice guideline and hypoglycemia treatment flow chart utilized in New Zealand may be found at www.fmhs.auckland.ac.nz/clinicalpracticeguidelines.

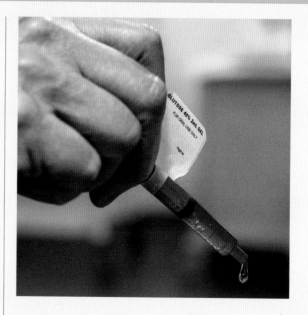

Note:

The referenced practice guideline and algorithm allows for up to six doses of dextrose gel in a 48-hour period. However, The S.T.A.B.L.E. Program recommends that no more than three doses of dextrose gel are given while concurrently deciding if supplementation, gavage feedings, and/or IV dextrose are necessary. Further doses of dextrose gel can be administered at the request of the medical team.

Let's Learn More... Intraosseous (IO) needle[210-222]

In a life-threatening emergency (e.g., shock or pre-cardiac arrest state), the IO route may be the quickest way to establish venous access. IO equipment and training should be available in all settings (rural through metropolitan) for use in neonatal emergencies when venous access is urgently needed or other attempts have failed. Medical staff in the emergency department are trained in IO insertion and can be a helpful resource.

In neonates, the IO insertion site is the medial aspect of the tibial bone just below the tibial tuberosity. Proper training is necessary to ensure the IO needle is inserted into the medullary portion of the bone and that care is taken to avoid the epiphyseal (growth) plate. Training should also include assessing for correct placement and monitoring for complications. As soon as other reliable IV access is established, the IO needle should be removed.

IO devices include an 18-gauge IO needle that requires a twisting motion to insert, a battery-operated drill, or a bone injection gun. Although not licensed for use as an IO needle, an 18- or 20-gauge short spinal needle with a stylet or a 21-gauge butterfly needle have been used in neonatal patients.[219] In preterm infants, the intramedullary diameter may be too small for IO needle insertion. Consult the tertiary neonatologist to discuss options for venous access.

If the patient is conscious or regains consciousness following resuscitation, infusion of fluids into the IO space can be painful because of the intense pressure felt within the bone. A small dose of lidocaine infused slowly into the bone marrow space can significantly help relieve pain. Follow all precautions and warnings associated with systemic lidocaine administration.[223,224]

What can be given via the IO route?

Any fluid, including crystalloids and colloids, blood, or medications that can be given in an IV line can also be given into the IO space.

Can laboratory testing be done on IO samples?[220]

To guide clinical care during an emergency, an IO sample can be analyzed using a point-of-care iStat® device. A blood culture may also be obtained from the IO site. For additional laboratory testing, it is important to first discuss the sample source with your lab because the sample can contain particulate matter (bone marrow contents) that can damage conventional laboratory equipment.

Pain control in the *conscious* infant who can feel pain and who has an IO in place

The following lidocaine administration process is from www.eziocomfort.com:

- Dose: 0.5 mg/kg of 1% or 2% preservative-free, epinephrine-free intravenous lidocaine.[225]

- Because of the small volume of lidocaine that will be in the syringe, add **NS 0.3 mL to the syringe** so that a slow infusion is possible.

- Connect the syringe with lidocaine and NS directly to the IO needle hub.

- Infuse **slowly** over 120 seconds.

- Allow the lidocaine to **dwell for at least 60 seconds** to allow numbing.

- Disconnect the 1 mL syringe and connect 2 mL of NS flush. Flush over at least 60 seconds while you assess for adequate pain control.

Umbilical Catheters

At times, it can be difficult to insert an IV, especially if the infant is in shock. If having difficulty inserting a peripheral IV, remember the **umbilical vein** can be used for delivering IV fluid and medications. The umbilical vein can usually be cannulated for up to 1 week after birth. However, even in newborns, the catheter may be difficult to insert. Table 1.5 on page 52 contains information about the correct UVC tip location and complications related to malposition. Table 1.6 on page 54 summarizes UVC placement indications, catheter size, infusion solutions, heparin dose, medication administration, and contraindications. Table 1.7 on page 55 contains mathematical formulas for both umbilical artery catheter (UAC) and UVC insertion depths. Figure 1.8 on page 52 shows the correct UVC tip location on X-ray. Figure 1.9 on page 57 explains how to secure an umbilical catheter.

Indications for Umbilical Vein Catheter (UVC) Insertion[63,213,226-228]

- Rapid IV access is required, and given the infant's condition, the UVC is the best option for administering emergency fluids and medications.

- Based on the infant's health status and condition, there is ongoing difficulty establishing a peripheral IV within a reasonable time or number of attempts.

- More than one intravenous line is required.

- To administer glucose concentrations exceeding 12.5% dextrose.*

- To administer total parenteral nutrition (TPN) with higher dextrose concentrations, amino acids, calcium, and phosphorus additives.

- To perform an exchange transfusion.

*Note:
Some centers will infuse $D_{15}W$ in a peripheral IV if there are no other ingredients (such as amino acids, calcium, etc.) in the IV fluid.

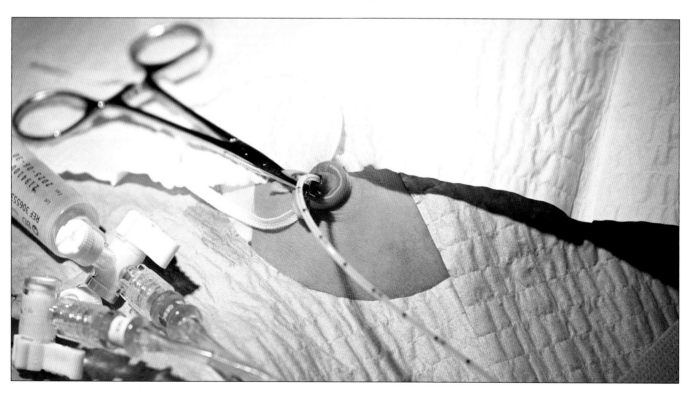

Table 1.5. Umbilical vein catheter (UVC) tip location and complications related to malposition.

Central Location[228-235]

On anteroposterior (AP) chest X-ray, the tip should be at the inferior vena cava/right atrial junction (IVC/RA junction). If unsure of the location of the tip, obtain a cross-table lateral chest X-ray. An ultrasound or echocardiogram may also help evaluate the catheter tip location.

Complications are reduced when the UVC tip is in a good position; however, they can still occur. Complications include bloodstream infection, thrombus formation, catheter migration to an undesirable location, pericardial tamponade, and supraventricular tachycardia.

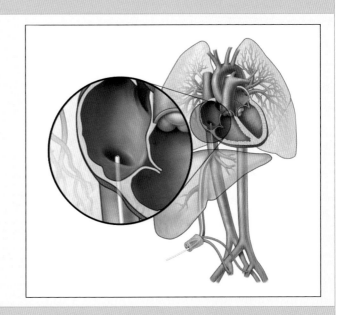

Emergency Placement[211,228,230,236]

In an emergency, the UVC can be inserted 2 to 4 cm (plus the length of the umbilical stump) until there is free-flow of blood. The insertion depth varies based on the size of the infant. This location is purposely low in the umbilical vein to reduce injury to the liver. A low-lying UVC can be used to administer resuscitation medications, normal saline volume infusions, and a glucose-containing solution pending the establishment of IV access.

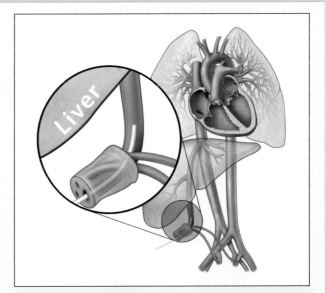

 In emergency situations, there may not be time to confirm the catheter tip location by X-ray before infusing hypertonic resuscitation medications. To avoid liver injury when hypertonic solutions are given, avoid placing the catheter tip in the liver or portal venous circulation.

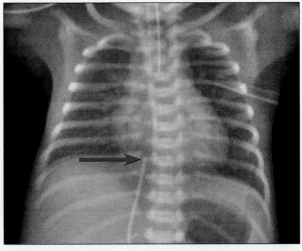

Figure 1.8. Chest X-ray of an infant showing the UVC tip (blue arrow) positioned correctly at the IVC/ RA junction. The ET tube is also in a correct position in the mid-trachea.

Complications of Malposition in the Heart[228,237-240]

- Arrhythmias
- Intracardiac thrombus formation
- Heart perforation
- Pericardial effusion
- Cardiac tamponade
- Pulmonary and systemic emboli; infected emboli may cause abscess formation
- Endocarditis
- Pulmonary infarction
- Pulmonary hemorrhage

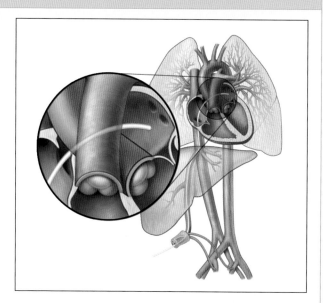

 Avoid placement in the right atrium because the tip may cross the foramen ovale into the left atrium and increase the risk for perforation, emboli, or malposition in a pulmonary vein.

Complications of Malposition in the Liver or Portal Venous System[228,237,241-244]

- Liver necrosis following thrombus formation or infusion of hypertonic or vasoactive solutions into the liver
- Liver abscess formation
- Chronic portal hypertension
- Ascites (secondary to extravasation of fluid into the abdomen)
- Peritoneal perforation
- Intestinal ischemia
- Hepatic vessel perforation and hematoma formation, followed by calcification when the hematoma resolves
- Intravascular thrombus formation
- Emboli released into the liver

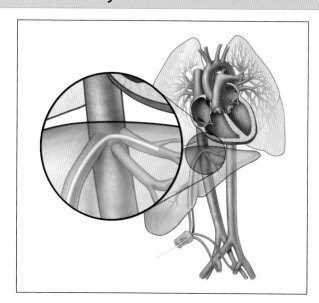

Umbilical Vein Catheter (UVC)

Indications for Placement[236,237]	Catheter Size[237]	Infusion Solutions[245]	Heparin Dose [63,236] (units per mL IV fluid)	Medication Administration [216,228,245]	Contraindications for UVC Placement[228,230]
1. To provide emergency fluids and medications during resuscitation 2. Unable to start a peripheral IV in a reasonable time or number of attempts 3. To provide a glucose concentration greater than $D_{12.5}W$* or hyperosmotic solutions (such as total parenteral nutrition) 4. When additional IV access is required for fluids or medications 5. Exchange or partial exchange transfusion 6. Central venous pressure monitoring	<1.5 kg: 3.5 French >1.5 kg: 5 French Single-lumen and double-lumen catheters are available. A double-lumen catheter is commonly used with preterm and sick infants to allow simultaneous administration of medications and total parenteral nutrition.	5 to 20% dextrose solution (D_5W to $D_{20}W$) is appropriate if the catheter tip is in a good position. **Note:** A dextrose concentration >20% may need to be infused in the UVC for some circumstances (i.e., to significantly restrict fluid administration or treat severe hypoglycemia).	0.25 to 1 unit per mL of IV fluid **Note:** Not all centers add heparin to the IV fluid. Consult your tertiary center for their recommendation.	If the catheter tip is properly positioned at the IVC/RA junction, then all medications, including vasopressors (dopamine, dobutamine, epinephrine), may be given in the UVC.	Omphalitis Omphalocele Peritonitis **Note:** Some centers also exclude UVC insertion when an infant has necrotizing enterocolitis.

*Note: Some centers will infuse $D_{15}W$ in a peripheral IV if there are no other ingredients (such as amino acids, calcium, etc.) in the IV fluid.

✓ **Clinical Tip**

A "bouncing back" feeling of resistance during placement usually indicates the catheter tip is malpositioned in the liver or portal venous system.

Table 1.6. Umbilical vein catheter: Indications for placement, catheter size, infusion solutions, heparin dose, medication administration, and contraindications for UVC placement.

Umbilical Artery Catheter (UAC)[63,213,246,247]	Umbilical Venous Catheter (UVC)[228-230]
High UAC The tip is located between thoracic vertebrae 6 and 9 (T6 and T9). > **UA catheter length** (in centimeters) = (3 X birth weight [in kilograms]) + 9[248] *For infants <1,500 grams,* the following calculation method[249] may be more precise:* > **UA catheter length** (in centimeters) = (4 x birth weight [in kilograms]) + 7 *The Wright study evaluated this formula to locate the UAC tip between T6 and T10. The S.T.A.B.L.E. Program recommends a high UAC tip location between T6 and T9.	The tip is located at the junction of the inferior vena cava and right atrium (cavoatrial junction). > **UV catheter length** (in centimeters) = (0.5 X *high line UAC insertion length*** [in centimeters]) + 1[213] Add the length of the umbilical stump (in centimeters) to the calculation. **This number is derived from the upper formula in the high UAC column.
Low UAC A low UAC location may be necessary if a high UAC position is not possible. The catheter tip should be located between lumbar vertebrae 3 and 4 (L3 and L4). This location usually places the catheter tip just above the aortic bifurcation.	

Table 1.7. UAC and UVC insertion depth calculations.

Mathematical formulas for catheter insertion depth only provide estimates. No one mathematical formula has proven to be 100% accurate. Confirm all catheter placement (or repositioning of catheters) with an X-ray. It may be necessary to evaluate both a chest and abdominal X-ray to determine whether the catheter was inserted into the umbilical artery or vein. If unsure of the tip location, a cross-table lateral view X-ray may provide additional helpful information. Ultrasound can also help with identifying catheter placement. If the UAC is located too deep or not deep enough, refer to the information in Table 1.10 on page 61 for guidance on how to correct a malpositioned UAC line.

Heparin Safety

Heparin, a blood anticoagulant, is frequently added to central line fluids to reduce catheter occlusion by thrombus formation.[230] Heparin is supplied in different concentrations; therefore, each time a heparin vial is opened, double check that the correct concentration was selected. If caregivers have little to no experience using heparin, consult the tertiary center to discuss if they prefer to add the heparin after the infant is transported.

Heparin Dose: 0.25 to 1 unit per milliliter of IV fluid (0.25 to 1 unit heparin per mL IV fluid)[250]

 Ideally, commercially prepared IV fluid containing heparin should be utilized. However, when this is not available, the IV fluid should be prepared in the pharmacy under strict aseptic conditions. If this is not possible, the heparin dose (how much was drawn up and the heparin concentration in the vial) should be checked by two registered nurses prior to adding to the IV fluid.

 Accidental overdose is a potential hazard when administering heparin. Be aware that it only takes 50 to 100 units of heparin per kilogram of body weight to "heparinize" an infant, which may lead to excessive bleeding. If a pharmacist is not available to measure and add the heparin to the IV fluid, be certain to double-check the following:

- The heparin concentration
- The dose and amount that is drawn into the syringe
- The heparin is being added to the correct IV fluid volume

Heparin vials may resemble other medication vials used in the nursery; therefore, it is recommended that you discard the heparin vial after use.

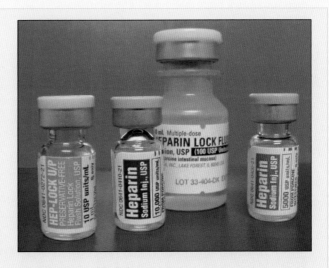

Photo courtesy of Institute for Safe Medication Practices (ISMP)

Figure 1.9. Directions for securing an umbilical catheter using a semipermeable transparent sterile dressing.

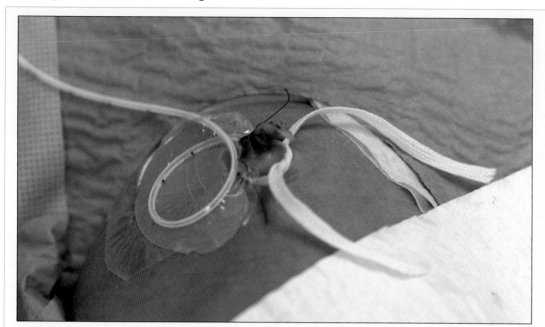

When possible, first apply a hydrocolloid base layer under the transparent dressing to protect the abdominal skin. This protective layer is especially important for premature infants who have immature, fragile skin.

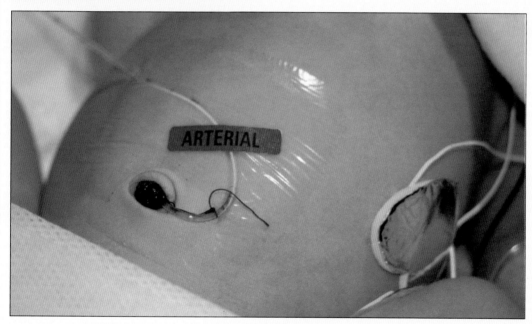

Step 1 While the protective backing is still on the transparent dressing, cut a semicircle in the top edge of the dressing so that it is applied as close to the umbilical stump as possible.

Step 2 Remove the central backing from the dressing. Position the catheter so it is looped slightly on the abdomen. Hold the catheter in place while the dressing is pressed onto the skin. Remove the edges of the backing. The catheter should be held securely under the dressing with as little of the catheter protruding from the umbilical stump as possible to help prevent accidental dislodgment.

Step 3 Extra dressing or tape may be used to reinforce the original dressing.

Step 4 To identify the type of catheter in place, apply a venous and/or arterial label over the dressing or on the IV tubing.

Umbilical Venous Catheter Safety Guidelines

1 Central line evidence-based bundles should be incorporated into your unit practice to prevent central line-associated bloodstream infection (CLABSI) and catheter-related complications.[251,252]

2 Use sterile technique when placing lines, setting up infusion tubing, drawing labs, and administering IV fluids and medications.

3 Once the sterile field is disassembled, do not advance the umbilical catheter.

4 If the umbilical catheter is repositioned, a chest or abdominal X-ray should be repeated to confirm the catheter tip is in a correct location.

5 Catheter tip migration is common. Note the centimeter marking at the umbilicus after the UVC is secured. During nursing assessments, check the marking to detect any unplanned movement of the UVC. Report any concerns to the medical care team. Obtain a surveillance X-ray 24 hours after UVC insertion to monitor for catheter migration to an incorrect location. Consider using ultrasound to determine tip location since ultrasound does not use radiation and it can be more sensitive and accurate than X-ray evaluation.[220,253,254]

6 Use caution when connecting IV fluids or medications to the central line or when drawing labs from the line to avoid contaminating the sterile system.

7 Maintain an air-tight system. Do not allow air bubbles to infuse into the infant's bloodstream.

8 Check connections to make sure they are tight. Rapid, life-threatening blood loss can occur with inadvertent disconnection of the tubing, especially with arterial lines.

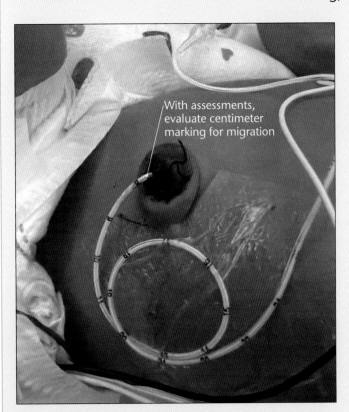

With assessments, evaluate centimeter marking for migration

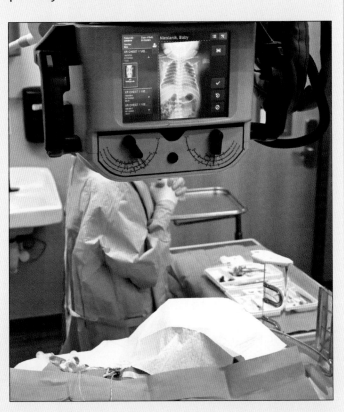

Additional Information for Neonatal Intensive Care Unit (NICU) Staff

Indications for Umbilical Artery Catheter (UAC) or Peripheral Arterial (Radial/Posterior Tibial) Line Insertion[246,247,255]

An arterial line is selected for

- Continuous arterial blood pressure monitoring

- Arterial blood gas evaluation and monitoring

If unable to insert a UAC, additional options include cannulation of the radial or posterior tibial artery. Table 1.7 on page 55 explains how to calculate UAC and UVC insertion depths, and Table 1.8 summarizes high and low UAC tip locations and the rationale for those locations. Table 1.9 on page 60 includes indications for placement of a UAC, catheter size, infusion solutions, heparin dose, medication administration, and contraindications for use, and Table 1.10 on page 61 provides guidance for resolving UAC malpositions.

Umbilical Artery Catheter (UAC)	Tip Location	Rationale for This Location
High Line[63,213,246,247]	On anteroposterior (AP) chest X-ray, the tip should be between thoracic vertebrae 6 and 9 (T6 and T9).	To avoid ischemic injury to organs and tissues served by the celiac and superior mesenteric arteries, and to arteries that come off the aorta in the upper chest • The celiac artery originates at the aortic level of T11 • The superior mesenteric artery originates at the aortic level of T11 to T12 • The aortic arch and carotid and subclavian arteries are located above T5
Low Line[63,230,246]	On abdominal X-ray, the tip should be in the abdominal aorta, between lumbar vertebrae 3 and 4 (L3 and L4) and above the bifurcation of the iliac arteries.	To avoid injury to organs and tissues served by the renal and inferior mesenteric arteries • The renal artery originates at the aortic level of L1 • The inferior mesenteric artery originates at the aortic level of L2 • The bifurcation of the aorta and iliac arteries is at approximately L4 to L5

Table 1.8. Umbilical artery catheter (UAC) tip location.

Umbilical Artery Catheter (UAC)

Indications for Placement[237,246]	Catheter Size[230,237,246,247]	Infusion Solutions[247,256-258]	Heparin Dose [63,246] (Units per mL IV fluid)	Medication Administration [245,246,259,260]	Contraindications for UAC Placement[213,246]
1. To monitor arterial blood pressure 2. To allow arterial blood gas evaluation and monitoring	<1.5 kg: 3.5 French >1.5 kg: 5 French	**UAC and peripheral arterial lines:** 0.9% sodium chloride (normal saline) or 0.45% sodium chloride (half normal saline) **UAC only*** (not recommended for peripheral arterial line): D_5W to $D_{15}W$, with or without amino acids and with 0.5 to 1 unit of heparin per mL of IV solution *Evidence is lacking regarding the effects related to administration of parenteral nutrition, calcium, and medications (including antibiotics) through the UAC. Consult your hospital pharmacist and neonatology leadership for guidance.	0.25 to 1 unit per mL IV fluid The dose varies by institutional preference, and if you are unsure which option to select, consult your tertiary center.	The UAC is not recommended for medications or blood administration. **!** *Do not infuse vasopressors (dopamine, dobutamine, or epinephrine), calcium boluses, or blood in the UAC or any arterial line.*	Omphalitis Peritonitis Omphalocele Gastroschisis Vascular compromise in the lower limbs or buttocks Acute abdominal pathology (may include necrotizing enterocolitis)

Table 1.9. Umbilical artery catheter: Indications for placement, catheter size, infusion solutions, heparin dose, medication administration, and contraindications for UAC placement.

Catheter Position[215,246,247]	Malposition	What to Do to Correct the Malposition
High-Positioned UAC Correct placement is between T6 and T9 --- **Note:** Some neonatologists will accept a tip located at T10.	The UAC tip is higher than T6	Pull the UAC back until it is between T6 and T9.
	UAC is curved back upon itself	Try to pull back on the catheter to see if it will straighten out. Repeat the chest X-ray, and if the catheter is still curved upon itself, further attempts to reposition it will most likely be unsuccessful. The catheter should be removed, and a new catheter inserted using sterile technique.
	UAC tip is below T9	Pull the catheter back until it is at the level of L3 to L4 (i.e., convert the catheter from a "high" line to a "low" line).
Low-Positioned UAC Correct placement is between L3 and L4	UAC tip is too high for a low line (the tip is located somewhere between L2 and T10) --- **Note:** Some neonatologists will accept a tip located at T10.	The UAC needs to be repositioned to a LOW line at L3 to L4. Once the catheter has been repositioned, repeat an abdominal X-ray to confirm the tip is in a correct position.
	UAC is curved back upon itself	Try to pull back on the catheter to see if it will straighten out. Repeat the abdominal X-ray, and if the catheter is still curved upon itself, further attempts to reposition it will most likely be unsuccessful. The catheter should be removed, and a new catheter should be inserted using sterile technique.
	UAC is going down the leg	Remove the UAC and reinsert a new catheter using sterile technique.
	UAC tip is below L4	The UAC tip may now be in the iliac artery rather than in the aorta. If the sterile field has been disassembled, do not advance the catheter! Remove the catheter and reinsert a new one using sterile technique.

Table 1.10. Actions to take to when the UAC is malpositioned. Once a catheter is repositioned, repeat the abdominal or chest X-ray (as applicable) to verify the tip is in the correct position.

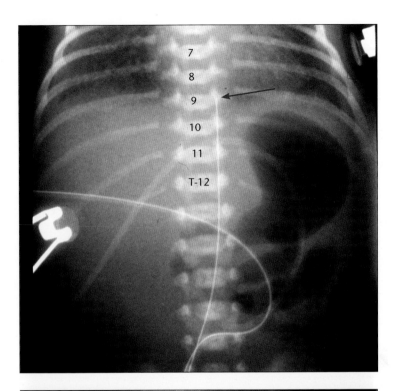

Figures 1.10 and 1.11 are X-rays of correctly positioned umbilical lines. Figure 1.12 is a cross-table lateral X-ray that shows the pathway of umbilical venous and arterial catheters.

Figure 1.10. Abdominal X-ray of a term infant showing the UAC tip in good position at T9.

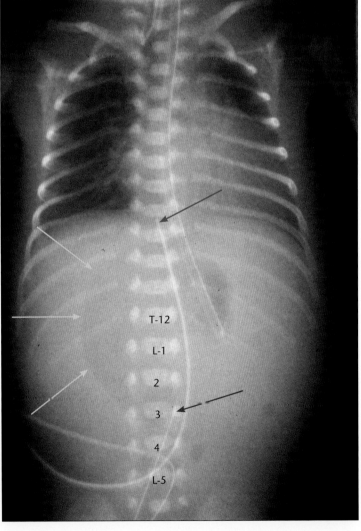

Figure 1.11. Chest and abdominal X-ray of a preterm infant with a UVC and UAC in correct position. The UVC tip (blue arrow) is located at the IVC/RA junction and the UAC tip (red arrow) is located at L3. This infant also had a pneumoperitoneum secondary to an intestinal perforation. The yellow arrows are pointing at the air collection.

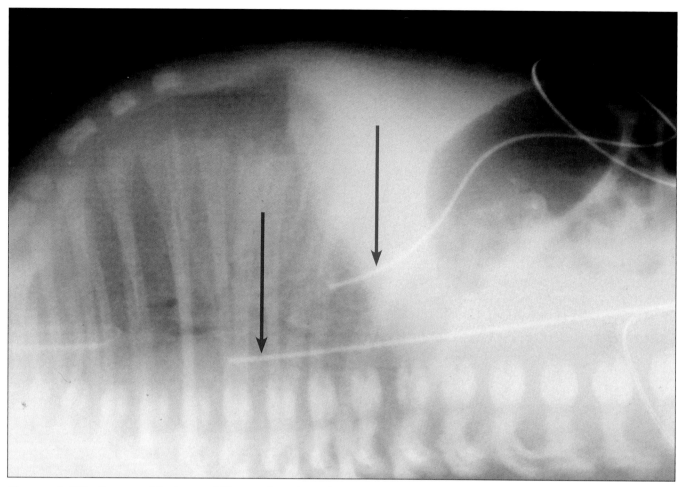

Figure 1.12. Cross table lateral X-ray showing the pathway of umbilical catheters. The UAC (red arrow) is in the aorta, and the UVC (blue arrow) is in the inferior vena cava. Both catheters are in good position, although it is possible that the UVC is in the right atrium. Ultrasound investigation may be necessary when uncertain about the UVC tip location.

Umbilical Artery Catheter (UAC) or Peripheral Arterial Line (PAL) Safety Guidelines

In addition to the other umbilical catheter safety guidelines previously discussed, the following information applies to care of an infant with a UAC or PAL.

1. The UAC or PAL should always be attached to a transducer. A dampened or flattened arterial waveform may indicate presence of an air bubble in the system, disconnection, development of a thrombus in or around the catheter tip, or hypotension.

2. When a UAC is in use, monitor the temperature and color of the infant's toes, legs, groin, abdomen, and buttocks for signs of arterial spasm, clot, or emboli.[261] Any abnormalities in the assessment of the lower body should be reported to the infant's care team. These complications can occur at any time while the UAC is in place, including just after insertion.

3. When a PAL is in use, monitor the temperature and color of the infant's feet and toes (posterior tibial artery placement) or temperature and color of the infant's hand and fingers (radial artery placement).

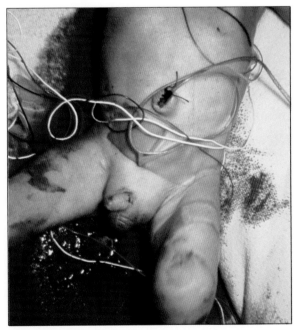

Massive hemorrhage secondary to accidental disconnection of the arterial line.

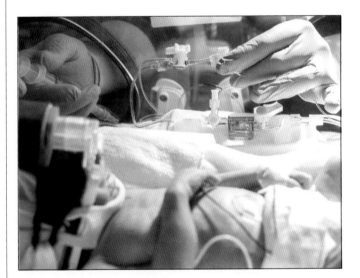

Arterial line transducer.

✓ Clinical Tip

What complications should I watch for when a UAC or PAL are in place?[230,246,255,261-263]

Arterial spasm or development of emboli from small blood clots that form on the tip or in the circulation adjacent to the catheter tip may occur when a UAC or PAL is in use. The area distal to the spasm or clot may show signs of impaired skin perfusion. Therefore, monitor the infant frequently for white, blue, or black discoloration of the skin on the back, buttocks, groin, abdomen, legs, feet, or toes. If the PAL is in the radial or ulnar artery, observe the hand and fingers for adequate perfusion and equal warmth. A cooler hand or fingers (or foot/toes) compared to the other side may indicate decreased perfusion secondary to impaired blood flow. In milder cases where no skin necrosis is evident, warming the contralateral limb may be useful to improve perfusion and should be considered.[263]

Document your assessment and include the presence of both normal and abnormal findings. If the catheter stops functioning correctly or evidence of vasospasm persists, there may be a thrombus at or near the catheter tip. Following catheter removal, monitor closely for improved perfusion. If perfusion does not improve, additional diagnostic studies and treatments should be considered, including ultrasound, Doppler assessment, angiography, application of systemic or topical vasodilators, and/or treatment with tissue plasminogen activator.[262,263]

 Notify the infant's medical team promptly to discuss actions that may be necessary, including line removal.

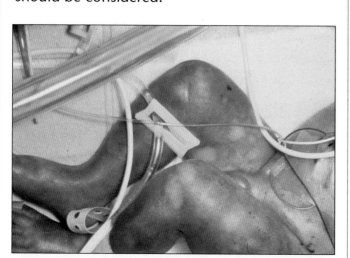

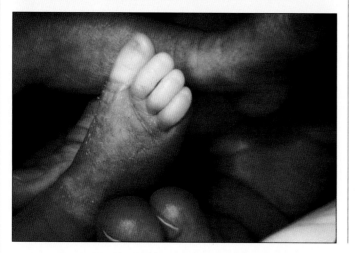

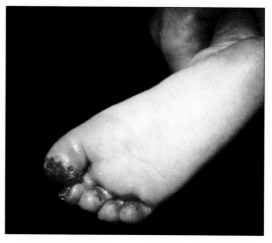

Examples of impaired perfusion related to arterial lines.

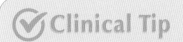

Clinical Tip

How fast should I withdraw blood from a high-positioned UAC, and how fast should I return blood and flush?

Studies have demonstrated changes in cerebral saturation and blood volume with arterial withdrawal of blood, even over intervals of 80 seconds. The clinical significance of these decreases in cerebral desaturation and cerebral blood volume, particularly regarding initiating or worsening intraventricular hemorrhage, has not been established. In light of these concerns, it is advised to review your unit protocol and establish a parameter for the speed with which blood should be withdrawn and returned through a UAC. Future studies are needed to evaluate the safest way to sample from the UAC and to determine any impacts on short- or long-term neurodevelopmental outcomes.

The studies of interest are summarized as follows:

Schulz et al.[264] found that withdrawing 2.5 mL of blood from a high-positioned UAC (tip between T6 and T9) over a 40-second interval prevented cerebral hemoglobin desaturation, whereas withdrawing the same volume of blood over a 20-second interval resulted in cerebral hemoglobin desaturation.

Roll et al.[265] evaluated 40 and 80-second withdrawal sampling times in a population of preterm infants who were smaller and more immature than Schulz's study patients. Both the 40 and 80 second withdrawal rates resulted in similar declines in cerebral desaturation and cerebral blood volume. A re-instillation time of 36 seconds was used to return the 1.6 mL draw-up volume and the 0.6 mL line flushing volume.

Two more recent studies by Mintzer and colleagues[266,267] examined changes in cerebral O_2 saturation ($CrSO_2$) during UAC blood sampling in 500 to 1,250-gram neonates and found significant declines in $CrSO_2$, as well as variable and, at times, prolonged recovery to baseline with UAC blood draws. The individual nursing process and blood withdrawal time was not controlled for.

Butt et al.[268] found that returning fluid and volume into a low-positioned UAC (catheter tip located between L3 to L4) at a rate of 0.5 mL per 5 seconds prevented retrograde aortic blood flow and elevation of blood pressure, whereas retrograde aortic blood flow and elevation of blood pressure were observed when faster return times were used.

If possible, use a commercially available sterile sampling device designed to reduce sampling volume and decrease the risk of contamination. If this equipment is not available, the removal and return volume from a UAC is usually between 1 and 3 mL per lab draw. Davies et al.[269] demonstrated a 1.6 mL withdrawal volume increased the accuracy of electrolyte lab values.

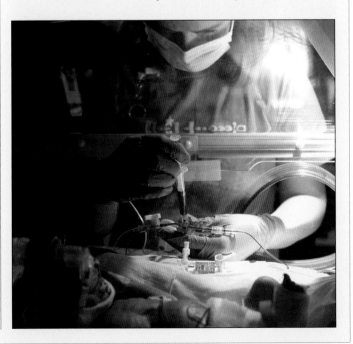

Appendix 1.1 Bowel Obstruction[35,39,40,42]

A maternal history of excessive amniotic fluid, or **polyhydramnios**, may be a sign that there is a bowel obstruction because of the inability of the fetal gut to absorb amniotic fluid. Other causes of polyhydramnios include but are not limited to genitourinary tract abnormalities (excessive urine output or polyuria), neurologic disorders (poor ability to swallow amniotic fluid), twin-to-twin transfusion syndrome (recipient twin becomes polyuric), and maternal diabetes (polyuria secondary to fetal hyperglycemia).[270,271]

Anatomical causes of a bowel obstruction include stenosis (narrowing of the lumen) or atresia (complete obstruction) anywhere in the intestinal tract: esophagus, duodenum, jejunum, ileum, anus, or secondary to an incarcerated hernia. If the infant has excessive drooling, frothy saliva, or is coughing or choking with feedings, then esophageal atresia and tracheoesophageal fistula should be suspected.

Functional causes of bowel obstruction include Hirschsprung's disease (absent ganglion cells in a section of the colon which interferes with normal peristaltic movement of stool), meconium plug syndrome, septic ileus, meconium ileus, and hypothyroidism.

Acquired causes of bowel obstruction include necrotizing enterocolitis (an intestinal infection that primarily affects preterm infants) and peritoneal adhesions that may develop following intestinal infection or surgery. Adhesions can also be congenital; they are usually called "bands."

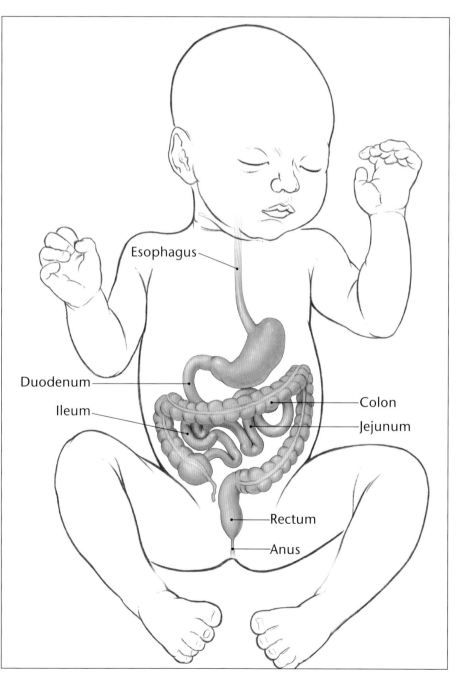

Anatomical locations where bowel obstruction may occur.

Appendix 1.1 **Bowel Obstruction** *(Continued)*

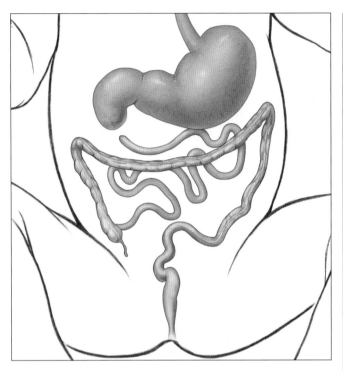

Duodenal atresia: complete atresia.

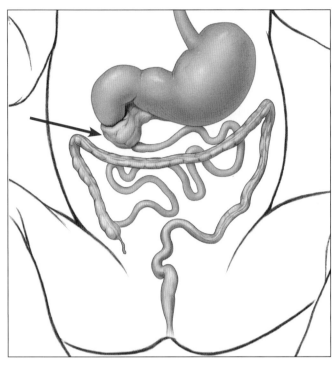

The duodenum may be partially or completely obstructed secondary to an annular pancreas (blue arrow).

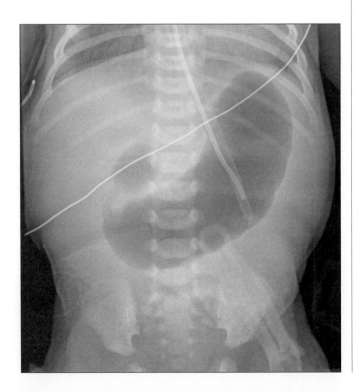

Abdominal X-ray of an infant with Trisomy 21 (Down syndrome) and duodenal atresia. The classic "double-bubble" sign from the dilated stomach and obstructed portion of the duodenum are shown as follows: a distended gas filled stomach, gas in the pyloric channel, and a small amount of gas filling the duodenal bulb. There is no intestinal gas after the atretic area.

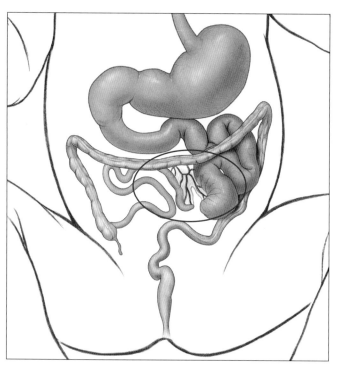

Jejunoileal atresia. Atresia may be in the ileum, jejunum, or both. There are various forms of jejunoileal atresia. One of the more common (type IIIa) is illustrated here. Notice the two ends of atretic bowel are separated by a "V" shaped defect in the mesentery. The small bowel is dilated with gas prior to the area of atresia.

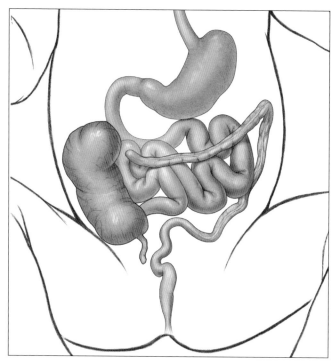

Colonic atresia. Notice the dilated small intestine and colon up to the area of atresia in the colon.

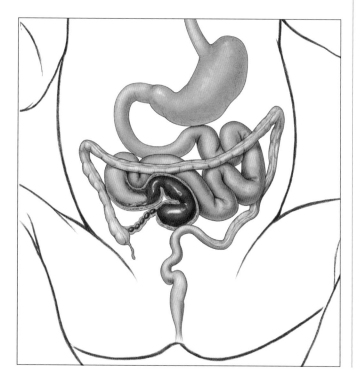

Meconium ileus. Thick viscid meconium obstructs the terminal ileum just prior to the ileocecal valve. Notice the pellets of thick meconium that prevent the passing of any gas or stool. In the majority of cases, the problem occurs because of a lack of pancreatic enzymes that are necessary to digest intestinal contents. Therefore, these infants should be assessed for cystic fibrosis. If an abdominal X-ray reveals calcifications, this means the infant experienced intestinal perforation in utero.

Appendix 1.1 Bowel Obstruction *(Continued)*

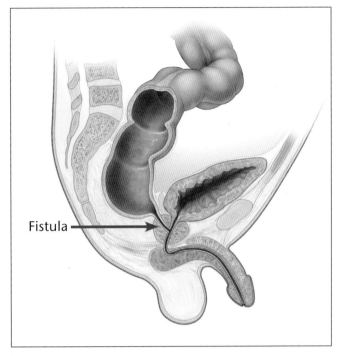

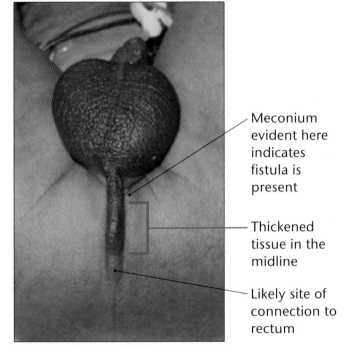

Meconium evident here indicates fistula is present

Thickened tissue in the midline

Likely site of connection to rectum

Imperforate anus in a male infant. Notice there is a rectoprostatic fistula between the distal bowel and the urethra (blue arrow).

Photos of two male infants with high imperforate anus. The most common lesion in a male that would require diversion is the rectoprostatic fistula. Signs of this and more proximal lesions would include the absence of any meconium in the perineum (photo on left), a flat bottom and abnormal sacrum (photo on right), and meconium in the urine or at the tip of the penis (bottom photo). The flat bottom, especially if the sacrum is abnormal, is virtually diagnostic of a proximally located rectum that would require diversion.

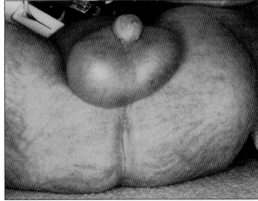

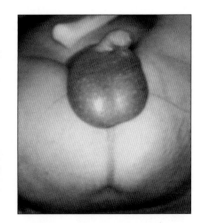

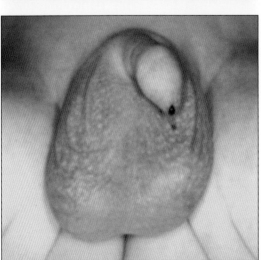

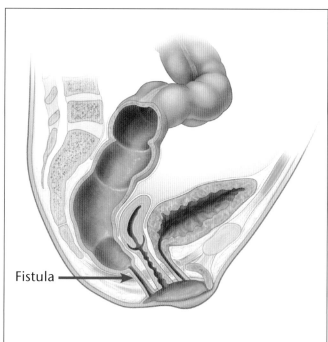

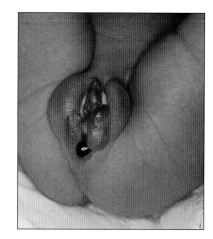

These photos are of two female infants with a rectovestibular fistula. Notice meconium is exiting via a fistula that connects the rectum to the lower aspect of the vaginal opening.

Fistula

Imperforate anus with rectovestibular fistula in a female infant. The illustration shows a rectovestibular fistula, which is the most common type of imperforate anus in females. There is a connection between the rectum and the posterior aspect of the introitus (the external opening of the vaginal canal) but external to the hymen. Stool will drain from the vaginal area.

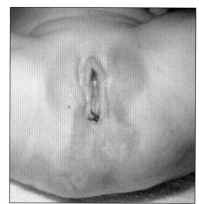

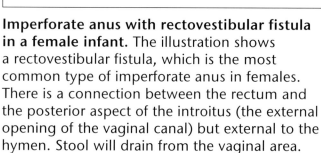

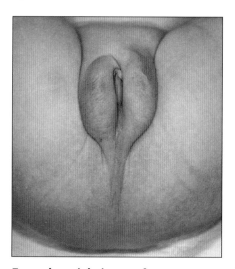

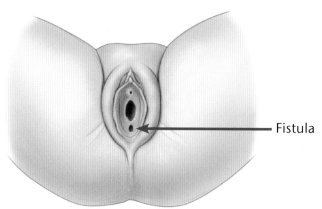

Fistula

Female with imperforate anus. There is no evidence of a fistula at this time (i.e., there is no meconium seen exiting the vaginal area). For this infant, the differential diagnosis would include a rectovestibular fistula (described above) or a cloaca. A cloaca is when the urinary tract, vagina, and rectum all meet in a common channel, and the rectal fistula is proximal to the hymen. With both of these variants, meconium might be seen draining from the vagina.

Appendix 1.2 Intrauterine Growth Curves: Female

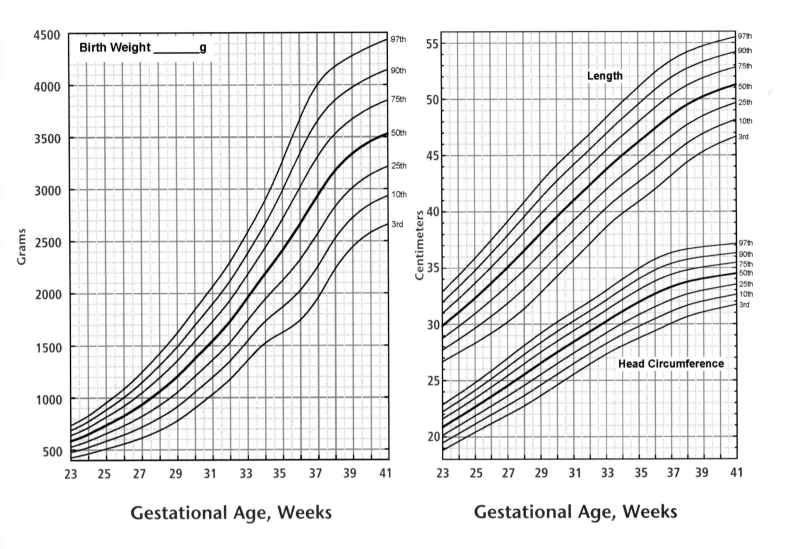

BIRTH ASSESSMENT: Classification of Infant	Weight (grams)	Length (cm)	Head (cm)
LGA: Large for Gestational Age (>90th percentile)			
AGA: Appropriate for Gestational Age (10th to 90th percentile)			
SGA: Small for Gestational Age (<10th percentile)			

Directions: Place an "X" in the appropriate box for the infant's weight, length, and head circumference. At times, an infant's measurements may be in the LGA, AGA, or SGA box, not necessarily always in the same weight classification box.

The 3rd and 97th percentiles on all curves for 23 weeks should be interpreted cautiously given the small sample size.

Reproduced with permission from Pediatrics, Volume 125, Pages e214-e244, Copyright 2010 by the American Academy of Pediatrics.[128]

Appendix 1.3 **Intrauterine Growth Curves: Male**

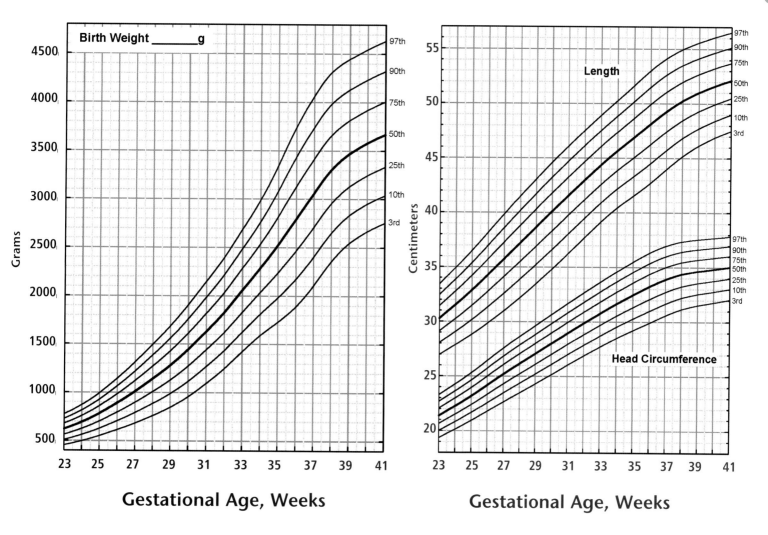

BIRTH ASSESSMENT: Classification of Infant	Weight (grams)	Length (cm)	Head (cm)
LGA: Large for Gestational Age (>90th percentile)			
AGA: Appropriate for Gestational Age (10th to 90th percentile)			
SGA: Small for Gestational Age (<10th percentile)			

Directions: Place an "X" in the appropriate box for the infant's weight, length, and head circumference. At times, an infant's measurements may be in the LGA, AGA, or SGA box, not necessarily always in the same weight classification box.

The 3rd and 97th percentiles on all curves for 23 weeks should be interpreted cautiously given the small sample size. For boys' HC curve at 24 weeks, all percentiles should be interpreted cautiously because the distribution of data is skewed left.

Reproduced with permission from Pediatrics, Volume 125, Pages e214-e244, Copyright 2010 by the American Academy of Pediatrics.[128]

Appendix 1.4 Dextrose Preparation Chart for IV Infusion

At times, a higher or lower dextrose concentration is required for IV infusion. Ideally, commercially prepared IV fluid should be used. However, in some settings, such as on transport or in a rural hospital, it may be necessary to prepare the IV fluid. In these tables, the Dextrose 50% for Injection

	Mixing Instructions Using a 250 mL Bag of $D_{10}W$ or D_5W			
	Note: In this chart, there is a 20 mL overfill when using a 250 mL bag; therefore, the starting volume is 270 mL[a]			
To Make	**Dextrose 50% for injection (mL)**	**$D_{10}W$ (mL)**	**D_5W (mL)**	**Final Volume (mL)**
Add Dextrose 50% to D_5W IV Fluid				
D_6W	6	-	270	276
D_7W	13	-	270	283
$D_{7.5}W$	16	-	270	286
D_8W	19	-	270	289
D_9W	26	-	270	296
Add Dextrose 50% to $D_{10}W$ IV Fluid				
$D_{11}W$	7	270	-	277
D12W	14	270	-	284
$D_{12.5}W$	18	270	-	288
Dextrose concentrations exceeding $D_{12.5}W$ should be infused via a central line*				
$D_{13}W$	22	270	-	292
$D_{14}W$	30	270	-	300
$D_{15}W$	39	270	-	309
$D_{16}W$	48	270	-	318
$D_{17}W$	57	270	-	327
$D_{17.5}W$	62	270	-	332
$D_{18}W$	68	270	-	338
$D_{19}W$	78	270	-	348
$D_{20}W$	90	270	-	360

[a]The overfill volume of 20 mLs is based on IV solution bags from Hospira®. If the IV bag is from a different manufacturer, check how much overfill (if any) there is and make appropriate adjustments to the Dextrose 50% volume that is required to make the correct dextrose concentration.

medication is added to either $D_{10}W$ or D_5W, and it should not be given full strength. Whenever possible, a pharmacist should mix the IV fluid.

	Mixing Instructions Using $D_{10}W$ or D_5W Because of the smaller final volume, do not round numbers. This chart may be utilized if infusing the fluids through a syringe pump using a 50 or 60 mL syringe.			
To Make	Dextrose 50% for injection (mL)	$D_{10}W$ (mL)	D_5W (mL)	Final Volume (mL)
Add Dextrose 50% to D_5W IV Fluid				
D_6W	1.1	-	48.9	50
D_7W	2.2	-	47.8	50
$D_{7.5}W$	2.8	-	47.2	50
D_8W	3.3	-	46.7	50
D_9W	4.4	-	45.6	50
Add Dextrose 50% to $D_{10}W$ IV Fluid				
$D_{11}W$	1.3	48.7	-	50
$D_{12}W$	2.5	47.5	-	50
$D_{12.5}W$	3.1	46.9	-	50
Dextrose concentrations exceeding $D_{12.5}W$ should be infused via a central line*				
$D_{13}W$	3.8	46.2	-	50
$D_{14}W$	5	45	-	50
$D_{15}W$	6.3	43.7	-	50
$D_{16}W$	7.5	42.5	-	50
$D_{17}W$	8.8	41.2	-	50
$D_{17.5}W$	9.4	40.6	-	50
$D_{18}W$	10	40	-	50
$D_{19}W$	11.3	38.7	-	50
$D_{20}W$	12.5	37.5	-	50

*Some centers will infuse $D_{15}W$ in a peripheral IV if there are no other ingredients (such as amino acids, calcium, etc.) in the IV fluid.

Temperature Module

Sugar

Temperature

Airway

Blood Pressure

Lab Work

Emotional Support

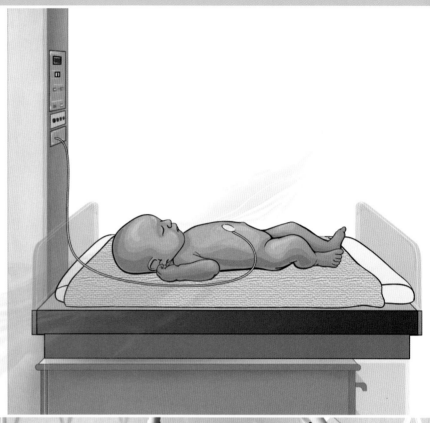

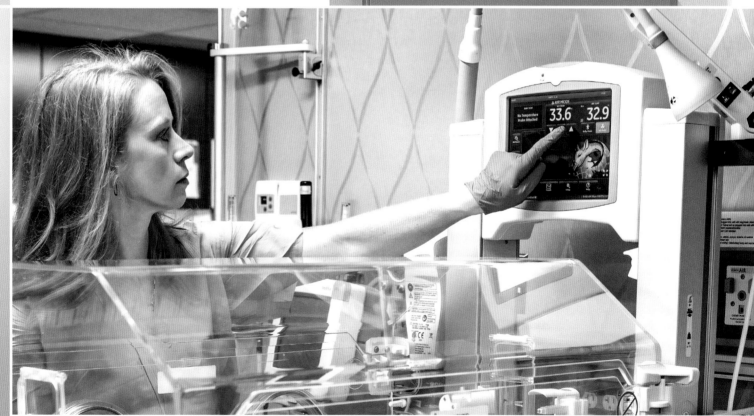

Temperature—Module Objectives

Upon completion of this module, participants will gain an increased understanding of:

1. Infants who are at increased risk for hypothermia.

2. The physiologic response to cold stress for term and late preterm infants.

3. Mechanisms of heat loss: conduction, convection, evaporation, and radiation.

4. The detrimental effects of hypothermia for term and preterm infants.

5. Methods to rewarm infants after accidental hypothermia.

Introduction

Hypothermia is a **preventable** condition that has a known impact on morbidity and mortality, especially in preterm infants.[1,2] Therefore, assisting the infant to maintain a normal body temperature and preventing hypothermia and hyperthermia during resuscitation and stabilization are critically important.[3,4]

Thermoregulation—Key Concepts

1 Maintenance of a Normal Body Temperature Must Be a Priority Whether Infants Are Well or Sick

Routine care following birth and throughout the neonatal period includes many activities aimed at preventing cold stress and hypothermia. For healthy infants, this includes drying the infant, removing wet linens, bundling in warm blankets, skin-to-skin holding, covering the head with a hat, and keeping the infant clothed.[5,6]

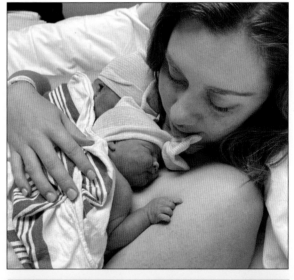

When infants are acutely sick or born preterm, thermoregulation is sometimes overlooked. Normal care procedures are replaced with activities aimed at resuscitation and stabilization. Infants are placed undressed on open radiant warming beds to permit observation and performance of intensive care procedures. The risk of cold stress and hypothermia increase dramatically; therefore, extra attention should be directed at preventing hypothermia.[7-13]

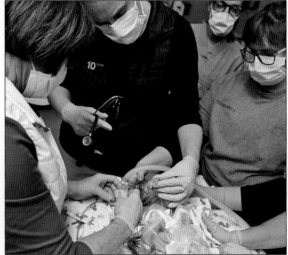

Normal and Hypothermic Body Temperature[14-16]

A normal core temperature is between 36.5 and 37.5°C (97.7 and 99.5°F). For infants, the World Health Organization defines levels of mild, moderate, and severe hypothermia as follows:

- **Mild hypothermia:** Core temperature is between 36 and 36.4°C (96.8 and 97.6°F)

- **Moderate hypothermia:** Core temperature is between 32 and 35.9°C (89.6 and 96.6°F)

- **Severe hypothermia:** Core temperature is <32°C (<89.6°F)

Preterm infants experience the effects of hypothermia sooner than term infants; however, preterm-specific ranges for mild, moderate, and severe hypothermia have not been defined. In small preterm infants (<1,000 grams) the lower end of the thermal range that defines severe hypothermia may start at ≤35°C.[17,18] In addition, infants with concurrent illnesses such as sepsis, respiratory distress, hypoxia, or shock may experience the negative effects of hypothermia more quickly, even before they reach the severely hypothermic range.[10,19]

Protect the infant from heat loss at all times! If the infant is healthy, follow your hospital guideline for how often to check the temperature. If the infant is unwell, check the temperature every 15 to 30 minutes until it is within a normal range and then at least every hour until the infant is transported or transferred to the neonatal intensive care unit (NICU).

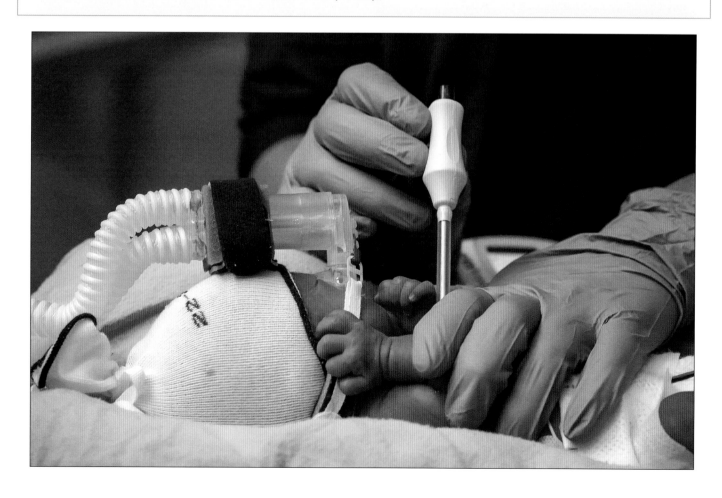

2 Infants at the Highest Risk for Hypothermia

Preterm and Small for Gestational Age Infants[10,14,20-24]

The most vulnerable for becoming hypothermic are preterm and small for gestational age infants because of the following characteristics:

- Relatively large head. *Impact:* the head is a prominent source of heat loss.

- A larger skin surface area-to-body weight ratio. *Impact:* increased water/evaporative heat loss.

- Thinner immature skin. *Impact:* increases water/evaporative heat loss.

- Poor ability to vasoconstrict peripheral blood vessels in the first 48 hours after birth. *Impact:* the inability to vasoconstrict allows the blood vessels to easily release heat through the thin skin.

- Decreased amounts of insulating subcutaneous fat. *Impact:* allows heat loss through the blood vessels that are near the skin surface.

- Reduced amounts of brown fat or no brown fat. *Impact:* there is limited or no ability to produce heat by chemical thermogenesis.

- Weak muscle tone and poor ability to hold a flexed position. *Impact:* extended extremities increase the surface area for heat loss.

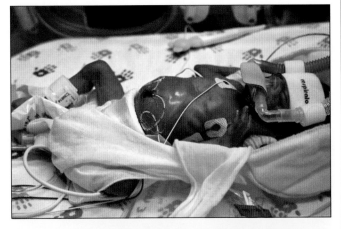

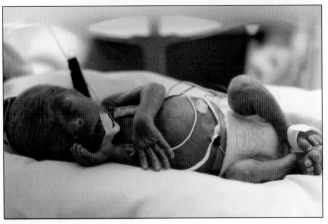

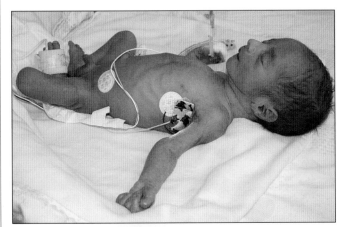

 If not protected from heat loss, the infant's body temperature may drop as quickly as 0.2 to 1°C (0.5 to 1.7°F) per minute.

Infants Who Require Prolonged Resuscitation[14,17]

Infants who require resuscitation are often hypoxic (i.e., not enough oxygen is delivered to the tissues). Oxygen is required to metabolize brown fat; therefore, during periods of hypoxia, this thermoregulatory mechanism is inactivated. During resuscitation, the infant is exposed to many thermal stressors, such as drafts, cool hands, and equipment that touches their body. Cold respiratory gases that have not yet been heated and humidified also contribute to cold stress.

Infants Who Require Transport[13,25,26]

Infants who require transport to a higher level of care because of respiratory, cardiac, infectious, neurologic, surgical, and metabolic problems are exposed to different environments with wide variations in temperature and humidity. If the infant is hypothermic upon arrival of the transport team, it can be challenging, and sometimes not possible, to rewarm the infant during transport, especially if the infant is low birth weight (<1,500 grams) or requires respiratory support. In preterm infants, the use of an exothermic (chemical) warming mattress and/or polyethylene plastic bag or wrap can help decrease the risk for hypothermia.

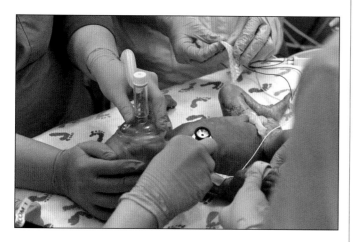

 Infants who experience perinatal asphyxia and require assessment for therapeutic hypothermia (whole-body cooling) require additional close attention and care. Appendix 2.1 on pages 103 to 110 explains hypoxic-ischemic encephalopathy and therapeutic hypothermia, along with important precautions to take, such as avoiding hyperthermia, hypoglycemia, and acid-base disturbances.

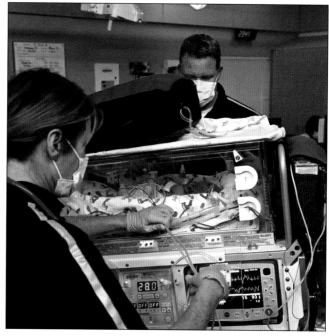

Infants With Abdominal Wall or Open Neural Tube Defects[27-29]

Especially vulnerable are infants with *gastroschisis* (bowel and potentially stomach and liver are herniated through a hole in the abdominal wall adjacent to the umbilicus), *omphalocele* (bowel and potentially other organs are herniated through the umbilicus and covered by a thin membrane or sac), or *myelomeningocele* (open spinal neural tube defect usually in the lower part of the back, with herniation of the spinal cord and nerves at the site of the defect). With these defects, the blood vessels are in close proximity to the environment where heat loss can occur. Preventing hypothermia can be very challenging while extraordinary care is undertaken to stabilize the infant.

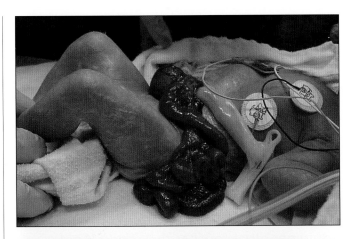

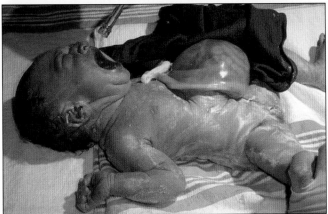

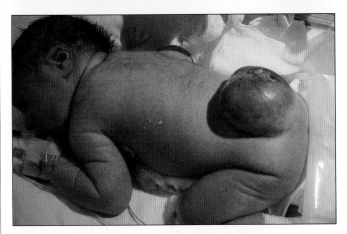

Gastroschisis (top photo), omphalocele (middle photo), myelocystocele (bottom photo).

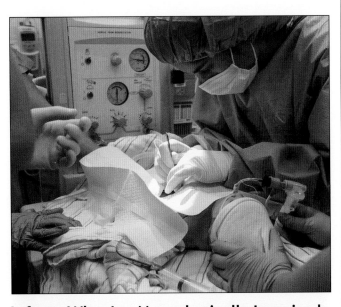

Infants Who Are Neurologically Impaired and/or Hypotonic From Sedatives, Analgesics, Paralytics, or Anesthetics[30-32]

Critically ill infants, such as those with persistent pulmonary hypertension of the newborn, often require deep sedation and analgesia during their care. Thermoregulation is entirely dependent upon the caregiver. Monitor the infant's temperature closely and provide extra vigilance during procedures or operations. Anesthesia significantly inhibits thermoregulation and increases the risk for hypothermia during surgery unless active measures are taken to protect the infant from heat loss.

3 In Term and Late Preterm Infants, Cold Stress Stimulates a Physiologic Response to Generate Heat and Decrease Heat Loss[10,17,22,33-35]

Cold and warm temperature receptors in the skin and deep tissues play an integral role in the maintenance of a normal body temperature. When receptors sense a low temperature, they stimulate the sympathetic nervous system to release norepinephrine. A series of reactions are then activated for the purpose of decreasing ongoing heat loss and increasing heat production.

These reactions include constriction of blood vessels in the arms and legs (peripheral vasoconstriction), metabolism of brown fat, and increased muscle flexion and activity (to decrease surface area for heat loss and generate heat by moving the muscles). Other impacts of norepinephrine release include increased oxygen and glucose consumption (related to an increase in metabolic rate) and pulmonary vasoconstriction (lung blood vessels constrict and increase pulmonary vascular resistance).

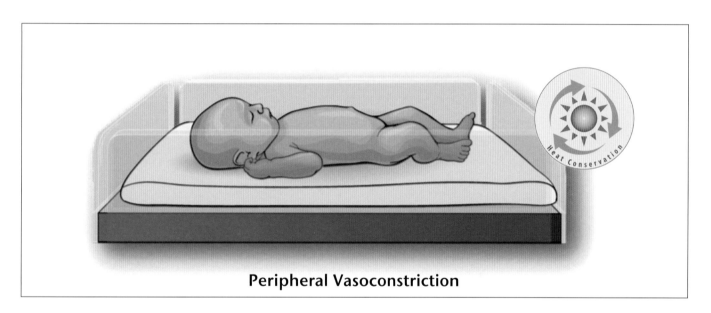

Peripheral Vasoconstriction

Physiologic Response to Cold Stress

Peripheral Vasoconstriction → Decreases Heat Loss[24,34,36,37]

When an infant experiences cold stress, blood vessels in the arms and legs constrict. Vasoconstriction prevents blood from reaching the skin surface where heat loss occurs. Prolonged vasoconstriction can reduce perfusion and oxygen delivery to the tissues.

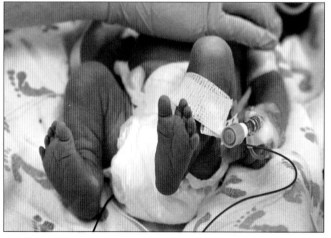

Acrocyanosis (blue color in the feet secondary to reduced perfusion and oxygen delivery) in a mildly hypothermic infant.

Brown Fat Metabolism → Increases Heat Production[10,17,35,38,39]

When brown fat is metabolized, it produces heat in the core regions of the body and warms the blood as it flows past those areas. This process of generating heat is called "chemical or non-shivering thermogenesis."

Brown fat begins to form at 25 to 26 weeks gestation, but there are no appreciable brown fat stores until the latter part of the third trimester.

Where Is Brown Fat Located?

Brown fat is located in the core regions of the body in the midscapular region: in the nape of the neck and under the clavicles and extending into the axillae, in the mediastinum (paraspinal and around the heart and great vessels), and around the kidneys and adrenal glands.

How Is Brown Fat Stimulated to Metabolize?

When cold receptors in the skin detect a cooling stimulus, such as a draft, they send a signal to the hypothalamus (the part of the brain that regulates temperature) that then responds by releasing norepinephrine into the nerve endings adjacent to brown fat. Norepinephrine release triggers a complex chemical reaction that causes brown fat to be metabolized or "burned." If the infant is neurologically impaired, the hypothalamus may not respond appropriately and fail to signal brown fat to burn or blood vessels to constrict.

Substrates Necessary for Brown Fat Metabolism

Brown fat metabolism requires oxygen and glucose as substrates. Infants who are hypoglycemic, have low or depleted glycogen stores, and/or are hypoxic are therefore unable to metabolize brown fat.

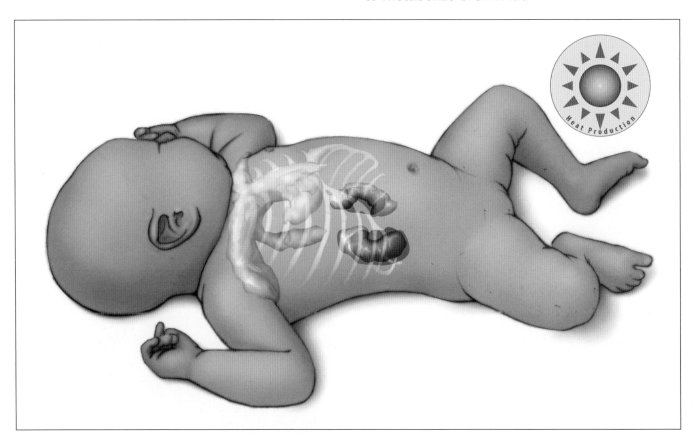

Increased Muscle Activity and Flexion → Increases Heat Production and Decreases Heat Loss[17,34,35]

Cold-stressed infants have limited to no capacity to shiver. Instead, infants increase their activity level by crying and flexing their arms and legs, which generates some heat in the muscles. Flexion of the arms and legs also reduces the surface area for heat loss. Depressed, severely ill, and preterm infants are often hypotonic and flaccid and lay with their limbs extended. This posture increases the surface area for heat loss.

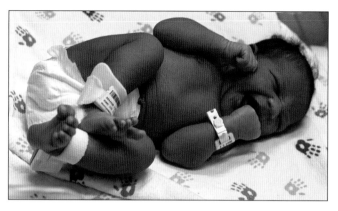

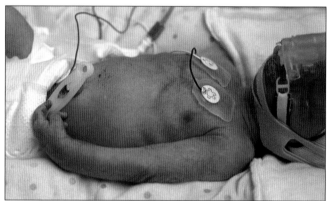

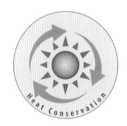 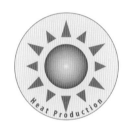

Mechanisms of Heat Loss[10,14,34-37]

Body temperature is lost (and gained) via four mechanisms: conduction, convection, evaporation, and radiation. However, there are two important concepts to understand prior to discussing mechanisms of heat loss.

Concept 1

Heat is lost on a gradient from warmer to cooler. **The larger the gradient, the faster heat is lost.** For example, a baby dressed only in a diaper and laying on an exam table will lose heat much faster if the room is 18°C (65°F) compared to a room that is 24°C (75°F).

Concept 2

Heat loss is faster when there is more than one mechanism of heat loss present. For example, a baby who is bathed in a room that is cool and drafty will become cold much faster than a baby who is bathed in a warm room with no drafts.

Heat Loss by Conduction[14,15,34,35,37,40-44]

Conductive heat loss involves the transfer of heat between two solid objects that are in contact with each other; for example, the infant's body and another solid object like a mattress, scale, or X-ray plate. The larger the temperature gradient between the two surfaces, the faster the heat loss.

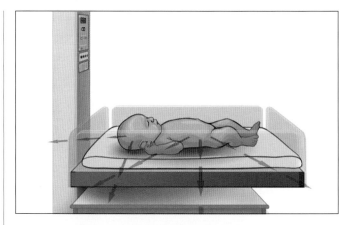

How to Reduce Conductive Heat Loss

- Pre-warm objects before they come in contact with the infant. These include the mattress, your hands, stethoscope, X-ray plates, and blankets.

- Cover the scale with a warm blanket or towel before weighing the infant.

- Clothing and hats serve as good insulators. However, critically ill infants are usually undressed to allow close observation. Keep the infant clothed as much as is practical and possible.

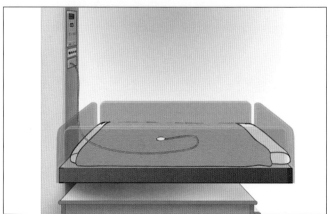

Preterm infants (<32 weeks)

- Place preterm infants on an exothermic (chemical) mattress to help with conductive heat gain. An exothermic mattress releases heat when it is activated. The risk for hyperthermia (temperature >37.5°C; 99.5°F) is greater when both a polyethylene plastic bag (or plastic wrap) and a thermal mattress are used, so monitor closely to prevent hyperthermia. Follow the manufacturer's recommendation for safe use.

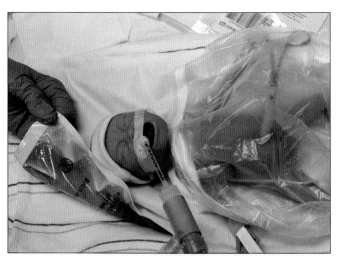

Premature manikin placed on an exothermic mattress and covered with a plastic wrap.

- Early skin-to-skin holding (also called Kangaroo Care) can effectively prevent hypothermia from conductive

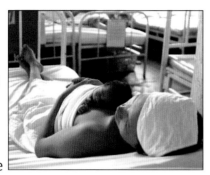

and convective heat loss. In resource-limited settings, early skin-to-skin holding and ongoing skin-to-skin contact was found to reduce mortality by 25% in preterm infants.[43]

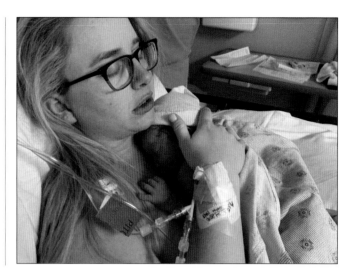

To Reduce the Risk of HYPERthermia and Burns

- *Use radiant warmers in skin servo-control mode once the infant is laid on the warmer.*
- *Do not overheat surfaces or place an infant on a surface hotter than the infant's skin temperature. The exception is when using an exothermic mattress (e.g., Infatherm® warming mattress, Porta-Warm™ transport mattress, TransWarmer®, etc.), which can warm to 40°C (104°F). Follow the manufacturer's guidelines for safe use.*
- *Never place hot water bottles or gloves filled with hot water next to the infant's skin.*
- *Do not apply heat directly to extremities that are poorly perfused.*

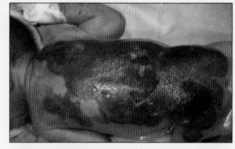
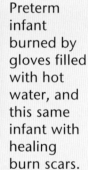
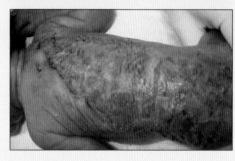

Preterm infant burned by gloves filled with hot water, and this same infant with healing burn scars.

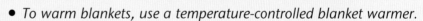

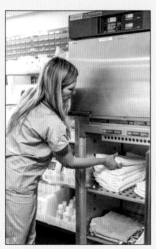

- *To warm blankets, use a temperature-controlled blanket warmer.*
- *Heat distribution is uneven, and the risk of fire or burns are increased when:*
  - *Blankets are 'warmed' on the top of an older model radiant warmer heating unit. **Do not place a blanket in that location for any reason.***
  - *Blankets are heated in a microwave. **Never use a microwave to warm a blanket.***
- *Microwave heating may superheat liquids, significantly increasing the risk of scald injury to staff or infants. In addition, there is uneven heat distribution when fluid is heated in a microwave. Therefore, a microwave should not be used to heat the infant's milk or anything that will touch the infant.*

Heat Loss by Convection[10,14,16,34,35,43-54]

Convective heat loss occurs when the infant's body heat is swept away by air currents, such as when the infant is exposed to drafts from open incubator portholes, air vents, air conditioners, windows, doors, fans, and movement of caregivers near the infant. Heat loss will be accelerated when the environmental air temperature is colder and/or when the velocity of air flow is higher.

How to Reduce Convective Heat Loss

- Keep warmer sides up during resuscitation and stabilization. When the warmer sides are down, air currents pass over the baby's skin and stimulate the cold receptors that in turn activate a cold stress response.

- When using an incubator, keep the portholes closed as much as possible. If available, use the incubator's "heat boost" function when opening portholes.

- Keep the infant dressed or covered as much as possible, including during diaper changes or following a bath.

- Avoid blowing dry, cold gases on the infant's face, as this will stimulate cold receptors and norepinephrine release, which will increase metabolic rate and oxygen consumption.

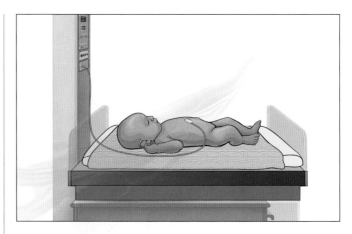

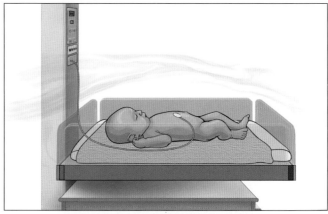

- Dry, cold gases (oxygen/air) used for respiratory support cool the blood flowing through the lungs and increase the risk for hypothermia, especially if the infant is preterm or resuscitation is prolonged. Use a heated, humidified system as soon as possible.

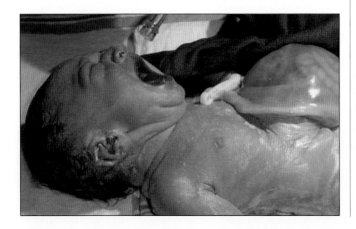

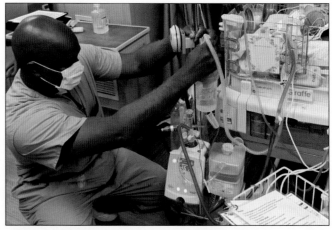

Late preterm infant with an omphalocele, receiving blow-by oxygen (left photo). Humidification system used to warm respiratory gases (top photo).

Preterm infants (<32 weeks)

- Increase the delivery or resuscitation room temperature to 26°C (79°F).[35,52] Other neonatal resources recommend a room temperature between 23 to 25°C (74 to 77°F).[16,53,54]

- Place a polyethylene plastic bag or wrap (without first drying) over the infant. The plastic covering helps reduce both convective and evaporative heat loss while still allowing the warmer radiant heat to reach the baby. Leave the bag or wrap in place as resuscitation and stabilization continue.

 Do not cover the head with the plastic. *If the infant is active, monitor closely to be sure the plastic does not get displaced over the face. Provide education to the family as to why the plastic covering is used and that this is a temporary measure to never be used outside the hospital.*

- Transport the sick and/or preterm infant between the delivery room and the nursery in a closed, pre-warmed incubator. If this equipment is not available, cover the infant with a pre-warmed blanket and a hat before moving them. This same principle applies for any movement of the infant from one location to another.

- An incubator reduces convective heat loss by providing a warmer environment within an enclosed space. Pre-warm the incubator before moving the infant into it.

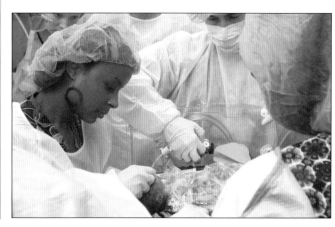

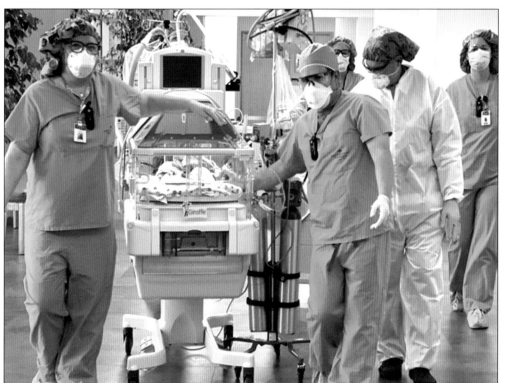

A preterm infant covered with plastic immediately following delivery (top photo). The neonatal resuscitation team transporting a newborn from the operating room to the NICU (left photo).

Heat Loss by Evaporation [10,14,16,20,22,35,45-48]

Evaporative heat loss occurs when water on the skin (such as after delivery or bathing) is converted to gas. The process of evaporation is always accompanied by a cooling effect. Infants also experience evaporative heat loss in the form of insensible losses, that is, passive evaporation from the skin and the respiratory tract. Insensible water loss is accentuated in preterm infants because of their thin, immature skin.

How to Reduce Evaporative Heat Loss

- Immediately after delivery or bathing, dry the infant with pre-warmed blankets or towels and promptly remove wet or damp linens. Dry the infant's head and apply a hat.

- If stable, the infant may be held skin-to-skin and covered with a warm blanket or towel.

- For all infants requiring respiratory support, heat and humidify the gases as soon as possible. Ventilating with cold gases will increase insensible water loss via the respiratory tract and will also cool the blood as it circulates through the lungs.

Preterm infants (<32 weeks)

- Immediately after delivery, place a polyethylene plastic bag or wrap (without first drying) up to the infant's neck. Monitor the infant's temperature closely to prevent hyperthermia.

- Eliminate drafts and increase the room temperature.

- Provide care in a heated, humidified incubator whenever possible. A radiant warmer significantly increases insensible water loss.

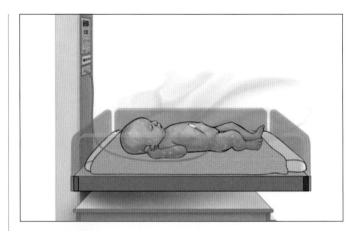

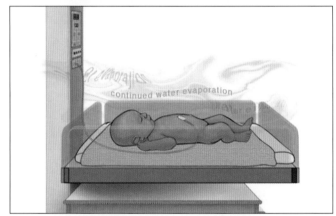

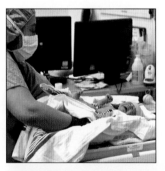

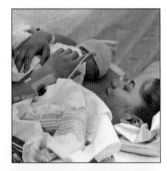

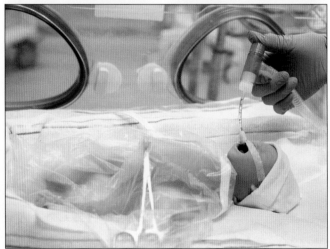

Do not bathe infants who are hypothermic or show other signs of instability. Cold stress and norepinephrine release cause pulmonary vasoconstriction and increase the risk for developing a clinical problem called **persistent pulmonary hypertension of the newborn** *(PPHN). See Figure 2.2 on page 97 for a description of* **right-to-left** *shunting of blood through the patent ductus arteriosus into the aorta, secondary to pulmonary vasoconstriction.*

☑ Clinical Tip

In healthy late preterm and term infants, when should the first bath be given?[55-62]

For healthy term infants, the bath can be given between 6 and 24 hours of age, and for healthy late preterm infants, the bath can be given after the infant is 12 hours old. In every case, the infant must first have thermal, cardiac, and respiratory stability, with a normal temperature on two consecutive routine evaluations and without the support of an external heat source when the temperatures were taken. An additional benefit of delaying the bath is to allow more time for vernix to be present on the skin since it inhibits the growth of pathogenic microorganisms and serves as an important moisturizer.

Limit the bath time to 5 minutes and close doors to reduce air movement that can increase convective heat loss.

- A room temperature of 26° C (77°F), or higher if possible, is recommended.

- Swaddle the infant before placing them in the water to improve comfort and decrease stress symptoms such as crying and agitation.

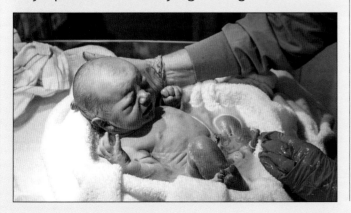

- A swaddle bath also improves the post-bath body temperature and is a commonly used method for preterm infants in the NICU.

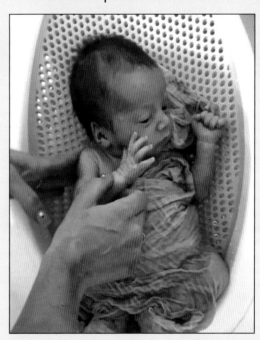

Maternal viral infections and when to bathe the infant soon after birth

If the mother has a hepatitis B or C viral infection, human immunodeficiency viral (HIV) infection, or active herpes simplex virus (HSV) genital lesions, a bath should be given as soon as possible after birth to remove maternal blood and body fluids. If possible, the bath should occur before any medications are injected in the thigh. However, if bathing is not possible, then the thigh should be thoroughly cleansed before the injection is given.

Heat Loss by Radiation[10,14,34,35]

Radiant heat loss is the transfer of heat between solid surfaces that are not in contact with each other. The infant's skin temperature is usually warmer than surrounding surfaces, so the direction of heat transfer will be from the exposed parts of the infant's body to the adjacent solid surfaces. The cooler those surfaces, the greater the heat loss. The size of the two solid surfaces also affects the amount of heat loss; therefore, it is easy to see why an infant would lose heat very quickly to a large window or wall.

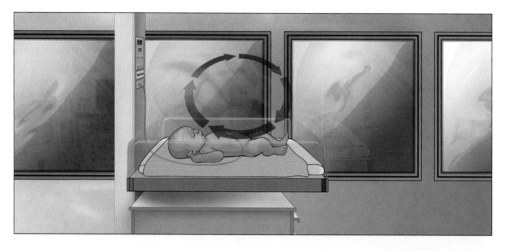

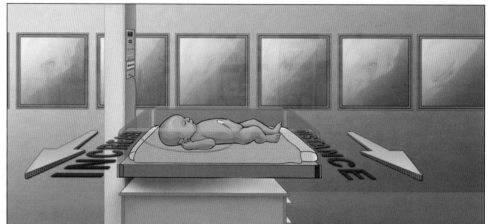

How to Reduce Radiant Heat Loss

- Move the infant away from windows or walls.

- Use thermal shades over windows.

- Cover the incubator to insulate it from nearby windows or walls.

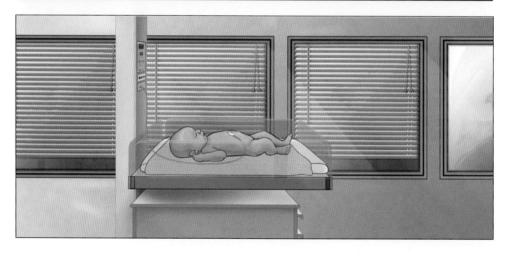

- Use a double-walled incubator to provide a warmer internal surface closest to the infant, and prewarm the incubator before placing the infant inside.

- Maintain a warm room temperature to decrease the gradient for heat loss.

- During resuscitation and stabilization, the radiant warmer heat element can be blocked by caregivers as they perform procedures or other activities. Remember to keep the area below the heater element clear.

Radiant Heat Gain[10,14,34,35]

Radiant heat gain occurs when the surrounding surfaces are warmer than the infant's skin temperature. For instance, when an infant is placed under a radiant warmer, the temperature beneath the heater element and projected over the infant's body and bed is higher than the temperature a few feet away from the warmer. Hyperthermia increases insensible water loss, metabolic rate, and oxygen consumption. If an elevated temperature is observed, assess whether the cause is environmental, iatrogenic, or secondary to infection.

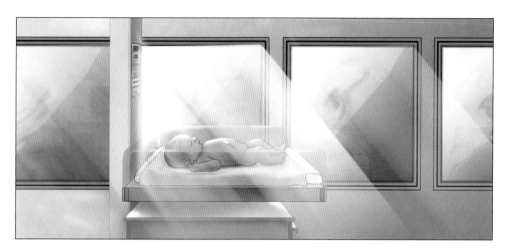

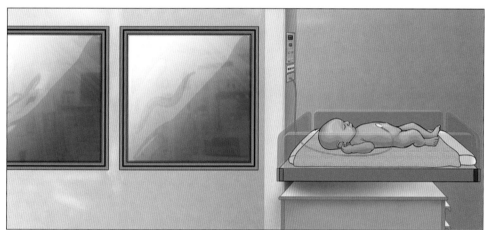

How to Reduce Unwanted Radiant Heat Gain

- When an infant is on the radiant warmer, ensure the skin temperature is set on servo-control mode, not the manual heat output setting.

- Ensure the temperature probe is attached securely to the skin. Loose contact will cause the radiant heater element to increase heat output and lead to overheating.

- Avoid direct sunlight on the infant or incubator.

Signs of hyperthermia include tachycardia, tachypnea, flushed skin and warmer than normal temperature of the skin over the extremities and abdomen (especially if there was iatrogenic overheating on a radiant warmer), increased activity and irritability, extended posture, and in older infants, sweating.

*Infrared heat lamp precautions. Although rarely used, if a radiant warmer is not available, an infrared heat lamp may be used **to warm the air near the baby**. The closer the infant is to the radiant heat lamp, the higher the temperature. Heat lamps are not servo-controlled to the infant's skin temperature. Therefore, **the risk that the infant can overheat or be burned is increased.** In addition, heat lamp bulbs have different wattages, with some capable of causing burns in a very short time. When a bulb is changed, ensure the bulb wattage is appropriate for infant use. Always remain vigilant to keep the lamp bulb a safe distance from the baby. Move the infant to an incubator or radiant warmer using servo-control mode as soon as possible.*

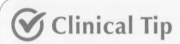 **Clinical Tip** *Skin temperature probe placement and precautions*[10,14,34,35]

- Secure the skin temperature sensor probe on the right upper quadrant of the abdomen (liver location). If the infant is not maintaining their temperature as expected or not rewarming in a timely manner, try an alternate temperature probe location, such as the lateral abdomen in the right axillary line between the ribs and the iliac crest.

- In late preterm and term infants, avoid placing the temperature probe over areas with brown fat, such as the axilla. However, preterm infants have little brown fat; therefore, this location is commonly used in the NICU.

- Ensure the temperature probe is attached securely to the skin.

- If the probe is not sticking well to the skin, wipe the skin with an alcohol swab.

- Cover the skin temperature probe with a manufacturer approved reflective probe cover. In addition to helping adhere the probe to the skin, the reflective foil on the cover helps provide a more accurate temperature reading by deflecting radiant and ambient heat. Preferably, the probe cover should be latex-free.

- Do not allow the infant to lie on the temperature probe. If the infant lies on the probe, the extra insulation and warmth created may signal the warmer to decrease the heater output and place the infant at risk for getting cold. In addition, do not cover the temperature probe with blankets.

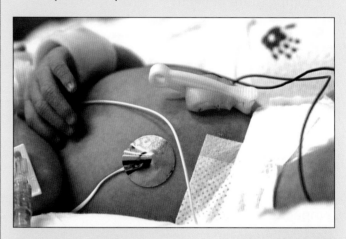

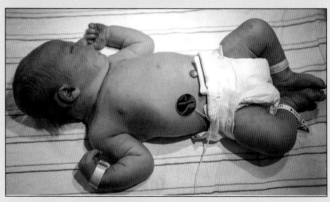

Temperature and Its Effect on Metabolic Rate and Oxygen Consumption[10,17,20,22,36,37]

With the onset of mild hypothermia, the infant will try to compensate to both produce and conserve heat. These compensatory mechanisms increase metabolic rate, which increases oxygen consumption and glucose utilization. If the infant is already experiencing respiratory distress, the increased oxygen demand can worsen hypoxemia (low blood oxygen levels) and lead to hypoxia (oxygen content in the tissues is lower than what the tissues need for normal function). Hypoxia and hypothermia eventually lead to a decrease in oxygen consumption that is thought to be an adaptive response to save oxygen that would otherwise be used to generate heat. With the onset of severe hypothermia (<32°C; 89.6°F), the hypothalamus ceases all ability to regulate temperature, and the risk of dying from hypothermia is very high unless reversed by careful rewarming. When the body temperature rises above 37.5°C (99.5°F), the metabolic rate and oxygen consumption also increase. Figure 2.1 illustrates the effect of body temperature on metabolic rate and oxygen consumption as the temperature increases and decreases.

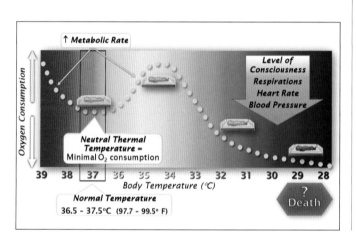

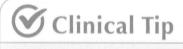

Figure 2.1. Effect of body temperature on metabolic rate and oxygen consumption.
As the body temperature increases or decreases outside of the normal range of 36.5 to 37.5°C (97.7 to 99.5°F), the metabolic rate and oxygen consumption increase. With progressive hypothermia, the infant will exhibit a decreased level of consciousness, hypoventilation, bradycardia, and hypotension. The risk for death increases as the body temperature further declines.

☑ Clinical Tip — *What is a neutral thermal environment?*[10,14,17,22,34-36]

A **neutral thermal temperature** is the body temperature at which minimal energy is expended by the infant to maintain a normal body temperature. When minimal energy is expended to stay warm, oxygen consumption is also lowest and energy may be used for other important functions, including growth.

Preterm infants require a higher environmental temperature to stay warm. A **neutral thermal environment** is the higher air temperature provided in an incubator that allows the preterm infant to expend the least amount of energy to stay at a normal body temperature. In the NICU, ensuring a thermoneutral environment will minimize the energy needed to stay warm and optimize the opportunity for growth. As the infant matures, the environmental temperature can be reduced, and eventually, the infant will be large and mature enough to grow and thrive outside of the incubator.

Detrimental Effects of Hypothermia: Term and Preterm Infants[8,10,14,17,30,34-37,63-65]

Norepinephrine ⟶ Effect on Vasoconstriction

In response to cold stress and progression to hypothermia, a cascade of events occur that explain the increased morbidity and mortality in these infants. When a cold stimulus is detected by the peripheral and core temperature receptors, a signal is sent to the hypothalamus that then activates the sympathetic nervous system to release norepinephrine. Norepinephrine stimulates brown fat metabolism (if there is any brown fat and the infant is not hypoxic), and it causes peripheral and pulmonary blood vessels to constrict.

Peripheral Vasoconstriction

Peripheral vasoconstriction keeps the blood in the core of the body and away from the skin where heat is dissipated. Evidence of peripheral vasoconstriction includes acrocyanosis (bluish discoloration of the hands and feet), cool hands and feet, and mottled skin. Prolonged vasoconstriction can impair tissue perfusion and oxygenation and lead to anaerobic metabolism. The consequences of anaerobic metabolism include accelerated glucose consumption, increased lactic acid production, and a drop in pH that leads to acidosis.

Pulmonary Vasoconstriction In Utero

In utero, the pulmonary arterioles are vasoconstricted because gas exchange is in the placenta, not the lungs. Ninety percent of the blood that is ejected from the right ventricle into the pulmonary artery flows directly into the fetal shunt vessel called the ductus arteriosus (DA), then into the aorta. After birth, when the umbilical cord is cut, the pulmonary arterioles begin to relax and dilate. If transition proceeds normally, all the blood ejected from the right ventricle enters the pulmonary artery, then into the lungs where gas exchange occurs.

Pulmonary Vasoconstriction and Cold Stress

In response to cold stress, norepinephrine is released and causes the pulmonary arterioles to constrict, which increases pulmonary vascular resistance (PVR). In healthy infants, mild pulmonary vasoconstriction usually has minimal, if any, impact on the infant's cardiorespiratory status. In sick infants or moderate to severely hypothermic infants, pulmonary vasoconstriction can have a very negative impact. The increased pulmonary vascular resistance causes the deoxygenated blood to shunt via the pathway of least resistance, through the patent ductus arteriosus (PDA) into the aorta. This pattern of blood flow is called a **right**-to-**left** shunt. The oxygen content in the aorta will be reduced (hypoxemia) and if severe enough, and/or if hypothermia is prolonged, the tissues will not receive enough oxygen for normal cell function (hypoxia). This state of hypoxia causes a conversion to anaerobic metabolism. The resulting acidosis and any ongoing hypoxemia will trigger or aggravate pulmonary vasoconstriction and increase the PVR. Figure 2.2 illustrates the **right**-to-**left** shunting of blood through the PDA when there is pulmonary vasoconstriction and an elevated PVR.

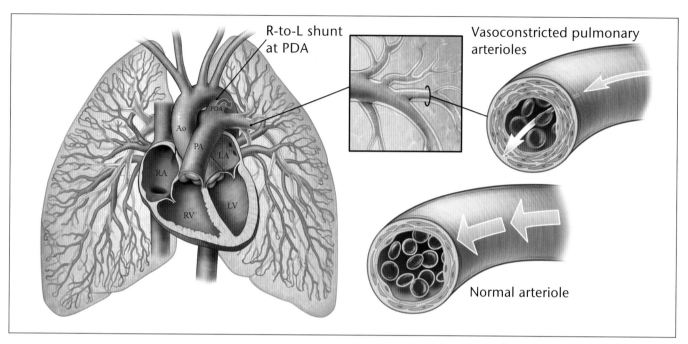

Figure 2.2. Illustration of a right-to-left shunt through the patent ductus arteriosus (PDA) secondary to vasoconstricted pulmonary arterioles and increased PVR. Because of increased PVR, blood shunts via the pathway of least resistance, right-to-left through the PDA, then into the aorta.

Summary

If the infant is already experiencing respiratory distress, there may not be enough oxygen to satisfy tissue demands. The resulting hypoxemia or hypoxia can trigger or aggravate pulmonary vasoconstriction. During hypothermia, hypoglycemia may result from increased glucose utilization and depletion of glycogen stores. Since glucose is the primary energy source for the brain, the infant's level of consciousness may decline, respiratory rate slow down, and hypoxia worsen as anaerobic metabolism increases.

For both term and preterm infants, the detrimental effects of hypothermia are similar:

- Increased metabolic rate and oxygen consumption

- Development of anaerobic metabolism

- Pulmonary vasoconstriction that worsens oxygenation

- Increased glucose utilization

Survivors of hypothermia may experience additional harmful side effects:

- Impaired immune function (increased risk for infection)

- Impaired coagulation (increased risk for brain and pulmonary hemorrhage)

- Impaired surfactant production (increased risk for respiratory distress syndrome in preterm infants)

- Acute renal failure (impaired kidney function)

Rewarming the Hypothermic Infant After Accidental Hypothermia[14,34,35]

Following therapeutic hypothermia for hypoxic-ischemic encephalopathy (a treatment reserved for infants >36 weeks gestation), the recommended rewarming speed is 0.5°C per hour to avoid sudden vasodilatation and resultant hypotension. However, rewarming an infant at a rate of 0.5°C per hour after *accidental hypothermia* may be too slow or impractical. The optimal speed to rewarm an infant after unintentional (accidental) hypothermia has not been established.

Preterm Infants[14,22,66-68]

Preterm infants, especially if born at home or requiring transport to a higher level of care, are the most vulnerable to becoming moderately to severely hypothermic. Slow versus rapid rewarming of preterm infants has been studied but definitive evidence to guide a recommendation is still lacking. Two studies of preterm infants with moderate hypothermia (32° to 35.9°C) on NICU admission evaluated a slow (<0.5° C/hour) versus rapid (>0.5°C/hour) rewarming rate.[67,68] There were no differences in neonatal outcomes except in one study—the incidence of respiratory distress syndrome was lower in the preterm infants who were warmed rapidly (>0.5 C per hour).[67] These two studies provide some guidance on how rapidly to rewarm a moderately to severely hypothermic infant, but more research is needed.

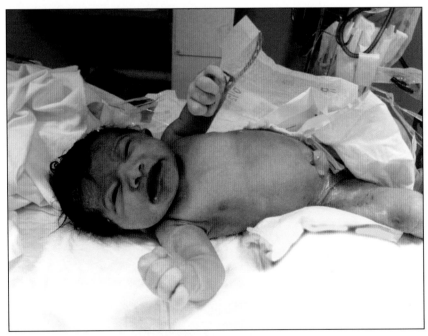

Infant delivered unexpectedly at home and was moderately hypothermic upon admission to the hospital.

 Individual patient circumstances, including the gestational age, cardiovascular state, and severity of the hypothermia need to be considered each time rewarming is necessary. In the setting of profound hypothermia (≤32°C), an even more cautious approach to rewarming should be considered.[66]

Rewarming Guidelines

There is a paucity of prospective research on how fast to rewarm an accidentally hypothermic infant. Establish an individualized rewarming plan with your medical team that includes the best device to use (warmer versus incubator), the speed of rewarming, and how the temperature will be monitored. Then, rewarm the infant at a steady pace while continuously monitoring:

- Temperature
- Heart rate and rhythm
- Blood pressure
- Respiratory rate and effort
- Oxygen saturation
- Neurologic status

Assessment of pulses and perfusion should occur at least every 15 minutes, and blood gas evaluation should occur as necessary to assist interpretation of exam findings.

Signs of Deterioration During Rewarming

- Tachycardia or sudden increase in baseline heart rate ⟶ may be in response to a decrease in cardiac output
- Hypotension or evidence of decreased perfusion (delayed capillary refill time)
- Onset of a cardiac arrhythmia
- Worsening respiratory distress
  - Hypoxemia or increased oxygen requirement (desaturation and cyanosis)
  - Apnea, tachypnea, grunting, retractions
- Worsening acidosis (metabolic or mixed metabolic and respiratory acidosis)
- Bleeding secondary to impaired coagulation (a detrimental effect of hypothermia)

Table 2.1. Signs of deterioration that may be observed when rewarming a severely hypothermic infant.

The following concepts will help guide the rewarming of infants with moderate to severe hypothermia.

1 **Speed of rewarming.** Rewarming too rapidly can result in clinical deterioration because of vasodilation that leads to hypotension.[37,69] Table 2.1 summarizes signs of deterioration during rewarming.

2 **Temperature measurement (axillary versus rectal).** In normothermic infants, the rectal temperature may be 0.3 to 0.4°C higher than the axillary temperature.[34] However, with severe hypothermia (<32°C), the skin temperature may be higher than the rectal temperature, especially if there is a heat source being used. In late preterm and term infants who are **severely** hypothermic, rectal temperature measurement can be used during rewarming, but care must be taken to avoid rectal injury.[14,34,40] Esophageal temperature measurement represents true core temperature but is rarely used except for special circumstances, such as during therapeutic hypothermia. In preterm infants, the axillary temperature correlates well with both normothermia and hypothermia, but not hyperthermia (temperature >37.5° C);[70] therefore, in most cases, the axillary temperature should be used.

3 **Rewarming device.** An incubator or a radiant warmer can be used for rewarming the infant; however, an incubator allows for better control over the rewarming rate. In either case, undress the infant, remove any blankets, and remove the hat to allow for maximum exposure of the infant's body surface area to the applied heat. See pages 100 to 101 for more information.

Incubator Method of Rewarming

- Attach the servo-control temperature probe to the upper right abdomen to monitor the skin temperature.

- Select the "air temperature" mode setting.

- Undress the infant and remove any blankets and the hat if not done already. The diaper can remain on.

- Set the air temperature so that it is 1 to 1.5°C above the infant's axillary or rectal temperature in Celsius.

- Some infants may need a higher gradient (i.e., a higher air temperature set point) before their core temperature will begin to rise.

- Adding humidity inside the incubator helps reduce ongoing heat loss from evaporation, and most modern incubators allow for additional ambient humidity.[14] Once normothermia has been achieved, humidification can be reduced to a level appropriate for that infant's gestational and postnatal age.[40,71]

- As the infant's core or axillary temperature reaches the air temperature set point, and there are no signs of deterioration from overly rapid rewarming (see Table 2.1 on page 99), increase the air temperature again by 1 to 1.5°C above the infant's core or axillary temperature (in Celsius) until their temperature is in the normal range.

- If not done already, evaluate the blood glucose and blood gas once rewarming is achieved.

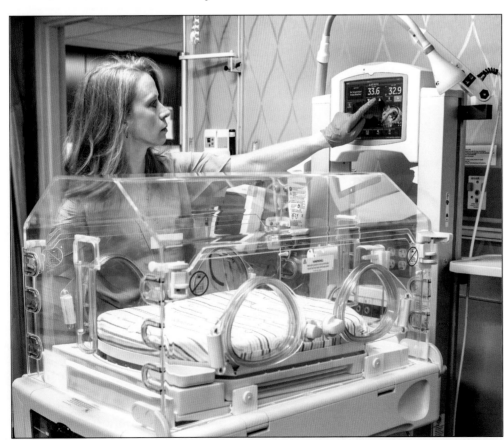

Radiant Warmer Method of Rewarming

- Undress the infant and remove any blankets and the hat if not done already. The diaper can remain on.

- Place the infant supine on a radiant warmer with the temperature probe located over the liver and the servo-control temperature set to 36.5°C.[14,34]

- Alternatively, to slow the rate of rewarming, set the servo-control temperature 1°C higher than the body temperature.[14] However, the lowest servo-control temperature setting on a radiant warmer may not be low enough to reach 1°C higher than the body temperature.

- Another strategy is to use a hypothermia blanket to control the rewarming rate, as is the process used to rewarm an infant after therapeutic (neuroprotective) hypothermia.

*One risk of rewarming an infant with a radiant warmer in servo-control mode (set to 36.5°C) is that the warmer will detect the low skin temperature and then significantly increase the heat output. The skin temperature receptors are very sensitive to externally applied heat. In response to full radiant heat output, the blood vessels may suddenly dilate and cause a rapid drop in blood pressure. Therefore, **monitor the heart rate closely and be alert to any abrupt increase,** as this may signal a decline in cardiac output. Administration of a normal saline fluid bolus (10 mL/kg) may be necessary if concerned about hypotension. In addition, the rate of rewarming may need to be slowed if the infant is decompensating. Also, **be alert to any signs of hemorrhage** (pulmonary, intracranial), as hypothermia can impair coagulation.*

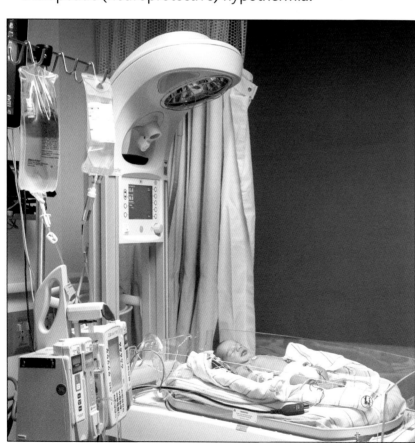

Temperature—Key Points

Be vigilant—prevent hypothermia in the first place!

Infants who are most vulnerable for becoming hypothermic include

- Preterm and small for gestational age infants
- Infants who require prolonged resuscitation
- Infants who become acutely ill and/or require transport
- Infants with abdominal wall or open neural tube defects
- Infants who are neurologically impaired
- Infants who are hypotonic from sedatives, analgesics, paralytics, or anesthetics

Remember the basics!

- Ensure a warm environment at all times
- Do not bathe the infant if hypothermic or even mildly unstable
- Use a radiant warmer on servo-control, not manual
- Prevent heat loss from conduction, convection, evaporation, or radiation
- Use warm, humidified gases (oxygen/air) as soon as possible

Rewarm hypothermic infants cautiously, monitor them closely, and be prepared to resuscitate during or after rewarming.

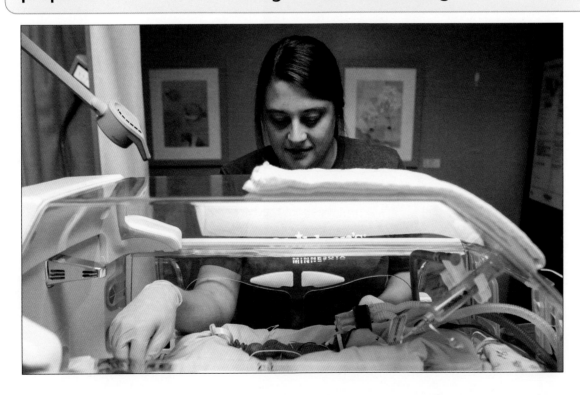

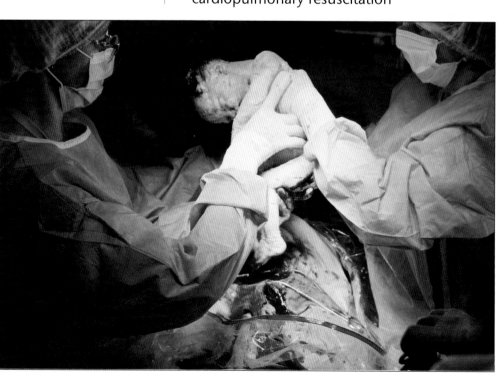

Appendix 2.1 Hypoxic-Ischemic Encephalopathy (HIE) and Therapeutic/Neuroprotective Hypothermia (Cooling)[72-82]

Neonatal Encephalopathy

The term encephalopathy is a broad term to describe altered brain function. Neonatal encephalopathy is clinically defined as an altered neurological function in late preterm and term infants. Causes of neonatal encephalopathy include significant hypoxia and/or ischemia during labor and/or delivery (i.e., hypoxic-ischemic encephalopathy), perinatal stroke, significant cardiorespiratory illness or sepsis, brain infection (meningitis, encephalitis), significant and/or persistent hypoglycemia, severe unconjugated hyperbilirubinemia (kernicterus), brain trauma (subdural hematoma), brain hemorrhage (hemorrhagic infarction, subgaleal hemorrhage), acute hydrocephalus, brain malformations, inborn errors of metabolism, and congenital neuromuscular disorders.

Encephalopathic infants may present with one or more of the following signs:

- Change in level of consciousness (decreased or hyperalert)

- Seizures

- Depressed tone and reflexes

- Brainstem impairment (impaired respiratory function such as hypoventilation or apnea)

Hypoxic-Ischemic Encephalopathy (HIE)

An acute perinatal event during labor and/or delivery can impair placental/fetal gas exchange. Three examples of perinatal events are shown in Figure 2.3 on page 104. Perinatal events include but are not limited to the following:

- Fetal heart rate abnormalities signifying fetal distress and hypoxia

  o Sudden and sustained fetal bradycardia

  o Absent fetal heart rate variability combined with persistent, late, or variable decelerations

- Prolapsed, ruptured, or tight nuchal cord

- Prolonged shoulder dystocia

- Uterine rupture

- Maternal hemorrhage/placental abruption

- Maternal collapse that requires cardiopulmonary resuscitation

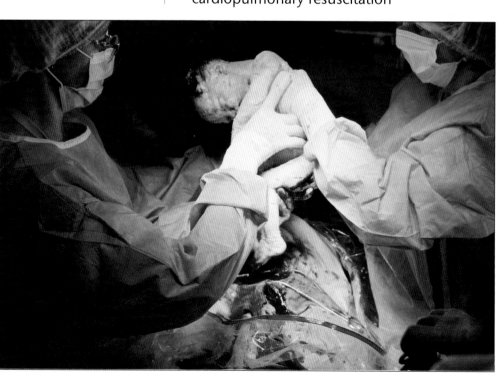

In utero, inadequate delivery of oxygen and removal of carbon dioxide and hydrogen ions leads to fetal acidosis, hypoxia, and hypercarbia. *Perinatal asphyxia* is the term used to describe impaired intrauterine gas exchange. The term *ischemia* refers to reduced blood flow and delivery of oxygen and glucose to the organs, including the vulnerable immature brain. The brain injury that occurs is called *hypoxic-ischemic encephalopathy* or HIE.

The acute phase of poor brain perfusion that leads to HIE is shown in Figure 2.4. Maternal medical conditions that increase the risk for impaired placental-fetal perfusion include chronic or acute hypertension, preeclampsia, diabetes, autoimmune diseases, and placental inflammatory changes from chorioamnionitis, villitis, vasculitis, funisitis, and intrauterine cocaine exposure.

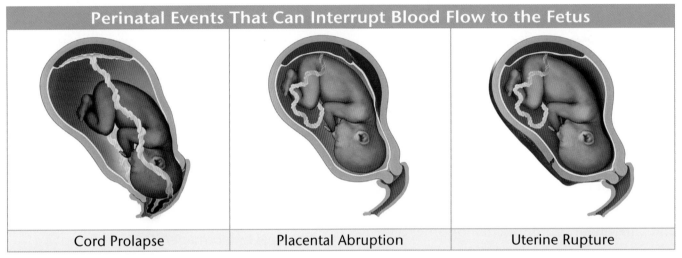

Perinatal Events That Can Interrupt Blood Flow to the Fetus

| Cord Prolapse | Placental Abruption | Uterine Rupture |

Figure 2.3. Examples of three perinatal events that can interrupt blood flow to the fetus.

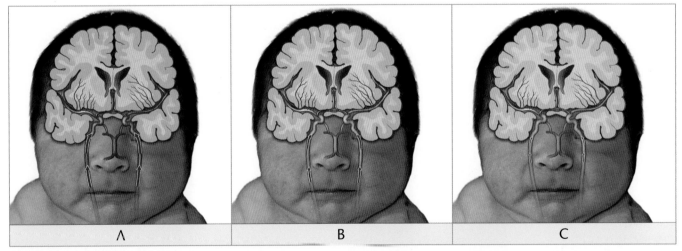

A   B   C

Figure 2.4. An acute perinatal event can interrupt blood flow and oxygen delivery to the brain and lead to ischemic brain injury. From left-to-right, A) Normal blood flow to the brain and adequate oxygenation, B) Onset of perinatal event: cerebral desaturation and reduced blood flow to the brain tissue, and C) Severely decreased cerebral blood flow and oxygenation following an acute perinatal event. Severely hypoxemic blood and poor perfusion lead to ischemic brain injury.

Incidence of HIE

HIE is the most common cause of neonatal encephalopathy. The incidence of HIE in developed countries is approximately 1 to 3 per 1,000 term or near-term live births. In low-resource settings where obstetric and perinatal care is less available and/or inadequate, the cases of HIE are appreciably higher at 26 to 31 per 1,000 live births. Each year, HIE affects 2 million infants, and as many as 20 to 50% of infants with HIE die in the neonatal period. For survivors of HIE, the neurological impact can include cerebral palsy, cognitive and motor deficits, epilepsy, deafness, and later learning problems.

Therapeutic Hypothermia (TH)

TH is the only evidence-based therapy available for clinical use to prevent/ameliorate brain injury and improve neurologic outcome in newborns with HIE. Therefore, all who attend deliveries or care for the recently born should be aware of HIE and TH. HIE brain injury occurs in two phases. **The first phase** is when brain tissue is injured by hypoxemia (low oxygen levels) and acidosis. If cooling is not initiated, **the second phase** of injury occurs between 6 and 16 hours after birth as oxygenation and perfusion are restored and multiple chemical reactions further damage brain tissue (i.e., reperfusion injury). Therefore, the optimal window for therapeutic hypothermia, also known as 'cooling,' is before 6 hours of age. It should be noted, however, that one study evaluated cooling beyond 6 hours but before 24 hours of age and found some benefit. For this reason, some centers may also offer therapeutic hypothermia beyond 6 hours after birth, especially if the initial 6-hour window was missed due to late identification, or the infant exhibited a significant neurological decline or started having seizures after 6 hours of age.[83]

Moderate hypothermia to a core temperature of 33.5°C for 72 hours, with rewarming over 6 hours, is now considered the standard of care for newborns with moderate to severe HIE and has been shown to both increase survival and reduce disability in survivors.

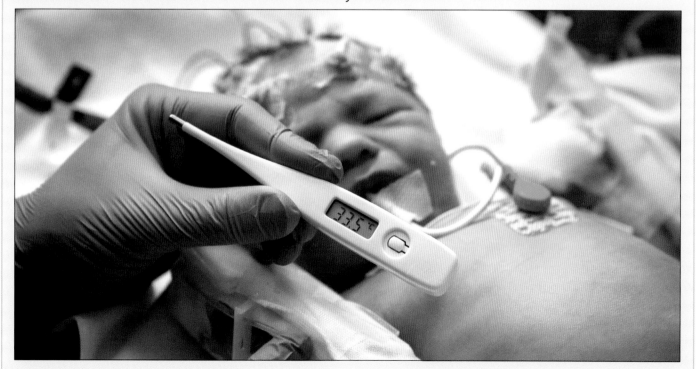

Eligibility for Therapeutic Hypothermia

TH must be started **within 6 hours of birth** and is limited to **infants who are >36 weeks gestation**. To commence TH, infants must also have an abnormal neurological exam as evidence of evolving and/or existing encephalopathy. Figure 2.5 is a checklist to help evaluate candidacy (eligibility) for cooling, and Figure 2.6 is designed to help guide the neurological exam. If possible, complete both forms prior to calling the tertiary cooling center, as this will help comprehensively discuss the infant's eligibility for cooling. If the infant meets historical (perinatal event, resuscitation, or Apgar scores) and biochemical (blood gas) criteria for cooling, perform the first neurological exam at approximately 1 hour of age.

Many centers that provide TH utilize criteria for eligibility that are identical or very similar to those used in the National Institute of Child Health and Human Development (NICHD) Neonatal Research Network study of TH in term infants. If the infant does not meet the neurological exam criteria for TH but does meet the other eligibility criteria, repeat and document the neurological exam every 1 to 2 hours until the infant is 6 hours old. This exam can be very subjective and can change from one time point to another. If, however, a decision is made to offer TH (because cooling eligibility criteria were met), and then the neurological examination improves, S.T.A.B.L.E. recommends that you continue with the plan to cool the infant. However, individual patient circumstances may arise that alter the plan of care. As needed, consult your tertiary center to discuss cooling eligibility and examination findings.

Each tertiary cooling center has specific inclusion and exclusion criteria, and some centers may be involved in TH studies that evaluate other aspects of this therapy, such as cooling infants with mild encephalopathy. Implementation of TH is time-sensitive, and it takes time to arrange and complete a transport, so it is important to quickly consult your tertiary center to discuss patient circumstances and eligibility for cooling.

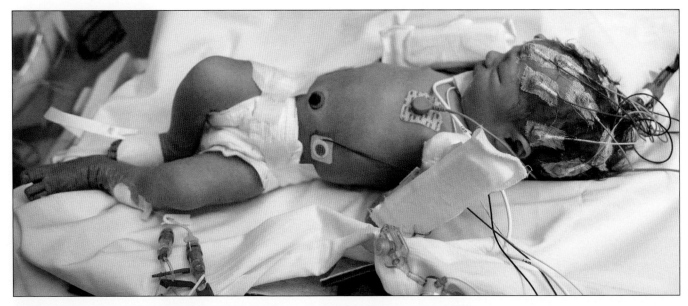

6-hour-old, 39-week gestation infant being cooled for treatment of HIE.

Eligibility for Cooling (Neuroprotective Hypothermia)

TIME of birth: _____ a.m./p.m.   **CURRENT AGE in hours/minutes:** _____ h. _____ min.

If current age is > 6 hours, but less than 24 hours, contact your tertiary center to discuss candidacy for cooling.

Clinical information	Criteria		Instructions
Gestation	**1** ≥ 36 weeks gestation	☐	Go to ➡ **2** *Weight*
	< 36 weeks gestation	☐	Ask tertiary center
Weight	**2** ≥ 1800 grams	☐	Go to ➡ **3** *Blood gas*
	< 1800 grams	☐	Ask tertiary center
Blood gas pH = _____ Base deficit = _____ Source: Cord A ☐ or V ☐ *Enter the worst blood gas results from the cord or the 1 hour of age gas* — — — — — — — — — — **Or 1st baby blood gas at < 1 hour of age** Time obtained: _____ : _____ ☐ Arterial ☐ Capillary ☐ Venous	**3** pH ≤ 7.0 *or* Base deficit ≥ –16	☐ ☐	Criteria met thus far, Go to **EXAM***
	No gas obtained	☐	
	Or pH 7.01 to 7.15	☐	Go to ➡ **4** *History of acute perinatal event*
	Or Base deficit –10 to –15.9	☐	
	pH > 7.15 or Base deficit < –10	☐	May not be eligible, Go to ➡ **4** *History of acute perinatal event*
Acute perinatal event *(check all that apply)*	**4** Variable/late fetal HR decelerations Severe fetal bradycardia Prolapsed/ruptured or tight nuchal cord Prolonged shoulder dystocia Uterine rupture Maternal hemorrhage/placental abruption Maternal trauma (e.g. vehicle accident) Mother received CPR/cardiovascular collapse	☐ ☐ ☐ ☐ ☐ ☐ ☐ ☐	Any checked, Go to ➡ **5** *Apgar score*
	No perinatal event *Or* Indeterminate what the event was because of home birth or missing information		May not be eligible, Go to ➡ **5** *Apgar score*
Apgar score at 1 minute _____ 5 minutes _____ 10 minutes _____	**5** Apgar ≤ 5 at 10 minutes **(yes)**	☐	Criteria met thus far, Go to **EXAM***
	Apgar ≥ 6 at 10 minutes **(yes)**	☐	Go to ➡ **6** *Resuscitation after delivery*
Resuscitation after delivery *(check all that apply)* ___ PPV/intubated at 10 minutes ___ CPR ___ Epinephrine administered	**6** Continued need for PPV or intubated at 10 minutes? **(yes)**	☐	Criteria met thus far, Go to **EXAM***
	PPV/intubated at 10 minutes? **(no)**	☐	May not be eligible, Go to **EXAM***

***Seizures:** If the infant is <6 hours old and meets the gestation, weight, and blood gas criteria and has a clinically recognized and/or electrographic seizure, the patient is eligible for hypothermia regardless of additional exam findings. However, complete the checklist so that complete information is provided. Consult the tertiary center where cooling is offered to discuss any questions or concerns.

Figure 2.5. Evaluating candidacy (eligibility) for therapeutic hypothermia/cooling. Start in the left column to complete the blood gas results. Then move to the middle column at the top and work through each numbered component. When directed to proceed to the neurological exam, refer to the exam found in Figure 2.6. If there is missing data, such as a known perinatal event and/or Apgar scores, and/or you are in doubt whether the patient qualifies for cooling, consult the tertiary cooling center to discuss the patient. In most cases, cooling therapy must be initiated by 6 hours of age.

Neurological Exam to Evaluate Eligibility for Cooling

Time of Birth:	Current Age (in hours/minutes) Hours:			Minutes:	Determination (0, 1, 2, or 3)
Stage Circle findings for each domain. Patient is eligible for cooling if 3 or more domains with findings in stages 2 or 3.	**Normal (0)**	**Mild (1)**	**Moderate (2)**	**Severe (3)**	
Spontaneous Activity	Normal/active	Jittery/increased	Decreased	No activity	__ =
Posture	Normal (moves around and does not maintain only one position)	Slight extension of arms and legs, and/or slight flexion of wrists, ankles, fingers, or toes	Extension of arms and legs (including a "frog-legged" position) and/or strong flexion of the wrists, ankles, fingers or toes	Decerebrate (all extremities rigidly extended)	__ =
Level of Consciousness	Normal (arouses to an awake state and responds to external stimuli)	Hyperalert or inconsolable/irritable	*Lethargic* Can elicit a response with stimulation, but may be delayed	*Stupor/Comatose* Unresponsive or barely responsive to touch/external stimuli	__ =
Tone	Normal (resists passive motion)	Slightly increased	Hypertonic or hypotonic/floppy	Flaccid (like a rag doll)	__ =
Primitive Reflexes (select the **worst** item for suck or moro)	**Suck:** strong/rhythmic **Moro:** normal (extension of limbs, opening of hands, followed by adduction of upper extremities)	**Suck:** effective but uncoordinated **Moro:** hyperreactive (low threshold to elicit)	**Suck:** weak or biting **Moro:** incomplete	**Suck:** absent **Moro:** absent	**Select highest stage for primitive reflex for determination**
Autonomic Nervous System [ANS] (vital signs) Select the **worst** for the ANS findings. Ex: if infant is intubated, circle the severe respirations item (column 3)	**Respirations:** regular respiratory rate and spontaneous breathing with no abnormal pauses **Heart rate:** normal range for age and variable with movement, crying	**Respirations:** tachypnea **Heart rate:** tachycardia	**Respirations:** periodic or irregular breathing **Heart rate:** <100 bpm, but variable up to 120 bpm	**Respirations:** intubated or receiving PPV via mask or laryngeal mask airway (LMA) **Heart rate:** little variability in rate, may be irregular, may be bradycardic	**Select highest stage of the 3 ANS for determination** __ =
ANS (pupils)	**Pupils:** normal size, reactive to light	**Pupils:** mild dilation, but reactive to light	**Pupils:** constricted, but reactive to light	**Pupils:** dilated and either fixed or sluggishly reactive; asymmetric	

● Observe infant first   ✋ Hands on exam

Seizures: If the infant is <6 hours old and meets the gestation, weight, and blood gas criteria and has a clinically recognized and/or electrographic seizure, the patient is eligible for cooling regardless of the rest of the exam findings. However, complete the entire neurological exam to establish a baseline exam.

Figure 2.6. Neurological exam to evaluate eligibility for therapeutic hypothermia/cooling. If the infant meets historical (perinatal event, resuscitation, Apgar scores) and biochemical (blood gas) criteria for cooling, perform the first neurological exam at approximately 1 hour of age. Circle findings and then complete the determination column. If the infant does not meet the neurological exam criteria for cooling but does meet the other eligibility criteria, repeat the exam every 1 to 2 hours until the infant is 6 hours old.

Controlled Passive Cooling Prior to Transport

Inquire whether the tertiary cooling center wants passive cooling prior to transport. Passive cooling may include turning the radiant warmer heater off while continuously monitoring the skin temperature and the infant's axillary temperature at least every 15 minutes. In addition, closely monitor all vital signs for deterioration. Initiate passive cooling only if instructed to do so by the tertiary center, and providing there are personnel trained and available to closely monitor the infant's temperature and vital signs during this process. One significant risk with passive cooling is that the body temperature may drop precipitously to below 33.5°C (92.3°F).[84] A heat source may be required to prevent accidental severe hypothermia and its associated complications. Active measures to cool the infant, such as cold chemical packs, are usually not necessary.

Optimizing Neurologic Outcomes Before, During, and After Therapeutic Hypothermia

Prevent Hyperthermia[85-88]

During resuscitation and stabilization of the infant who has experienced an asphyxial insult, take extra care to **prevent hyperthermia** (temperature >37.5°C or 99.5°F) or to **reduce fever if it occurs** since an elevated body temperature may worsen damage to neurons. Careful temperature management includes before cooling is started, as well as during and after cooling therapy is completed.

Neurologic Outcomes and Hypoglycemia, Hyperglycemia, and/or Unstable Blood Glucose Levels[76,77,89-94]

Neurologic outcomes are worsened in infants with HIE who become hypoglycemic (<40 mg/dL; 2.2 mmol/L), hyperglycemic (>144 mg/dL; >8 mmol/L), or who have unstable blood glucose concentrations with at least one episode of hypoglycemia and one episode of hyperglycemia. Monitor the blood glucose closely and provide supplemental IV dextrose to maintain the blood glucose level (blood sugar) between 50 and 100 mg/dL (2.8 to 5.6 mmol/L).

Monitor for Metabolic Derangements and Detect and Treat Seizures[73,75,76,81]

To optimize outcomes before and during cooling, additional metabolic derangements should be monitored for and treated, including the following:

- Hypocalcemia

- Hyponatremia

- Hypomagnesemia

- Hypocarbia and hypercarbia

- Hypoxemia and hyperoxia

- Metabolic acidosis

Seizures can occur in up to 50% of infants with HIE, and in many cases, seizures are subclinical, meaning they are only seen using brain monitors, such as amplitude integrated electroencephalogram (aEEG) or video EEG. Seizures are usually observed within 24 hours after birth and are associated with worsened neurodevelopmental outcome. Therefore, it is important to utilize brain monitoring equipment and to treat seizures during and after cooling therapy.

Is Candidacy (Eligibility) for Therapeutic Hypothermia Evolving?

Preterm Infants

TH is currently intended for infants with moderate to severe HIE who are ≥36 weeks gestation, ≥1,800 grams, and ≤6 hours old, and who meet other blood gas, perinatal event, and/or resuscitation criteria.[77] However, many centers worldwide now offer cooling for infants who are ≥35 weeks gestation. A recently completed study that evaluated the safety and efficacy of TH in preterm infants (33 to 35 completed weeks of gestation) with moderate to severe neonatal encephalopathy reported a higher risk of death compared to preterm infants with HIE who were not cooled. In addition, there was no evidence that TH reduced the combined outcome of death or moderate/severe disability.[95] Therefore, The S.T.A.B.L.E. Program will continue to recommend TH for infants who are ≥36 weeks gestation.[77] We are awaiting formal publication of the Preemie Hypothermia for Neonatal Encephalopathy study results. Please follow the neonatal literature for this publication.
For more information, see
https://clinicaltrials.gov/study/NCT01793129.

Mild HIE

Infants with mild HIE are increasingly being offered TH despite a paucity of research that cooling infants with mild HIE is beneficial. However, there is emerging evidence that infants with mild HIE have lower cognitive scores compared to healthy infants.[96,97] A new study is underway to evaluate the safety and effectiveness of cooling infants with mild HIE (COOLPRIME: Comparative Effectiveness for Cooling Prospectively Infants With Mild Encephalopathy).[82] Results of this trial are expected in early 2029. To be eligible for study enrollment, the infant must be ≥35 weeks gestation, have perinatal acidosis, and mild encephalopathy on the neurological exam within 6 hours after birth (defined as the presence of at least two signs of mild, moderate, or severe encephalopathy with no more than two signs in the moderate or severe stage).
For more information, see
https://clinicaltrials.gov/study/NCT04621279.

Airway Module

Sugar

Temperature

Airway

Blood Pressure

Lab Work

Emotional Support

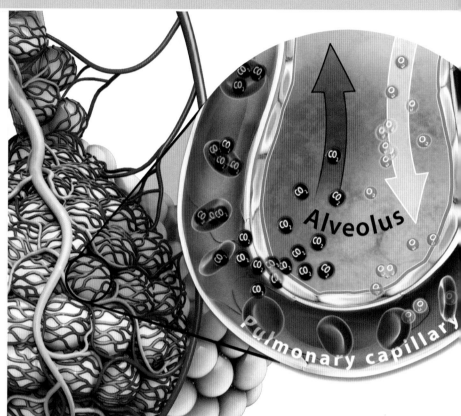

Alveolus

Pulmonary capillary

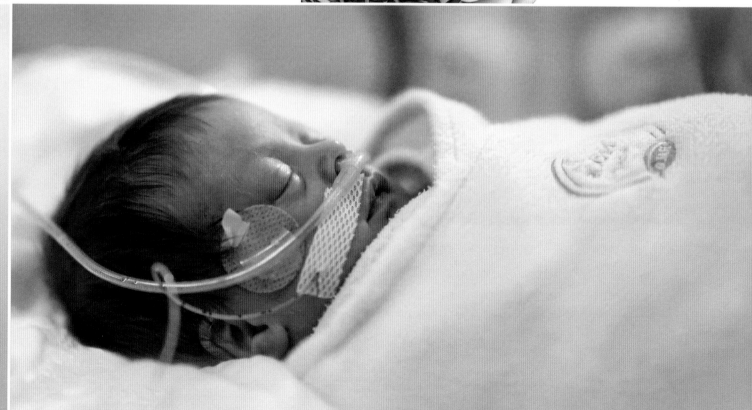

Airway—Module Objectives

Upon completion of this module, participants will gain an increased understanding of:

1. Labs and tests to obtain and items to monitor when evaluating and stabilizing a sick infant.

2. Signs of respiratory distress and how to distinguish between mild, moderate, and severe distress.

3. Blood gas interpretation and the treatment of respiratory and metabolic acidosis.

4. Signs of respiratory failure and when assisted ventilation may be necessary.

5. Principles of assisted ventilation, including candidates for continuous positive airway pressure, positive pressure ventilation, endotracheal intubation, and the initial ventilatory support to provide.

6. Respiratory illnesses and airway challenges that present in neonates.

Introduction

Infants with a variety of illnesses or conditions frequently present with respiratory distress. In all settings, continuously evaluate the degree of respiratory distress the infant is experiencing so that appropriate support can be provided. Promptly notify the medical care team if concerned about a worsening cardiorespiratory status.[1-3]

Airway—General Guidelines

▣1 Gather Information to Help Determine the Reason for Respiratory Distress[3-5]

In addition to a thorough physical examination, the following items can provide clues to the underlying problem:

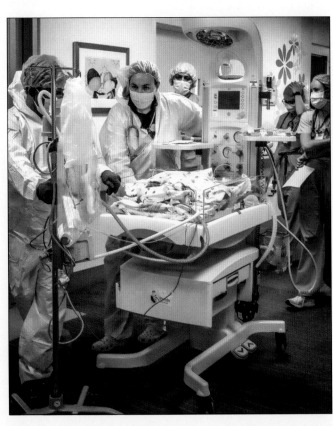

- Maternal history: pre-pregnancy, pregnancy, and labor and delivery.

- Infant history: gestational age and weight, the need for birth resuscitation, presenting signs, and timing of presentation (at birth, shortly after birth, hours or days after birth).

- Laboratory and X-ray evaluation. Obtain an ultrasound when indicated.

2 Provide Respiratory Support and Monitor for Deterioration

Providing an appropriate level of respiratory support can help prevent respiratory failure. Respiratory support ranges from giving supplemental oxygen via a nasal cannula to increased levels of support via high flow nasal cannula (HFNC), continuous positive airway pressure (CPAP), noninvasive positive pressure ventilation (NIPPV), or endotracheal intubation with positive pressure ventilation (PPV).[6-9] These modes of support are further explained starting on page 137.

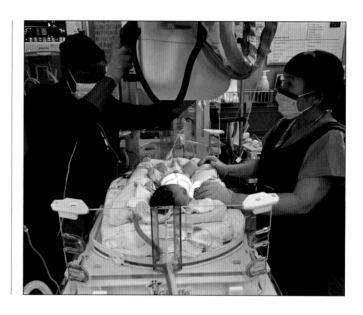

Assessment and Monitoring[2-4,9-13]

Table 3.1. lists the items to monitor and evaluate when an infant is sick. Assess the infant's condition frequently and record your observations. Some infants require re-assessment every few minutes, while others may be less ill and more stable and can be assessed every 1 to 3 hours.

Vital signs	Assess the following:
• Temperature	• Work of breathing (nasal flaring, grunting, retractions)
• Heart rate and rhythm	• Color and oxygen (O_2) saturation
• Respiratory rate	• How much oxygen is being provided, and how is the oxygen being delivered?
• Blood pressure	• Neurologic status
Laboratory and radiology tests	• Skin perfusion (capillary refill time, temperature of the hands and feet)
• Blood glucose	• Strength and equality of pulses in the brachial and femoral arteries
• Blood gas	• Urine output (declining or low)
• Complete blood count	
• Blood culture (if concerned about sepsis and prior to starting antibiotics)	
• Chest X-ray	
• Abdominal X-ray (if the infant has gastrointestinal signs such as abdominal distension, vomiting, or a history of not stooling)	

Table 3.1. Items to monitor, evaluate, and observe when an infant is sick and has respiratory distress.

Severity of Respiratory Distress: Mild, Moderate, Severe[2,10]

Respiratory distress is classified as mild, moderate, or severe.

Mild

- There is tachypnea (respiratory rate >60) with or without other signs of respiratory distress (any combination of nasal flaring, grunting, or mild retractions).

- The infant is on room air or needs <30% supplemental oxygen to maintain the oxygen (O_2) saturation >90%.

Moderate

- There are signs of respiratory distress, such as tachypnea, nasal flaring, grunting, and retractions.

- The infant is cyanotic on room air and requires >30% supplemental O_2 to maintain the O_2 saturation >90%.

Severe

The infant has all the following:

- The infant is working hard to breathe and has any combination of apnea, tachypnea, nasal flaring, grunting, or retractions.

- The O_2 requirement is increasing above 30% supplemental oxygen, or the infant has difficulty maintaining an O_2 saturation >90% on supplemental oxygen.

- There is respiratory acidosis and/or respiratory and metabolic acidosis indicative of respiratory failure and worsening hypoxia.

- There is an altered mental status (hypotonia and poor or no response to stimulation).

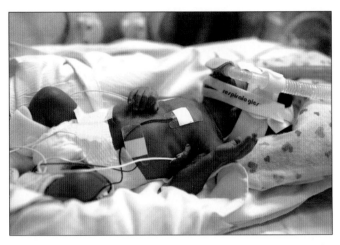

Former 28-week gestation, 4-week-old infant with both intercostal and subcostal retractions.

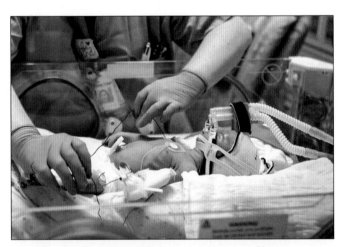

33-week gestation, 6-hour-old infant with moderate respiratory distress on CPAP.

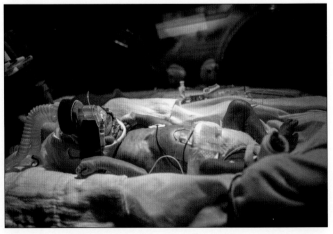

30-week gestation, 12-hour-old infant with severe subcostal retractions on CPAP.

Respiratory Rate[5,9,14,15]

A **normal respiratory rate** in infants is between 30 and 60 breaths per minute. The infant should be breathing easily and with no signs of respiratory distress, such as nasal flaring, grunting, retractions, or cyanosis. On auscultation, the breath sounds should be clear and equal bilaterally.

A **slow respiratory rate** of less than 30 breaths per minute is called **bradypnea**. In association with labored breathing, a slow respiratory rate may be a sign that the infant is becoming exhausted. A slow respiratory rate may be secondary to a decrease in central respiratory drive because of brain injury (e.g., hypoxic-ischemic encephalopathy, cerebral edema, or intracranial hemorrhage), a metabolic disorder, medications (e.g., opioids), neuromuscular disease, or severe shock. A very depressed or sick infant may start to gasp, which almost always progresses to apnea (breathing stops completely).

A **fast respiratory rate** greater than 60 breaths per minute is called **tachypnea**. Tachypnea occurs when an infant is trying to compensate for something abnormal in the blood gas—that is, an elevated carbon dioxide (PCO_2) level, a low oxygen (PO_2) level, and/or a low pH. Interference with effective ventilation because of lung disease or other pulmonary problems (e.g., pneumothorax) can lead to hypercarbia (an elevated PCO_2) and hypoxemia (a low PO_2). A state of shock leads to anaerobic metabolism and increased lactic acid production. To compensate for the low pH, the respiratory rate will increase to blow off CO_2, which can help raise the pH.

 Gasping is a sign of impending cardiorespiratory arrest! When an infant is gasping, ventilation and air exchange are ineffective. This extremely critical state should be treated the same as if the infant were apneic. Immediately provide positive pressure ventilation (PPV) via a bag and mask or T-piece resuscitator.[9,16]

 Let's Learn More... How does ventilation (inhalation and exhalation) help with alveolar gas exchange?[2,17-21]

Tidal volume (VT) is the amount of air (in milliliters; mL) inhaled or exhaled with each breath or respiratory cycle. When an infant is on volume mechanical ventilation, VT is discussed in mL per kilogram (mL/kg) of body weight. Minute ventilation is the volume of air inhaled or exhaled (VT) over a 1-minute period. When an infant has a respiratory illness, such as pneumonia, congestion in the alveoli decreases the tidal volume and the ability to exhale CO_2. Rising CO_2 levels in the blood stimulate the respiratory center (medulla oblongata) to increase the respiratory rate and volume of each breath. The faster respiratory rate and size of each breath (increased minute ventilation) may or may not sufficiently lower the PCO_2 level. Ineffective ventilation is one indication for offering respiratory support, such as continuous positive airway pressure (CPAP) or positive pressure ventilation (PPV). As mentioned earlier, an infant may also be tachypneic for non-pulmonary reasons. For example, if an infant is in shock and the pH is low, the respiratory center will be stimulated to increase minute ventilation (to breathe off CO_2) to help correct or compensate for metabolic acidosis.

Respiratory Distress[2,10,22,23]

In addition to an abnormal respiratory rate, other signs of respiratory distress include nasal flaring, grunting, stridor, retractions, and cyanosis.

Nasal flaring, or dilation of the nostrils, occurs when the alae nasi muscles contract. Nasal flaring increases the diameter of the nasal passage, which reduces resistance to air flow through the upper airways.

Grunting is heard when the infant exhales against partially closed vocal cords. The vocal cords open on inspiration to increase gas flow into the lungs. On expiration, the infant partially closes their vocal cords to trap air in the alveoli and increase functional residual capacity (lung volume), which helps prevent the alveoli from collapsing. Grunting may be intermittent or continuous. Until the infant tires out, grunting helps improve oxygenation and ventilation.

Older infants and children who grunt are usually severely ill; however, this rule may not apply to all newborns who grunt. Most late preterm and term infants who begin to grunt will do so within 30 minutes after birth and will stop grunting by 2 hours of age.[24] If grunting does not stop within a few hours of age, or if grunting appears for the first time several hours or more after birth, and especially if accompanied by other signs of respiratory distress, this is a warning sign that requires further evaluation since the infant may be sick.

Stridor is a high-pitched sound heard with inspiration but may also be heard on inspiration and expiration with the same breath. When heard on expiration only, a tracheal obstruction should be considered. Inspiratory stridor is commonly caused by laryngomalacia, but stridor may be heard with vocal cord paralysis, tracheomalacia, or subglottic stenosis. Stridor is worse when lying supine, when the infant is agitated, or when the head is flexed forward. Figure 3.1 is a photo of swollen vocal cords taken during laryngoscopy in a former 3-month-old preterm infant who subsequently required a tracheostomy.

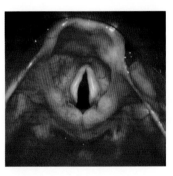
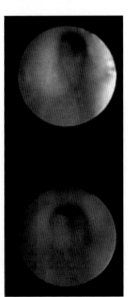

Figure 3.1. Swollen vocal cords in a 3-month-old former preterm infant (right photo). For comparison, a photo of a normal larynx is shown above.

Reproduced with permission of American Academy of Pediatrics via Copyright Clearance Center; Textbook of Pediatric Care, McInerny TK, Adams HM, © 2012.

Retractions occur with inspiration and reflect the abnormal inward movement of the chest wall as the infant tries to increase tidal volume (the amount of air breathed in and out with each breath). Retractions become evident because of a combination of diaphragm contraction and accessory use of respiratory muscles. They are graded as *mild, moderate,* or *severe* to communicate the degree to which accessory muscles are used. Varying degrees of lung disease cause the lungs to become stiffer, and the stiffer the lungs (less compliant), the worse the retractions.

Intercostal retractions alone usually signal mild respiratory distress. When retractions become severe (deeper and/or more areas are involved), the infant should be thoroughly assessed for causes, including airway obstruction, pneumothorax, displaced or plugged endotracheal tube, or worsening atelectasis (collapse of alveoli) because of worsening lung disease (e.g., pneumonia or respiratory distress syndrome).

Severe substernal retraction seen in a late preterm newborn.

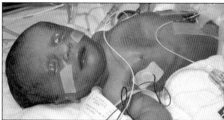

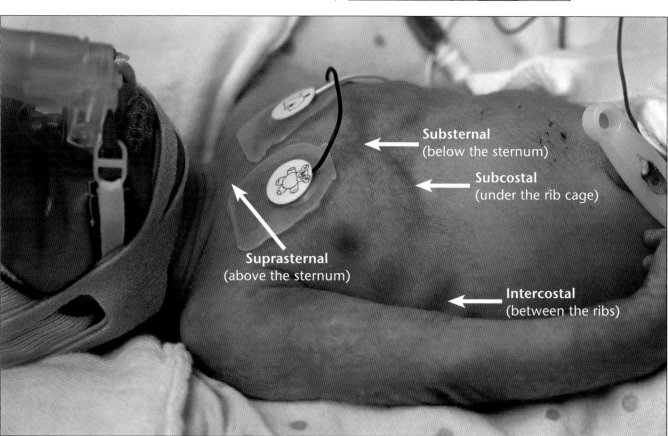

Locations where retractions may be seen.

Oxygen Requirement

Cyanosis is a bluish discoloration of the skin that is seen when desaturated arterial blood circulates from the heart to the body. *Central cyanosis* is present when the tongue and oral mucosa are cyanotic because of impaired oxygenation of the arterial blood secondary to respiratory and/or cardiac dysfunction.[2]

Acrocyanosis is the term used when just the hands and/or feet are cyanotic. Acrocyanosis may be seen in the first day or two after birth in healthy infants; however, it can occur in response to shock or cold stress because of peripheral vasoconstriction.[25]

Significantly anemic patients may not appear cyanotic even with a low PO_2 and O_2 saturation. Infants with polycythemia (i.e., a hematocrit >65%) may appear cyanotic even though they have a normal PO_2 and only mild desaturation. However, polycythemic infants are at increased risk for hyperviscosity, which can compromise blood flow to vital organs and cause end-organ injury.[26]

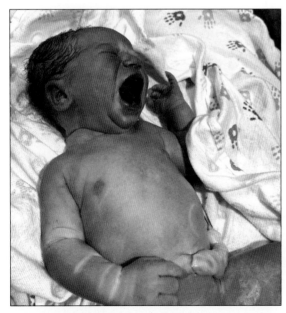

Newborn infant with expected cyanosis shortly after birth.

Responding to the Cyanotic Infant[27,28]

Immediately after birth, cyanosis is normal. However, in the post-resuscitation period, if the infant is cyanotic when breathing room air, evaluate the O_2 saturation and give the infant supplemental oxygen. Whenever possible, administer oxygen using humidified blended gases of oxygen and air. Starting with 21% O_2, slowly increase the amount of inspired O_2 until the saturation remains between 91 to 95%. If oxygen administration via nasal cannula is not improving oxygenation, consider additional respiratory support, such as CPAP or PPV. Remember, O_2 is a drug, and administration should follow the same rules and precautions as any drug. That is, side effects can occur from using more O_2 than is necessary (e.g., retinopathy of prematurity in preterm infants and hyperoxic injury to the organs in all infants),[29] and the amount administered should be regulated and monitored by pulse oximetry or blood gas analysis while in use.[9]

 A rapidly increasing O_2 requirement may be a sign of impending respiratory or cardiac failure and should be reported immediately to the medical care team. If the oxygen concentration reaches 100% and the infant's O_2 saturation does not rise to 90%, **cyanotic congenital heart disease (CHD) or persistent pulmonary hypertension of the newborn (PPHN)** *may be the reason. In cases of ductal-dependent cyanotic CHD, a prostaglandin E1 (PGE) infusion can be lifesaving. Consult a neonatologist or pediatric cardiologist if the infant is not improving satisfactorily.[30-33]*

Hypoxemia, Hypoxia, and Anaerobic Metabolism[16,34,35]

Hypoxemia is the term used to describe a low level of oxygen in the arterial blood. Hypoxemia, combined with poor cardiac output or the presence of factors cited in Table 3.2, can lead to hypoxia.

Hypoxia is the term used when there is an inadequate amount of O_2 in the tissues, below what the tissues need for normal cell function. Cells can survive with reduced or no oxygen supply for a short period by relying on **anaerobic metabolism**. During periods of anaerobic metabolism, tremendous amounts of glucose are consumed (thus increasing the risk for hypoglycemia), and significant amounts of lactic acid accumulate in the blood. Severe hypoxia and acidosis increase the risk of organ damage and death. See Figures 1.6 and 1.7 on page 39 for illustrations of aerobic and anaerobic metabolism.

Hypoxemia	Hypoxia
Low level of oxygen in the arterial blood secondary to a respiratory and/or cardiac problem	Inadequate amount of oxygen in the tissues, below what is needed for normal cell function

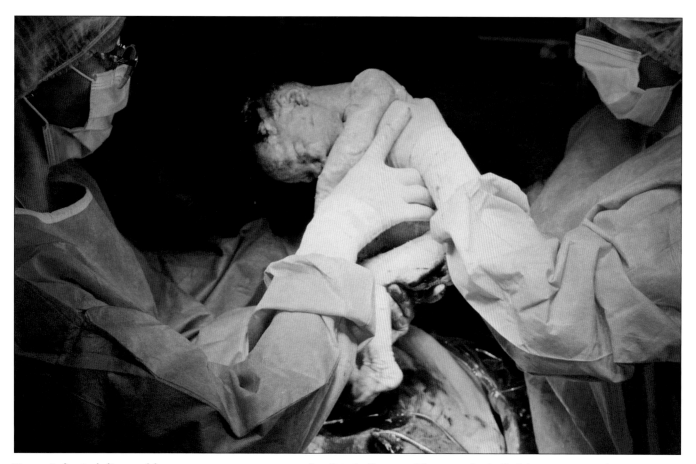

Term infant delivered by emergency cesarean for fetal distress. The amniotic fluid was meconium stained and there were three nuchal cords. This severely hypoxic and depressed infant required extensive resuscitation.

Table 3.2. Factors that interfere with oxygenation and O_2 delivery to the tissues.[2,16,31,33,34]

Tissue hypoxia can result from many causes, including the following:

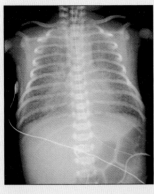

Lung disease: Gas exchange occurs in the lungs. Interference with oxygenation and ventilation because of pneumonia, meconium aspiration syndrome, respiratory distress syndrome, and other respiratory illnesses causes poorly oxygenated blood to return to the heart, where it is then pumped to the body. The low O_2 content in the blood may be insufficient to satisfy tissue demands.

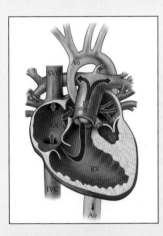

Heart failure: When the left ventricle can't effectively pump blood through the aorta and out to the body, the tissues receive less oxygen than they need for a healthy metabolism. Heart failure can also lead to pulmonary edema and congestive heart failure, which further impairs gas exchange in the alveoli. Heart failure can occur because of cardiomyopathy, myocarditis, post-asphyxia cardiac dysfunction, and left-sided obstructive heart lesions such as hypoplastic left heart syndrome (shown in the illustration and with a closing ductus arteriosus).

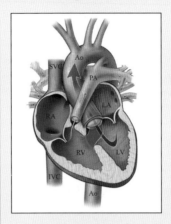

Intracardiac mixing of blood: Normally, deoxygenated venous blood returns to the heart, where it is pumped to the lungs to become oxygenated. Then, the oxygenated blood is pumped through the aorta to the body. With an intracardiac shunt, some deoxygenated blood is shunted **right-to-left** into the left side of the heart instead of being pumped into the lungs. The degree of hypoxemia in the aortic blood depends on how much blood shunts **right-to-left**. Infants with cyanotic congenital heart disease, such as tetralogy of Fallot (shown in the illustration), are cyanotic because deoxygenated blood is being ejected through the aorta to the body.

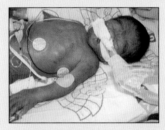

Increased metabolic rate or demand: Severe illnesses, such as sepsis, can significantly increase oxygen consumption at the cellular level. The photo is of a hypotensive preterm infant with sepsis.

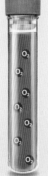

5 gm Hb

Low hemoglobin, altered ability of hemoglobin to bind with O_2, or an abnormal type of hemoglobin: The tissues require O_2 for normal cell function. Hemoglobin binds with O_2 in the lungs and delivers it to the tissues. If the hemoglobin level is low (anemia) or there is an abnormal type of hemoglobin, such as methemoglobin, the oxygen content in the blood is lower, which impairs tissue oxygenation.

Oxygen (O₂) Saturation[9,11,13,27,34,36-38]

Hemoglobin (Hb) is the molecule in red blood cells that binds to and carries oxygen to the tissues. **Oxygen saturation (SaO₂) is** the **percentage** of hemoglobin bound with oxygen and is measured at the bedside using **pulse oximetry.** When Hb is carrying oxygen, or "saturated with oxygen," the color of the red blood cell is **red**. When Hb is carrying little oxygen, or is "desaturated," the color of the red blood cell is **purple. Cyanosis** is apparent when 3 to 5 grams per deciliter (dL) of Hb is not carrying oxygen. For more information about hemoglobin levels, oxygen content, and cyanosis, see page 122, Let's Learn More... *How do hemoglobin levels affect oxygen content and the appearance of cyanosis?* It is important to realize that anemic infants will not appear cyanotic until they are more severely hypoxemic and desaturated than infants with normal or elevated hemoglobin levels. In addition, anemic patients have a lower O₂ content than infants with a normal Hb level.

Pulse Oximetry

Noninvasive monitoring using pulse oximetry provides a reliable measurement of arterial hemoglobin O₂ saturation. In addition to an O₂ saturation reading, the detected arterial pulsations show a heart rate on the monitor. If a cardiorespiratory monitor is in use, compare the two heart rates to ensure they match. The pulse oximeter probe can be attached to the palm, wrist, or foot. When the probe is attached to the right palm or wrist, the *preductal* O₂ saturation is reported. Healthy late preterm and term infants will have an O₂ saturation on room air between 95 and 99% (median 97%). As altitude increases, both barometric pressure and partial pressure of oxygen in the air decrease, which means as altitude increases, the O₂ saturation decreases.[39,40] Therefore, the O₂ saturation is lower for infants living at altitude than those living at sea level. When the O₂ saturation is in the upper 90s, and the infant is on oxygen, the arterial PO_2 may exceed 100 mmHg, so assessment of arterial PO_2 may be necessary to avoid hyperoxia. See Table 3.3 for factors that can alter the accuracy of pulse oximetry.

- Pulse oximetry relies on normal pulsatile flow beneath the sensor. Readings can be inaccurate when arterial pulsations are weak secondary to hypotension, with peripheral vasoconstriction secondary to hypothermia or vasopressor therapy, or if the probe is secured too tightly.

- Pulsations are not adequately detected because there is severe edema of the extremity where the probe is attached.

- Readings will be inaccurate if the probe is secured too loosely and light strikes the sensor, causing optical interference.

- There is motion artifact because of movement of the extremity where the probe is attached.

- There are abnormal forms of hemoglobin (i.e., methemoglobin, carboxyhemoglobin). The oximeter reading will be falsely high because these forms of hemoglobin are also included in the saturation calculation.

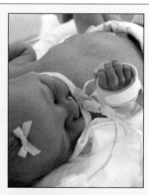

Table 3.3. Factors that can alter the accuracy of pulse oximetry.[9,11,36]

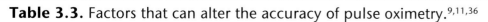

Let's Learn More... *How do hemoglobin levels affect oxygen content and the appearance of cyanosis?*[11,17,26,41]

O_2 saturation is measured using pulse oximetry. The appearance of cyanosis can be confusing when it is readily visible, but the O_2 saturation is not very low, as is the case when the Hb level is high. On the other hand, an anemic patient may not appear cyanotic until the O_2 saturation is low.

It is important to interpret O_2 saturation and O_2 content in the context of the infant's hemoglobin level.

- When an infant is *polycythemic* (Hb >22 grams or a venous hematocrit ≥65%), cyanosis will be apparent when the O_2 saturation is between 77 and 86%. Yet, the infant will have an adequate O_2 content since each gram of Hb binds 1.34 mL of O_2. The O_2 content in the blood with an 86% O_2 saturation will be 25 mL/dL of blood.

- When an infant is *anemic* (Hb ≤10 gm/dL or a hematocrit of ≤30%), they will not appear cyanotic until there is desaturation of at least 3 grams/dL of Hb (30% of the infant's total hemoglobin). Cyanosis will not be apparent until the O_2 saturation is 70%, and the O_2 content will only be 9.4 mL/dL.

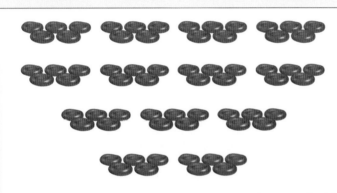

	Hb 20 gm/dL — O_2 saturation 100%, pink color, and no cyanosis is apparent
	Hb 20 gm/dL — O_2 saturation 75 to 85%, and cyanosis may be apparent
	Hb 15 gm/dL — O_2 saturation 67 to 80%, and cyanosis is apparent
	Hb 10 gm/dL — O_2 saturation 50 to 70%, and cyanosis is apparent

To determine the approximate O_2 saturation where cyanosis may be apparent, divide 3 or 5 by the grams of Hb. For example:	
3 gm Hb divided by 20 gm Hb = 15%	O_2 saturation 100% minus 15% = 85% O_2 saturation
5 gm Hb divided by 20 gm Hb = 25%	O_2 saturation 100% minus 25% = 75% O_2 saturation

Effects of Varying Hb Levels on O_2 Content

At 37° Celsius, 1 gram of Hb binds with 1.34 mL of O_2. When Hb is 100% saturated with O_2, the total O_2 content of the blood at varying Hb concentrations is displayed to the right. Under normal conditions, a negligible amount of O_2 is also dissolved in plasma and is not included in the calculation of O_2 content. To support normal metabolism, the tissues require approximately 5 mL of O_2 for every 100 mL of blood perfusing them.

At 37°C, 1 gm Hb x 1.34 mL O_2 = O_2 content per 100mL whole blood

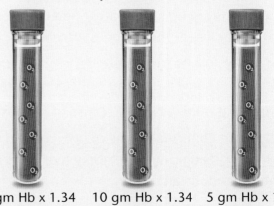

| 15 gm Hb x 1.34 = 20.1 ml O_2 | 10 gm Hb x 1.34 = 13.4 ml O_2 | 5 gm Hb x 1.34 = 6.7 ml O_2 |

Monitoring the Preductal and Postductal O₂ Saturation[1,2,11,16,33]

When concerned an infant may be shunting **deoxygenated** blood into the **systemic** circulation, as can occur with persistent pulmonary hypertension of the newborn (PPHN), the O_2 saturation is monitored in two locations simultaneously. The ductus arteriosus is a fetal shunt that connects the pulmonary artery to the aorta to allow blood to bypass the nonaerated lungs. A **preductal** site is the arterial branch (i.e., the right subclavian artery) off the aorta before the ductus arteriosus. A **postductal** site is anywhere in the descending aorta after the ductus arteriosus. The left subclavian artery branches off the aorta close to the ductus arteriosus, so the left hand is not considered a site for postductal monitoring. Figure 3.2 illustrates where to place oximeter probes for preductal and postductal monitoring. As shown in the illustration, a right radial artery blood gas would be from a preductal site, and an umbilical artery or posterior tibial artery blood gas would be from a postductal site.

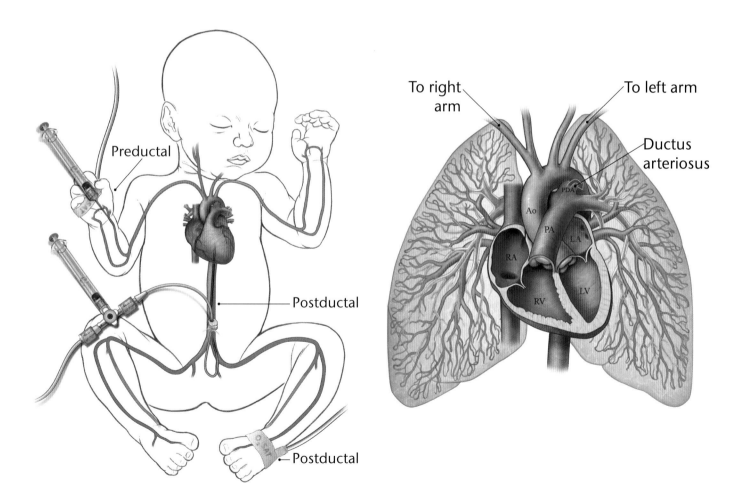

Figure 3.2. Preductal and postductal blood gas and O₂ saturation monitoring sites. Preductal O_2 saturation is monitored on the right hand, and a preductal arterial blood gas is obtained from the right radial artery. Postductal O_2 saturation is monitored on either foot, and a postductal arterial blood gas is obtained from the umbilical artery or the posterior tibial artery. The heart illustration shows the right-to-left shunt at the PDA and the location of the preductal right subclavian artery that branches off the aorta.

Procedure for Monitoring the Preductal and Postductal O$_2$ Saturation[2,3,11]

Two pulse oximeters are required; however, if two monitors are not available, place an oximeter probe on the right hand (preductal) and another probe on either foot. Using the single cable, record the preductal saturation values for several minutes, then change the cable to the postductal probe and record the saturation values for several minutes. **Right-to-left** ductal shunting is confirmed when the preductal O$_2$ saturation is 5 to 10% higher (or more) than the postductal O$_2$ saturation. In some cases of PPHN, blood also shunts **right-to-left** at the foramen ovale, which is a small opening between the right and left atrium. With **right**-to-**left** shunting at the foramen ovale, deoxygenated blood enters the left side of the heart, where it is ejected into the aorta. With **right**-to-**left** atrial shunting, there may be little difference between the pre- and postductal O$_2$ saturations, but there is still pulmonary hypertension causing the shunting. For more information, see the Clinical Tip—*Making sense of O$_2$ saturation values and shunting.*

Pulse Oximetry Screening (POS) for Critical Congenital Heart Disease (CCHD)[33]

POS screening for CCHD is being performed in many hospitals worldwide. The purpose of screening is to detect *lower-than-normal O$_2$ saturation values* secondary to previously undiagnosed CCHD. Healthy-appearing infants are screened prior to discharge home since there is a significant risk of morbidity or even mortality if the infant is home when the ductus arteriosus begins to close. Follow your hospital's protocol for how to perform CCHD screening since it varies between facilities and regions.

When is CCHD screening done? After birth, the transition from fetal to neonatal circulation involves the closure of fetal shunts (the foramen ovale and ductus arteriosus) and stabilization of O$_2$ saturation levels. To prevent false positive results (meaning it is determined there is a CCHD when, in fact, there is not), it is best to wait until the infant is at least 24 hours old to perform the screen. If the infant is discharged home prior to 24 hours, the screening can be done earlier. The seven primary and five secondary heart lesions that may be detected by CCHD screening include the following:

Primary

- Hypoplastic left heart syndrome
- Pulmonary atresia
- Tetralogy of Fallot
- Total anomalous pulmonary venous connection
- Transposition of the great arteries
- Tricuspid atresia
- Truncus arteriosus

Secondary

- Coarctation of the aorta
- Double-outlet right ventricle
- Ebstein anomaly
- Interrupted aortic arch
- Various forms of single ventricle CHD

Illustrations of critical (ductal-dependent) left-side obstructive heart defects are shown on page 189. Figure 4.6 on page 197 shows critical coarctation of the aorta with an open and closing ductus arteriosus. A prostaglandin E1 (PGE) infusion is lifesaving for infants with critical forms of CHD. Not all infants with a positive POS screen have CHD. Noncardiac problems that may be detected include:

- Infection (sepsis)
- Hypothermia
- PPHN
- Hemoglobinopathies
- Lung disease

| ☑ Clinical Tip | *Making sense of O₂ saturation values and "shunting"*[1-3,11,32,42] |

- **No evidence of right-to-left shunt at the ductus arteriosus:** Right hand and foot saturation values are in a normal range and are nearly equal; for example, there is a structurally normal heart and blood flow.

- **Evidence of right-to-left shunt at the ductus arteriosus:** Right hand saturation is 5 to 10% **higher** (or more) than the saturation in the foot; for example, with persistent pulmonary hypertension or left-side obstructive CHD (coarctation of the aorta or interrupted aortic arch).

- **Right-to-left shunt at the foramen ovale, with or without shunting at the ductus arteriosus:** Right hand and foot saturation values are **nearly equal, but both are lower than normal**; for example, there is persistent pulmonary hypertension with shunting at both locations or there is right-side structural obstructive CHD (tricuspid or pulmonary atresia).

- **Reverse differential cyanosis:** This finding describes a lower O₂ saturation in the right hand compared to the O₂ saturation in the foot and can be seen with a ductal-dependent cyanotic congenital heart defect called transposition of the great arteries (TGA). As shown in the illustration, with TGA, the aorta originates from the right ventricle, and the pulmonary artery originates from the left ventricle. While the ductus arteriosus is widely open (usually after starting a PGE infusion) and the pulmonary vascular resistance is still elevated, the O₂ saturation in the right hand may be lower than the O₂ saturation in the foot. This pattern of saturation (called reverse differential cyanosis) is the opposite of what is observed when there is a right-to-left shunt at the ductus arteriosus secondary to PPHN.[2]

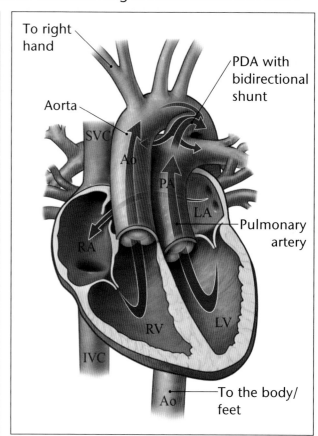

Reverse differential cyanosis secondary to TGA.

Blood Gas Evaluation[3,13,16,43-46]

Blood gas analysis helps evaluate the degree of cardiorespiratory distress an infant is experiencing and aids in the treatment of sick infants.

- **Arterial samples.** Acid-base status (pH and HCO3), ventilation (PCO2), and oxygenation (PO2) can be assessed from an arterial blood gas (ABG). Arterial blood drawn from an umbilical artery catheter or posterior tibial artery reflects postductal oxygenation, and blood drawn from a right radial artery catheter reflects preductal oxygenation.

- **Venous samples.** Acid-base status (pH and HCO3) and ventilation (PCO2) can be assessed from a venous blood gas (VBG), but the pH, on average, is 0.03 units lower and PCO2 5 to 8 mmHg higher than an arterial blood gas. Oxygenation is evaluated by pulse oximetry (O2 saturation).

- **Capillary samples.** A capillary blood gas (CBG) is obtained from a well-warmed heel to promote 'arterializing' the sample. It is useful to assess acid-base status (pH and HCO3) and ventilation (PCO2). Oxygenation is evaluated by pulse oximetry (O2 saturation). The CBG may be inaccurate if the infant is hypotensive or hypothermic (i.e., there is poor blood flow to the heel) or if the heel was not warmed properly.

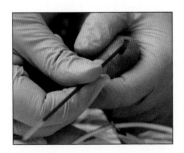 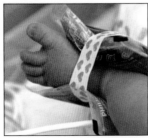

Table 3.4 summarizes blood gas values commonly observed in very young infants. Infants less than 48 hours old are slightly acidemic but with renal retention of bicarbonate, the pH rises to the normal range of 7.35 to 7.45 by approximately 48 hours of age. Figure 3.3 contains an acid-base alignment nomogram that is useful for interpreting blood gas results.[47]

	Arterial	Capillary
pH	7.35 – 7.45	7.35 – 7.45
PCO2	35 – 45 mmHg	35 – 50 mmHg
PO2 (on room air)	60 – 80 mmHg	—— (not useful for assessing oxygenation)
Bicarbonate (HCO3)	20 – 26 mEq/L	20 – 26 mEq/L
Base Excess	-3 to +3	-3 to +3

Table 3.4. Blood gas values in young infants.[12,16,48-52]

The following are normal blood gas values in kPa: PCO2 4.7 – 6, PO2 8 – 10.7

Notes:
- In the first 48 hours after birth, lower limits of normal for pH and bicarbonate (HCO3) values are 7.30 and 19, respectively. After 48 hours, the HCO3 rises, and the pH rises in response.
- Some practitioners prefer to use the term 'base deficit' instead of 'base excess' when referring to base levels with a negative value: "The base deficit is negative 4 [expressed in writing as -4). The base deficit provides valuable information about the severity of acidosis; the more negative the number, the more serious the base deficiency.
- Small air bubbles in a blood gas sample can cause significant errors in results (i.e., a falsely high PO2 and falsely low PCO2). As soon as the specimen is collected, any air bubbles should be promptly removed.
- Dilution of the blood gas sample with IV fluid may produce inaccurate results.
- If the blood gas cannot be analyzed immediately, place the sample on ice to slow down the ongoing O2 consumption and CO2 production that occurs once the sample is drawn.

Blood Gas Interpretation Using a Modified Acid-Base Alignment Nomogram and The S.T.A.B.L.E. Blood Gas Rules©

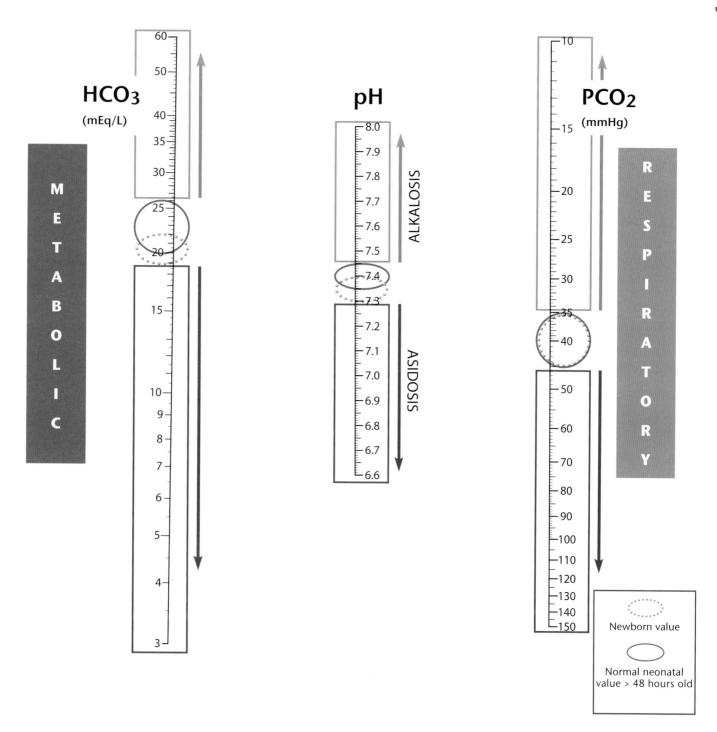

Figure 3.3. Acid-base alignment nomogram to guide blood gas interpretation.

Adapted with permission from Andersen OS. Blood acid-base alignment nomogram: Scales for pH, PCO2, base excess of whole blood of different hemoglobin concentrations, plasma bicarbonate, and plasma total-CO2. Scandinavian Journal of Clinical and Laboratory Investigation. 1963;(15):211-217.[47]

S.T.A.B.L.E. Blood Gas Rules

Accurate interpretation of a blood gas is important because it guides appropriate treatment. The following steps explain how to use the blood gas interpretation chart in Figure 3.3 on page 127.

Step 1. Obtain the baby's pH, PCO2 and HCO3 values from a blood gas measurement.

a. Put a dot on the nomogram for each of these values. Notice the HCO3 scale goes from high to low (top to bottom), and the PCO2 scale goes from low to high (top to bottom).

b. Using a ruler, draw a straight line through the three dots. **If the line is not straight**, then something is wrong with the blood gas result. For example, if there is too much heparin or other solutions in the sample, the pH will decrease, which affects the calculations for base excess and HCO3. In most cases, the test should be redrawn and analyzed.

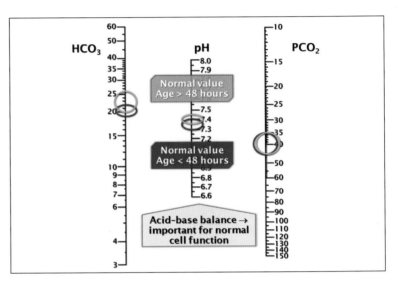

Step 2. Interpret the blood gas.

Read rules 1 through 5 and decide into which category the blood gas falls. These rules apply to very young infants and do not necessarily apply to older infants or children with metabolic derangements from multiple causes.

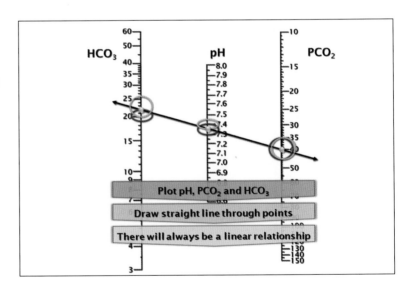

RULE 1

Think of carbon dioxide (CO_2) as an **acid**.

- CO_2 reflects the respiratory component of acid-base balance.

- The only way to remove CO_2 is to exhale it through the lungs.

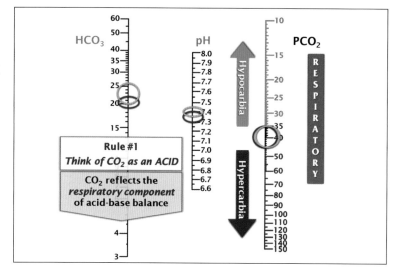

RULE 2

Think of bicarbonate (HCO_3) as a **base** (a hydrogen ion acceptor).

- Bicarbonate is consumed when neutralizing acids; therefore, changes in HCO_3 reflect the metabolic component of acid-base balance.

- To regulate acid-base balance, the kidney retains or excretes bicarbonate.

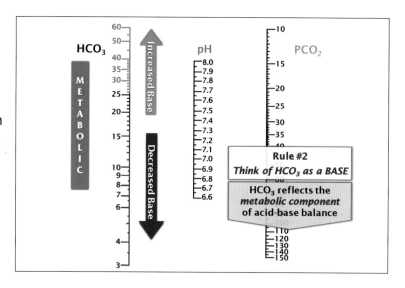

RULE 3

That which happens on the acid side (loss of or accumulation of acid or CO_2) will be balanced by the base side (HCO_3) and vice versa.

If the base side declines, the infant will try to blow off (exhale) CO_2 to balance out or "compensate" for the change on the base side.

- The overall purpose of this balancing act is to restore a normal pH value.

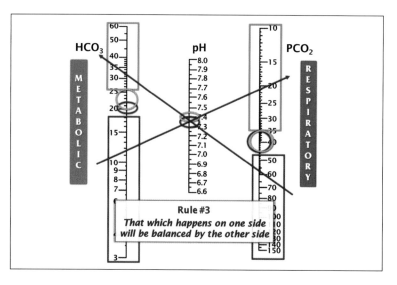

The red zone

If the blood gas dots are in the metabolic, respiratory, or both metabolic and respiratory **red** zones (the areas within the **red** boxes), then a **metabolic and/or respiratory abnormality** is the primary problem. For example, if a dot is in the metabolic **red** zone but not in the respiratory **red** zone, then the primary problem is metabolic.

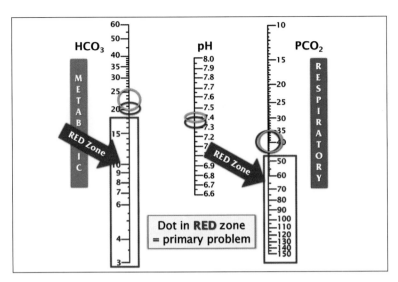

The green zone

The **green** zone is the area within the **green** boxes on the metabolic and respiratory scales. The **green** zone represents the **compensatory** area for both respiratory and metabolic components.

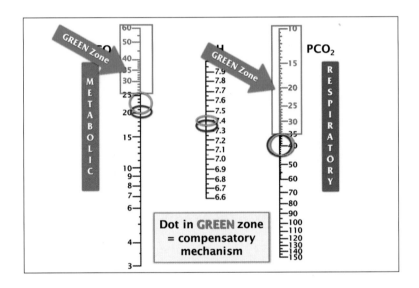

Interpreting the pH

- A dot in the pH **red** zone is "acidemia."

- A dot in the pH **green** zone is "alkalemia."

Identifying the underlying cause of the acidosis or alkalosis will guide the correct treatment.

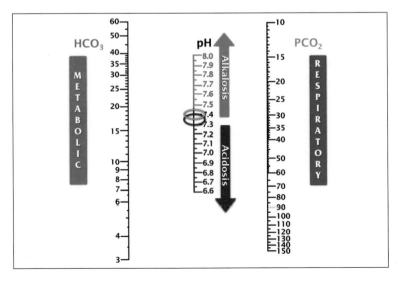

RULE 4

If the pH is normal, the blood gas is normal, *or* the blood gas is compensated.

- **Normal blood gas:** All three dots are within the three circles on the HCO₃, pH, and PCO₂ scales.

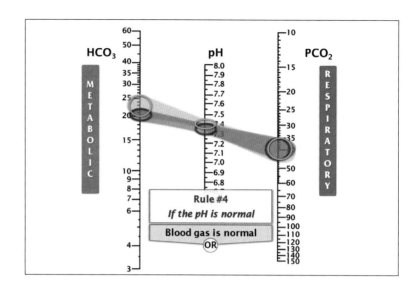

- Compensated **blood gas:**
  The pH will be in the circle, but there will be a dot in the **red** zone on either the HCO₃ (metabolic) or PCO₂ (respiratory) scale.*

The focus of this discussion is on acidemia since acidosis is more often observed in sick infants.

Example of compensated metabolic acidosis:

- A dot is in the metabolic **red** zone.
- A dot is in the pH normal circle area.
- A dot is in the respiratory **green** zone.

Example of compensated respiratory acidosis:

- A dot is in the respiratory **red** zone.
- A dot is in the pH normal circle area.
- A dot is in the metabolic **green** zone.

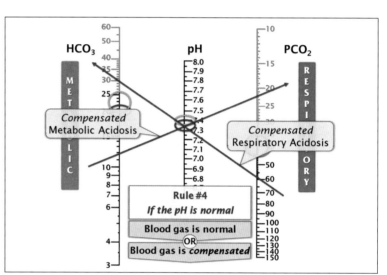

RULE 5

If the pH is low, the blood gas is **uncompensated**, secondary to metabolic and/or respiratory acidosis.

- The pH dot will be in the **red** (acidosis) zone.

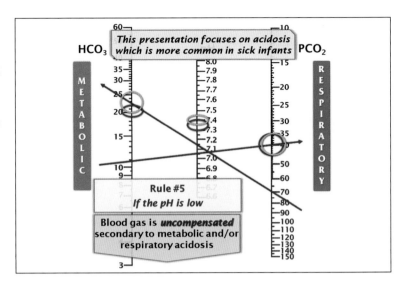

Example of uncompensated metabolic acidosis:

- A dot is in the metabolic **red** zone.
- A dot is in the pH **red** zone.
- A dot is in the circle (normal area) on the respiratory side.

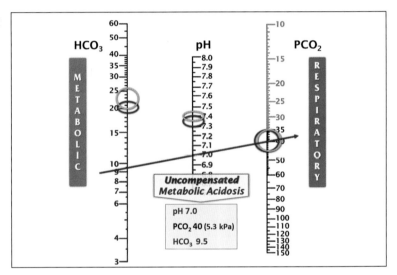

Example of uncompensated respiratory acidosis:

- A dot is in the respiratory **red** zone.
- A dot is in the pH **red** zone.
- A dot is in the circle (normal area) on the metabolic side.

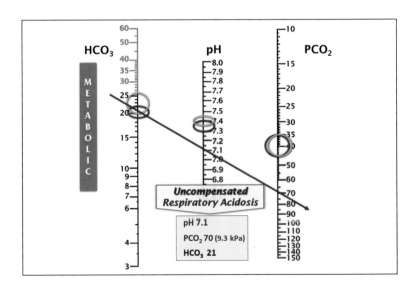

Example of uncompensated mixed metabolic and respiratory acidosis:

- A dot is in the metabolic red zone.

- A dot is in the respiratory red zone.

- A dot is in the pH red zone.

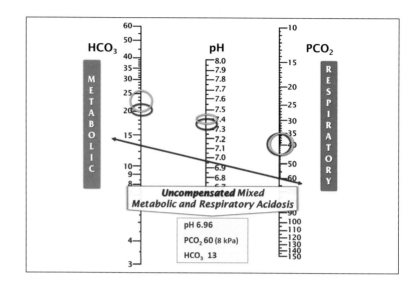

Uncompensated Mixed Metabolic and Respiratory Acidosis

pH 6.96

PCO₂ 60 (8 kPa)

HCO₃ 13

If the pH is high, the blood gas is uncompensated, secondary to metabolic and/or respiratory alkalosis.*

- The pH dot will be in the green (alkalosis) zone.

Example of uncompensated respiratory alkalosis:

- A dot is in the respiratory green zone.

- A dot is in the pH green zone.

- A dot is in the circle (normal area) on the metabolic (HCO₃) side.

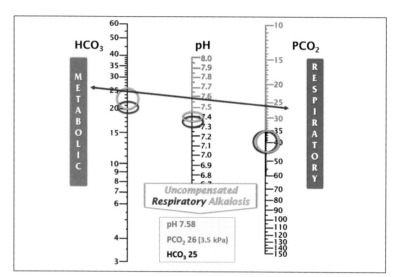

Uncompensated Respiratory Alkalosis

pH 7.58

PCO₂ 26 (3.5 kPa)

HCO₃ 25

---

*Note:

The treatment of alkalosis starts with determining the cause.

Respiratory alkalosis (low PCO_2 and elevated pH) is usually secondary to overventilation while on mechanical support. Reducing the ventilator rate or settings allows the PCO_2 to increase, which, in turn, restores the pH to a normal range.

Metabolic alkalosis (elevated HCO_3 and pH) can occur with excessive hydrogen ion loss from the gastrointestinal tract (prolonged vomiting, sustained suctioning of gastric secretions) or kidney (secondary to loop diuretics) or a base gain (administration of sodium acetate, sodium bicarbonate overdose).[49,53]

Causes of METABOLIC Acidosis[16,54-59]

Increased lactic acid production can be secondary to the following:

- Anaerobic metabolism secondary to:
  - Shock (i.e., poor tissue perfusion and oxygenation)
  - Hypothermia that is severe enough to result in anaerobic metabolism
  - Hypoglycemia that is severe enough to impair cardiac function and result in impaired O_2 and glucose delivery to the tissues
  - Severe forms of congenital heart disease that cause severe hypoxemia or left-sided heart obstruction
- Sepsis
- Inborn errors of metabolism (IEM)
  - Metabolic acidosis is seen with lactic or organic acidemia types of IEM.
  - Hyperammonemia is found with urea cycle defects and there are other IEM that do not have acidosis as a presenting sign.
  - In short, an IEM can be life-threatening because an enzyme deficiency leads to an accumulation of metabolites that have a toxic effect on cellular function.
  - Signs may not appear for a day or more and often follow the initiation of a milk intake. Signs can include poor feeding, lethargy, cardiorespiratory deterioration, neurologic abnormalities (i.e., encephalopathy and seizures), cardiomyopathy, hepatic dysfunction, sepsis, and hematologic abnormalities.[59]

Treatment of METABOLIC Acidosis[16,58,60]

Identify and treat the underlying problems:

- Hypoxia is treated by improving oxygenation, ventilation, and perfusion.
- It is not recommended that metabolic acidosis be treated with hyperventilation, as this is a temporary maneuver that will not treat the underlying problem and could potentially cause other problems.
- Hypotension and shock are treated with volume infusions, blood pressure medications, and correction of anemia as necessary.
- Heart failure is treated once the primary cause has been identified, such as infection, structural heart disease, arrhythmias, hypoglycemia, and electrolyte disturbances.
- Inborn errors of metabolism require an extensive workup and treatment to minimize the impact of toxins that accumulate and impair brain, heart, and other organ function.

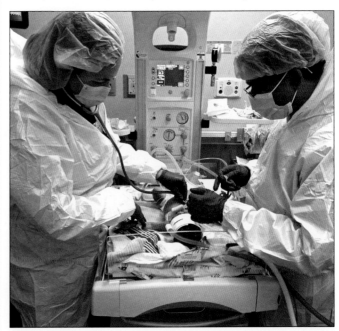

Resuscitation of a term infant following emergency cesarean delivery for fetal distress.

Causes of RESPIRATORY Acidosis[2,3,52,61]

Inadequate ventilation leads to increased levels of CO_2 in the blood. Causes may include the following:

Loss of Tidal Volume

- Lung disease (pneumonia, aspiration, surfactant deficiency)

- Pneumothorax

- Airway obstruction or malformations

- Mechanical interference with ventilation as occurs with chest wall deformities, hyperexpansion of the lungs in ventilated infants, pleural effusions, and compression of the lungs secondary to abdominal distention

Loss of Respiratory Drive

- Poor respiratory effort, which occurs most often in preterm or very sick infants

- Neurologic injury: hypoxic-ischemic encephalopathy, neonatal encephalopathy, neuromuscular disease, structural brain abnormalities, and ischemic or hemorrhagic stroke, which can lead to respiratory depression

- Apnea with concurrent hypoxemia that further depresses respirations

Treatment of Respiratory Acidosis[8,19,52,62-64]

- Retention of bicarbonate (renal compensation) for an elevated PCO_2 is a slow process that can take days.

- In most cases, the elevated PCO_2 will decline by providing continuous positive airway pressure (CPAP) or positive pressure ventilation (PPV) by bag and mask or intubation.

- Identify the cause of respiratory acidosis (lung disease, insufficient respiratory drive, etc.) and initiate therapies to treat the primary problem.

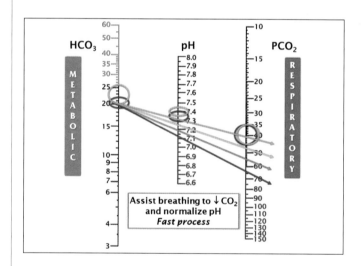

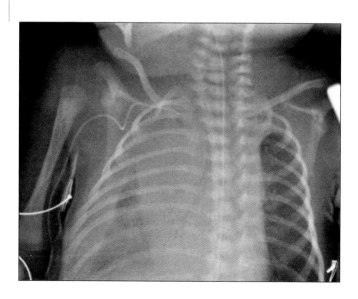

Chest X-ray of an infant who developed respiratory distress acutely. The percutaneously inserted central catheter (PICC) tip had eroded through the vein and total parenteral nutrition (TPN) infused into the pleural space, causing a pleural effusion on the right side. A chest tube was placed to drain the fluid.

✅ Clinical Tip — *Questions to ask when evaluating a blood gas*[65]

1. What degree of respiratory distress was the baby experiencing when the blood gas was drawn?

☐ Mild

☐ Moderate

☐ Severe

Respiratory failure rapidly leads to CO_2 retention, hypoxemia, and acidosis. If respiratory distress increases after the blood gas is drawn, obtain another blood gas for comparison.

2. Where was the blood gas obtained?

☐ Capillary (not useful for assessing oxygenation)

☐ Arterial

    ☐ Right radial artery (preductal)

    ☐ Left radial artery (near ductus; juxtaductal)

    ☐ Umbilical artery catheter (postductal)

    ☐ Posterior tibial artery (postductal)

☐ Venous (UVC) (not useful for assessing oxygenation)

3. Is the pH <7.30 and the PCO_2 >50?

If yes, this is respiratory acidosis and reflects inadequate ventilation (difficulty exhaling CO_2). Correlate the blood gas with the clinical exam and, if indicated, support breathing with continuous positive airway pressure (CPAP), positive pressure ventilation (PPV) with a bag and mask, or by placing an advanced airway (laryngeal mask airway or endotracheal intubation) and giving PPV.

Is the pH <7.30 and the bicarbonate (HCO_3) <19?

If yes, this is metabolic acidosis and means the infant is using bicarbonate to buffer (neutralize) lactic acid. The lower the pH and HCO_3, the worse the situation. A pH less than 7.20 is severe acidosis.

4. Is the pH <7.30, the PCO_2 >50, and the HCO_3 <19?

If yes, this is mixed respiratory and metabolic acidosis.

5. Is the arterial PO_2 <50 on >30% oxygen?

Evaluate the O_2 saturation, and if <85%, the infant is hypoxemic, and the oxygen concentration should be increased. If ≥50% oxygen is reached, this is a warning sign that should be reported to the medical care team.

Respiratory Support

Continuous Positive Airway Pressure (CPAP) and Positive Pressure Ventilation (PPV)[8,9,15,17,28,52,63,64,66-68]

The alveoli are tiny air sacs in the lungs where gas exchange occurs. The capillaries (blood vessels) in the lungs lie in very close proximity to the alveoli. With inhalation, air (that contains oxygen) enters the alveoli and then diffuses into the capillaries. The oxygenated blood flows to the heart, where it is pumped to the body. With exhalation, CO_2 diffuses the opposite way, from the capillaries into the alveoli, where it is breathed out. A healthy lung normally maintains some amount of gas in the lung at the end of expiration, commonly termed the functional residual volume (FRV). Surfactant lines the walls of the alveoli and, combined with air, prevents the alveoli from collapsing. Collapse of alveoli is called atelectasis and can be the result of surfactant deficiency which leads to insufficient FRV. Atelectatic lungs are stiff (poorly compliant), which makes breathing become labored. Gas exchange is also impaired, as there is difficulty exhaling CO_2 and inhaling O_2. Signs of worsening respiratory distress include retractions, tachypnea (or a dangerous slowing of respirations if the infant tires out), grunting, and cyanosis that requires higher amounts of oxygen to keep the O_2 saturation >90%.

A higher percentage of supplemental O_2 may be required at higher elevations; however, amounts exceeding 30% should raise concern that increased respiratory support may be needed to help recruit collapsed or congested alveoli. Depending on the degree of respiratory distress, the options for providing positive airway pressure include high-flow nasal cannula (HFNC), continuous positive airway pressure (CPAP), nasal intermittent positive pressure ventilation (NIPPV)*, or endotracheal intubation plus mechanical ventilation. If already on CPAP, additional options to improve oxygenation and ventilation include increasing the CPAP level, converting to NIPPV, or proceeding with endotracheal intubation.

*NIPPV (also called nasal intermittent mandatory ventilation or NIMV) involves delivering CPAP on a ventilator, then adding pressure and time-limited breaths that are either synchronized with the infant's breaths or not synchronized. When a rate is added, the term positive end-expiratory pressure (PEEP) is used instead of CPAP.

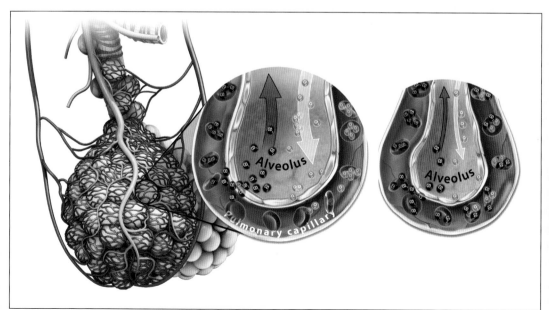

Well inflated alveolus with adequate surfactant and air (FRV) in the air sac (left illustration).

Alveolar collapse because of inadequate surfactant and/or air (FRV) in the air sac (right illustration).

Continuous Positive Airway Pressure (CPAP)

Using nasal prongs, a mask that covers the nose, or nasal cannulae, continuous CPAP support is usually delivered by three pressure-generating devices: a T-piece resuscitator, a bubble CPAP device, or a ventilator. CPAP is usually started at 5 to 6 cmH$_2$O pressure, but CPAP levels can be lower or higher depending on the respiratory condition and clinical exam. The goal is to use a pressure that helps improve oxygenation and ventilation yet avoid overdistension (which can cause a pneumothorax) and underinflation (that leads to atelectasis). See the notes below for device-specific information. Tables 3.5 and 3.6 identify infants who are and are not candidates for CPAP.

Notes:

- When CPAP is delivered by a cannula (such as the RAM Nasal Cannula offered by Neotech), the actual pressure reaching the lungs is lower than when delivering CPAP via prongs or a mask.
- HFNC therapy also delivers positive pressure to the airways and requires the use of a specific nasal cannula and flow delivery device with heated humidification. Gas flow (not pressure) between 2 and 8 liters/minute (L/min) is usually selected; the amount of delivered pressure increases as flow increases.
- A low-flow nasal cannula is used when <2 L/min is required to deliver oxygen.

- The infant must have an adequate respiratory effort to be a candidate for CPAP.

- There is persistent mild to moderate CO$_2$ retention and/or a persistent need for supplemental O$_2$ to maintain the O$_2$ saturation between 90 and 95%.

- There is an increased work of breathing and/or increasing O$_2$ requirement, but the infant does not meet the clinical or blood gas criteria that merit endotracheal intubation and mechanical support.

- There is increased frequency or severity of apnea; however, episodes are not severe enough to warrant endotracheal intubation with mechanical ventilation.

- To relieve airway obstruction secondary to laryngo- or tracheomalacia.

Table 3.5. Infants who *are* candidates for CPAP.

- There is a poor respiratory drive and/or those with severe apneic episodes that require vigorous stimulation and/or PPV to resolve.

- There is rapidly progressing respiratory failure and/or cardiovascular instability.

- Cleft lip/palate or other facial anomalies are not contraindications, but they may make CPAP application challenging.

- CPAP is usually ineffective if there is choanal atresia, and if bilateral, CPAP cannot be delivered past the area of obstruction.

- Avoid using CPAP with conditions that may be complicated by allowing air to enter the stomach (but recognizing initial resuscitation may necessitate the use of CPAP pending the placement of a gastric tube to remove air from the stomach). These conditions include gastroschisis, diaphragmatic hernia, unrepaired tracheoesophageal fistula, and intestinal perforation.

Table 3.6. Infants who are *not* candidates for CPAP.

Positive Pressure Ventilation (PPV) With Bag and Mask or T-Piece Resuscitator[64]

PPV is used to resuscitate the deteriorating infant or to help support an infant who requires assisted ventilation. Giving PPV correctly is an essential skill that takes practice to learn. Three resuscitation devices are used: a self-inflating bag, a flow-inflating (anesthesia) bag, or a T-piece resuscitator. Refer to the neonatal resuscitation program used by your facility for detailed information about the features of each device, mask selection, and the correct performance of PPV.

Indications for PPV include the following:

- Inadequate or no breathing effort

- Hypoxemia or bradycardia that is not responding to CPAP and oxygen administration

- Gasping

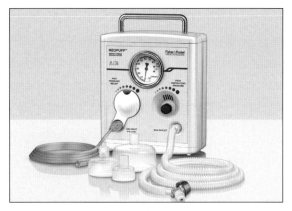

Neopuff™ Infant T-piece resuscitator
Photo courtesy of Fisher and Paykel, www.fphcare.com

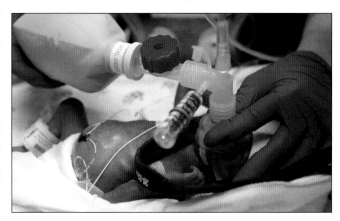

CPAP being given via an ambu bag.

 Gasping respirations are a sign of impending cardiorespiratory arrest!

With gasping, ventilation and air exchange are ineffective. If **the infant is not already intubated**, immediately give effective PPV using a bag and mask or T-piece resuscitator. If the infant's heart rate is low (<100 beats per minute) and not rising despite *effective* ventilation, insert a laryngeal mask airway or perform endotracheal intubation. Intravenous cardiac stimulant medications may also be necessary. PPV should continue until the infant's heart rate is >100 beats per minute and may need to continue even after the heart rate is >100. Further evaluation for treatable causes of respiratory deterioration (such as pneumothorax) should be ongoing.

If the infant is intubated, quickly assess the airway to determine whether the endotracheal tube is dislodged or obstructed. An acronym that helps troubleshoot respiratory distress in the intubated infant is **DOPE—D**isplaced, **O**bstructed, **P**neumothorax, **E**quipment failure.[69]

When delivering positive pressure ventilation (PPV) with or without chest compressions, all distractions should be minimized. The staff performing PPV or chest compressions should stay focused on the essential technical skills they are performing. Distraction when performing a skill leads to erratic and uncoordinated administration of breaths and/or compressions. If the team leader is performing a skill and other personnel are available, the performance of PPV and/or chest compressions should be delegated to others to allow the leader to communicate most effectively.

Using a Bag and Mask or T-Piece Resuscitator and Mask to Give CPAP or PPV[64]

- Apply a pulse oximeter to monitor oxygenation status and heart rate continuously. After confirming effective PPV is being given, placement of an advanced airway (endotracheal intubation or laryngeal mask airway) should be considered if there is no improvement in heart rate or there is persistent severe hypoxemia.

- A well-fitting, appropriately sized mask will help ensure a good seal. Position the face mask over the mouth and nose. If using an anatomically shaped mask, the bottom rim should cover the upper edge of the chin, and the top of the mask should not cover the eyes. If using a circular mask, the mouth and nose should be completely covered.

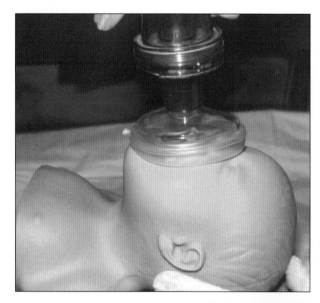
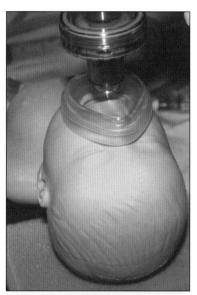

- A CO_2 detector may be used with a face mask and a laryngeal mask airway to monitor for exhaled CO_2.

- Hold the mask with your non-dominant hand and use your dominant hand to deliver breaths.

- Form a "C" with the thumb and index finger placed over the top of the mask and an "E" with the other three fingers. This method of holding the mask helps maintain a good seal and good control over the chin position. Use the fingers forming the "E" to lift the jaw up to the mask rather than push the mask down onto the face, which is uncomfortable for the baby and can cause facial bruising.

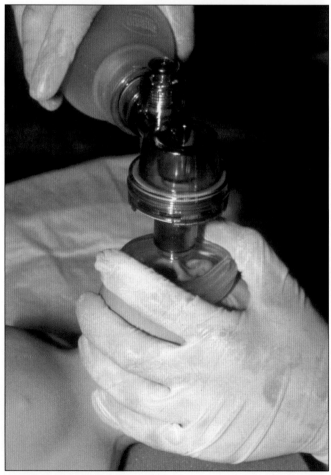

- **Precautions**

  - Avoid putting pressure on the trachea with the fingers that are forming the "E".

  - Avoid pressure over the eyes.

  - Don't press the infant's head into the mattress, which is especially possible with preterm infants.

  - If using a resuscitation bag, use a pressure manometer to monitor the inflating pressure being given.

  - If using a T-piece resuscitator, then the peak inspiratory pressure is set.

> ⚠ *If the infant was newly born, remember the possibility of a congenital diaphragmatic hernia in any newborn who deteriorates with bag/mask ventilation. Proceed with endotracheal intubation and CPAP or PPV (as indicated) if a diaphragmatic hernia is suspected. A pneumothorax may also be the reason for failure to improve.*

- Watch for chest rise while squeezing the bag. **Avoid excessive chest rise!** If the heart rate is not increasing or the chest does not rise:

  - Recheck the mask seal and ensure the correct mask size is being used.

  - Reposition the head to open the airway.

  - Suction the mouth (first) and then the nose to remove secretions that may block the airway.

  - Ensure the mouth is open.

  - Increase the inflating pressure.

  - Consider inserting an alternative airway: laryngeal mask airway or endotracheal tube (intubation).

- Watch for improvement in O_2 saturation or color. If improvement is not seen, increase the O_2 concentration.

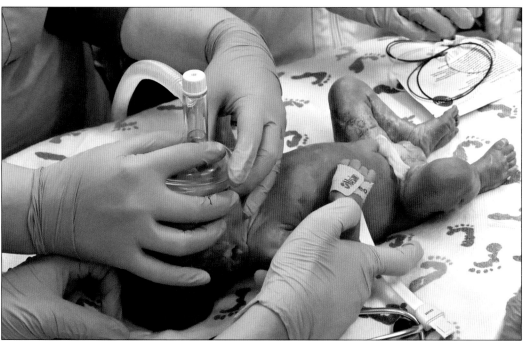

33-week gestation infant who was delivered precipitously and required CPAP for poor respiratory effort. The infant responded well and was then transitioned to bubble CPAP.

Pneumothorax[3,9,14,69-71]

Term or preterm infants can develop a pneumothorax, which can occur spontaneously in non-intubated infants with no history of assisted ventilation or as a complication of CPAP or PPV. A pneumothorax occurs when air escapes from the air sacs (alveoli) into the pleural cavity. Air collects in the pleural space (between the parietal and visceral pleura), and as air accumulates, it compresses the lung(s) and impairs oxygenation and ventilation. A tension pneumothorax is a large collection of air that compresses the lung(s) and heart so significantly that it impairs venous return to the heart and arterial blood flow out of the heart. A tension pneumothorax can be unilateral or bilateral. If time allows, a chest X-ray will provide details about the size and location of the pneumothorax. If, however, the infant is severely compromised, proceed with transillumination, and, if positive, evacuate the pneumothorax. Signs of a pneumothorax are listed in Table 3.7. The equipment to evacuate a pneumothorax is shown in Figure 3.4 on page 146.

Table 3.7. Signs of a pneumothorax.

Respiratory and Cardiovascular Deterioration	
<ul><li>Increased respiratory distress—cyanosis, tachypnea, retractions, grunting, nasal flaring</li><li>Acute onset of bradycardia or tachycardia</li><li>Irritability and restlessness</li><li>Hypotension</li><li>Blood gas may reveal a respiratory and/or metabolic acidosis and hypoxemia</li></ul>	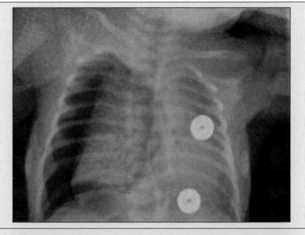
Evaluate for	
<ul><li>Positive transillumination of the chest</li><li>Chest asymmetry (one side appears higher than the other)</li><li>Asymmetric breath sounds (one side sounds quieter than the other)</li><li>Shift in point of maximum impulse (PMI)</li><li>Mottled appearance</li><li>Poor pulses (brachial and/or brachial and femoral)</li><li>Hypotension</li><li>Flattened or decreased QRS complex on ECG and if the infant has an arterial line, dampened arterial waveform</li></ul>	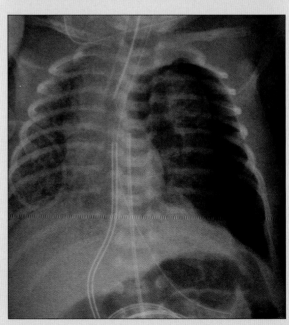

Transillumination for Pneumothorax Detection

Rapid preliminary detection of a pneumothorax can often be accomplished by transilluminating the chest using a cool, high-intensity fiberoptic light. To prevent burns, check that the transilluminator does not emit heat. Darken the room as much as possible. Lightly press the light source perpendicular into the chest and compare each side by moving the light from the right to the left chest, in the axillae, under the midclavicular areas, and under the subcostal regions.

Possible Transillumination Results

Negative transillumination means a pneumothorax is not present.

False negative transillumination (means a pneumothorax *is* present but is not detected by transillumination) may be seen if the room is not dark enough, the infant has a thick chest wall or darkly pigmented skin, or the transilluminator light source is too weak.

True positive transillumination (means a pneumothorax appears to be present and there is a pneumothorax) is when the glow of light transmits through the chest cavity on the side being evaluated, not just in the immediate region of the light source. If the pneumothorax is large, the entire hemithorax lights up.

False positive transillumination (means a pneumothorax appears to be present, but there is *no* pneumothorax) may be seen if the light source is not held perpendicular to the chest wall or if there is chest wall edema (as occurs with hydrops fetalis), subcutaneous air in the chest wall, a pneumomediastinum, or severe pulmonary interstitial emphysema. Small, preterm infants may also yield a falsely positive transillumination because of their small chests, thin skin, and easily transmitted light.

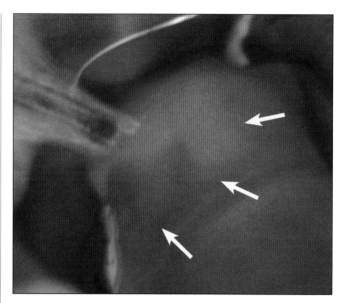

Example of a positive transillumination on the right side.

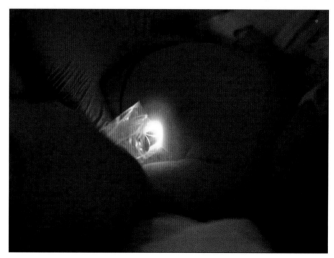

Example of a negative transillumination on the left side.

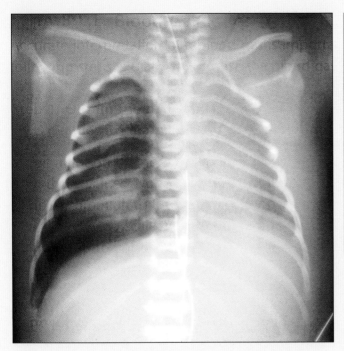

Right-sided pneumothorax with mediastinal shift to the left and left lung atelectasis. The ET tube is at T1, the UAC tip is at T6-T7, and the UVC tip is in good position at the IVC/RA junction or just in the right atrium.

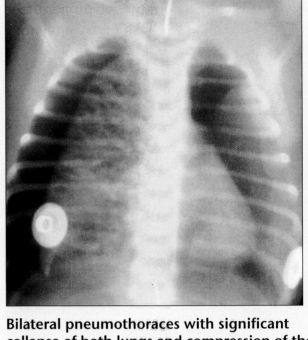

Bilateral pneumothoraces with significant collapse of both lungs and compression of the heart. This very lordotic projection makes the ET tube tip appear too high. With proper X-ray projection, the ET tube may be in a satisfactory position. The UAC tip is malpositioned at T11.

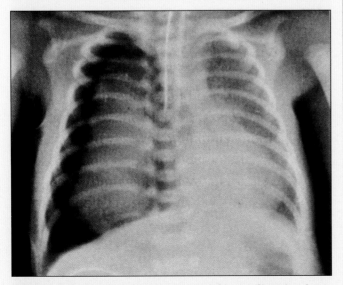

Right-sided pneumothorax with mediastinal shift to the left. The ET tube is in the right mainstem bronchus, and there is significant collapse of the right lung.

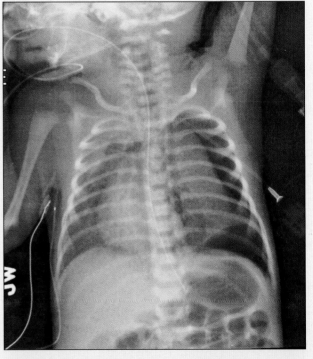

Tension pneumothorax on the left with complete collapse of the left lung and a mediastinal shift to the right. An angiocatheter is visible in the pleural space, but the air is still present.

Chest X-Ray for Pneumothorax Detection

A definitive diagnosis of a pneumothorax is made by evaluating an anteroposterior (AP) view chest X-ray. The X-ray should be taken if the infant is stable enough to tolerate the time it takes to complete the test. At times, a lateral decubitus chest X-ray is also required if the AP view chest X-ray is indeterminate to diagnose a pneumothorax.

Positioning the Infant for a Lateral Decubitus Chest X-ray

Turn the infant on their side for at least ten minutes (if the infant is stable) with the side of the suspected pneumothorax *up*. Maintain this position by placing a roll behind the back. The lateral decubitus X-ray is taken with the infant side-lying. When finished with the X-ray, turn the infant to their back (supine) to allow optimal lung inflation.

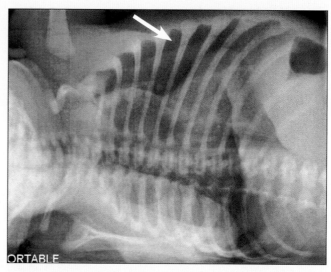

Right lateral decubitus X-ray. The infant is positioned on the right side to allow the air to rise. The arrow points to the free air in the pleural space in the left lung.

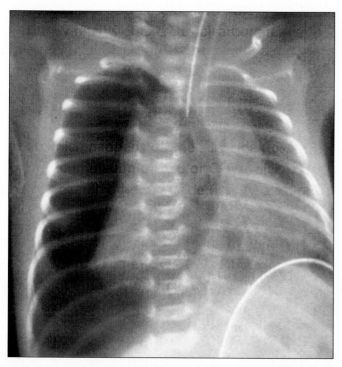

Massive tension pneumothorax on the right. The ET tube is in good position. Note, there is complete collapse of the right lung, mediastinal shift, and compression of the left lung.

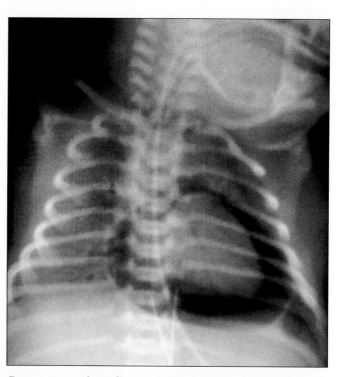

Pneumopericardium. Note the rim of air completely encircling and compressing the heart. The ET tube is in good position. Umbilical catheter tips are visible.

Needle Aspiration to Evacuate a Pneumothorax

In the late preterm or term infant, if mildly symptomatic, consider observing the infant to see if the pneumothorax resolves on its own. If there is respiratory and/or cardiovascular compromise, the pneumothorax should be evacuated. Needle aspiration may be attempted first and may be all that is necessary to resolve the pneumothorax. If, however, air continually accumulates or the infant fails to improve to a satisfactory level following needle aspiration, a chest tube should be inserted. Figure 3.4 identifies the equipment needed for needle aspiration. The Clinical Tip on page 147 explains how to connect a one-way Heimlich valve to a chest tube or angiocatheter to evacuate air that accumulates. Additional equipment includes sterile gloves for the person performing the procedure and an antiseptic solution to cleanse the skin before the needle is inserted.

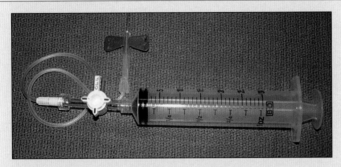

- 18 to 20-gauge angiocatheter (also called a catheter over needle device and intracatheter)
- T-connector or other short IV extension tubing
- Three-way stopcock
- 20 or 30 mL syringe

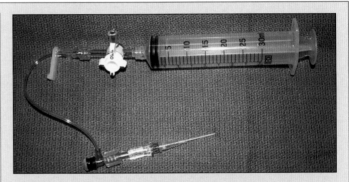

- 21 or 23-gauge butterfly needle (if an angiocatheter is not available)
- Three-way stopcock
- 20 or 30 mL syringe

Figure 3.4. Needle aspiration kits for pneumothorax evacuation. An IV angiocatheter is preferred since the soft catheter can be secured to the chest for ongoing air evacuation, but if an angiocatheter is not available, a butterfly needle can be used.

Pneumopericardium and Pericardial Effusion[3,72]

A pneumopericardium is a collection of air that becomes trapped in the pericardial sac that surrounds the heart, and it rarely occurs in the absence of mechanical ventilation. A pericardial effusion may also occur if fluid extravasates from a central line and accumulates in the pericardial sac. A pericardial effusion has the same restricting effect as air. As the air (or fluid) accumulates, it compresses the heart and acutely impairs cardiac output. Most occurrences of pneumopericardium or tamponade from fluid are symptomatic and require immediate detection and evacuation by needle aspiration (i.e., pericardiocentesis).

Signs can include the following:

- Sudden onset of severe cyanosis

- Muffled or inaudible heart sounds

- A flattened or decreased QRS complex (reduced cardiac voltage) on the electrocardiogram (ECG) tracing

Other signs include initial tachycardia followed by bradycardia, poor or absent pulses, and poor perfusion. If arterial monitoring is in progress, the waveform becomes acutely dampened as the pulse pressure narrows.

✓ Clinical Tip

What is a Heimlich one-way valve, and how do I connect it to a chest tube or angiocatheter?

A Heimlich valve can be connected directly to a chest tube for transport (top photo) or it can be connected to an angiocatheter needle aspiration set-up (bottom photo).

To connect the Heimlich valve to an angiocatheter, take a sterile suction connection tubing and, using sterile scissors, cut off the end (as shown). Attach the blue end of the tubing to the Heimlich valve. Attach the trimmed end of the suction tubing to a three-way stopcock. An IV tubing T-connector is then attached to the stopcock, which is attached to the angiocatheter in the chest. If the pneumothorax is under enough pressure, it will escape through the Heimlich valve. However, if the patient is unstable, turn the stopcock off to the Heimlich valve and gently aspirate using the three-way stopcock to evaluate for residual air. If direct aspiration does not help improve the patient's condition and pneumothorax is suspected as the cause, the patient may need a chest tube inserted emergently. Chest tube insertion should be performed by personnel with the proper training.

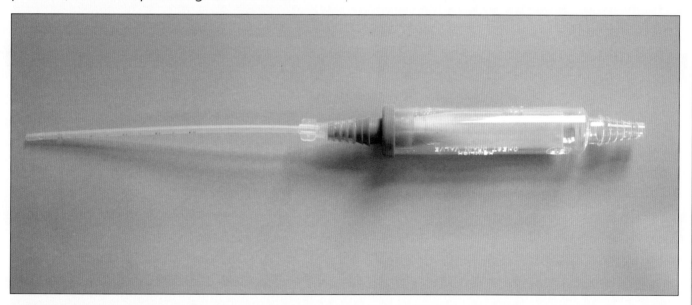

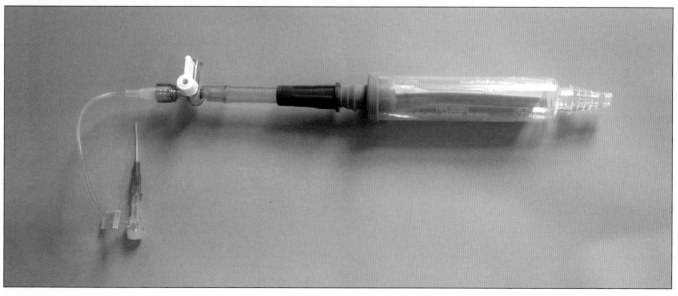

Respiratory Failure Warning Signs[63,67,73-75]

Respiratory failure with cardiovascular collapse can occur rapidly. Table 3.8 identifies the warning signs of respiratory failure and when to strongly consider endotracheal intubation with positive pressure ventilation.

PPV via an endotracheal tube or laryngeal mask airway should be considered in the following situations:

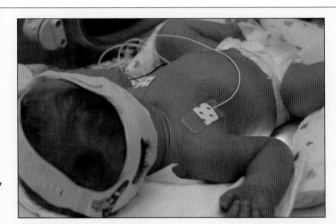

- The infant is gasping (give PPV immediately)

- There are periods of severe apnea and bradycardia needing PPV

- There is persistent bradycardia despite properly performed PPV

- There is labored respiratory effort—moderate to severe retractions, plus there may be grunting and flaring, persistent tachypnea, or slowing of respirations (bradypnea) because of exhaustion

- The PCO_2 is elevated (hypercarbia), and there is moderate to severe respiratory acidosis (low pH)

- You are unable to ventilate and/or oxygenate adequately with PPV, and the infant is not a candidate for CPAP

- The O_2 concentration is increasing rapidly to maintain the O_2 saturation >90%

- The infant has a diaphragmatic hernia and is in distress

- You are unable to maintain an acceptable O_2 saturation for the infant's suspected disease process

  - It should be noted that infants with cyanotic CHD often have an O_2 saturation <90%; however, they may have 'comfortable' tachypnea and no other signs of respiratory distress. If breathing is not labored, the decision to intubate should be at the discretion of a neonatologist, pediatric cardiologist, or a transport team that is following transport protocol. Close monitoring of the cyanotic CHD infant is required since severe hypoxemia may lead to hypoxia and cardiorespiratory failure.

Consult the tertiary center neonatal physician in the following situations:

- You are uncertain of the respiratory support to give: CPAP, NIPPV, or proceed with intubation

- You are unsure about the ventilatory support to provide once the infant is intubated

- The blood gas fails to improve after intubation

- The infant deteriorates after intubation

Table 3.8. Respiratory failure warning signs and when to strongly consider endotracheal intubation.

Endotracheal Intubation

Endotracheal intubation can be a technically challenging procedure, and prolonged or repeated intubation attempts can lead to hemodynamic instability, hypoxia, and even death. The smaller the infant and the less experienced the staff performing the intubation, the more likely a repeated intubation attempt will be necessary.[76,77]

Assisting With Endotracheal Intubation

Providing anticipatory support during intubation can increase the successful performance of the procedure. If possible, have two people assist the person performing the intubation (the "operator"). One assistant contains the infant and monitors the vital signs, and the other assistant prepares and hands equipment to the operator. An intubation equipment checklist and instructions on securing the ET tube with tape can be found in Appendix 3.1 on page 168. The following information guides how to prepare the infant for intubation and how to assist during intubation.

Before intubation—Prepare the infant and check the equipment[73,78]

- Unless the procedure is being performed during an emergency, do a "time-out" to correctly identify the patient.

- Attach a pulse oximeter and, if available, a cardiorespiratory monitor.

- If sedating medications are given, then cardiorespiratory monitoring must be used. Medications, including those used for "rapid sequence intubation (RSI)" may include any of the following combinations: an anticholinergic agent, an opioid medication, a sedative, and/or a paralytic.[76]

- Use a radiant warmer to protect from cold stress and hypothermia.

- Have the appropriate size endotracheal (ET) tube available (see Tables 3.9 and 3.10 for sizes).

  ○ Do not leave the tube on the warmer bed, or the tube will warm up and become too flexible.

  ○ The part of the ET tube that will be inserted into the trachea should be kept sterile while preparing it for use. The same is true for the part of the stylet that will be inserted into the tube if one is used.

- Ask the operator if they want a stylet inserted into the ET tube. A stylet makes the ET tube stiffer and allows for a slight curve of the ET tube before insertion.

  ○ If a stylet is used, ensure the tip does not extend past the end of the ET tube since the sharp tip can damage the trachea.

  ○ After inserting the stylet, add a bend at the inlet of the ET tube to keep the stylet from advancing into the tube.

  ○ The stylet is removed after the ET tube is in the trachea and before breaths are given.

- If a videolaryngoscope is available, prepare the equipment by powering it on and attaching the correct blade size.

- If using a traditional laryngoscope, choose the correct blade size for the infant's weight: Size 1 (term), 0 (preterm), 00 (extremely preterm).

  ○ Before starting, make sure the bulb is bright and screwed on tight.

  ○ Do not leave the bulb light on while waiting for the intubation to begin, as the light and blade may overheat.

- Prepare a resuscitation bag or T-piece resuscitator and an appropriate size face mask for the infant's weight.

- Attach the resuscitation bag or T-piece resuscitator to an oxygen source and blender (to enable adjustment of inspired oxygen concentration).

- Have a bulb syringe available and prepare suction equipment as follows:

  o Turn on and adjust the suction level to 80 to 100 mmHg when the suction tubing is occluded.

  o Attach a 10 Fr catheter to the suction tubing (for suctioning oral secretions). Have both an 8 Fr catheter and 5 or 6 Fr suction catheter available in case the ET tube needs to be suctioned.

- Prepare tape or an FT tube holder to secure the tube once inserted.

- Before starting the procedure, determine what the tube insertion depth will be (at the upper lip). For orotracheal intubation, refer to the insertion depth guidelines outlined in Tables 3.9 and 3.10.

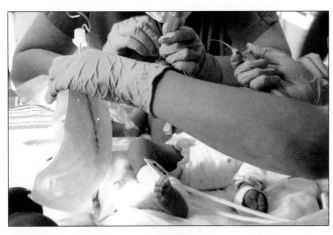

Assisting *during* intubation

- In many cases, CPAP and/or PPV are required before the procedure begins and between intubation attempts.

- Stabilize the head and provide comfort to the infant.

- Hand equipment to the operator as they request it: suction catheter (and occlude the suction finger hole when requested) and ET tube.

- Once the laryngoscope is inserted, provide equipment close to the operator's hand in their line of vision, so they don't have to take their eyes off the vocal cords.

- If the operator asks for 'cricoid pressure', gently apply pressure on the cricoid cartilage of the trachea and ask the operator if the applied pressure is helping them to visualize the vocal cords.

- Monitor the O_2 saturation, heart rate, and duration of the intubation attempt and communicate concerns to the operator.

Assisting *after* intubation

- To prevent accidental dislodgment of the tube, discuss who will be responsible for holding the tube securely once it is inserted.

  o Use a gloved finger to gently press the tube against the infant's palate until it is secured with tape or a holder. Do not let the infant turn their head.

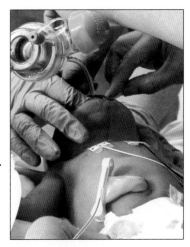

Hold the ET tube firmly on the palate following intubation until the tube is well secured.

- After the tube is inserted, **confirm the depth of the ET tube** and make adjustments before giving PPV.

- Attach the CO_2 detector or capnography device and provide breaths using the bag or T-piece resuscitator. Continue to provide CPAP or PPV once the tube is inserted.

- The color of the paper in the CO_2 detector should be blue or purple initially. If not, then it is defective and should be discarded. The CO_2 detector can *falsely* turn yellow if the following endotracheal medications touch the paper in the CO_2 detector: epinephrine, atropine, or surfactant. Gastric secretions can also cause the CO_2 detector to turn yellow. Replace the contaminated CO_2 detector with a new one.

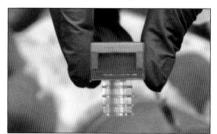

Purple or **blue** = negative CO_2

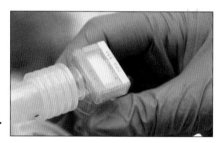

Yellow = positive CO_2

- A color change to yellow (from blue or purple) indicates adequate circulation of blood to and from the lungs such that CO_2 is being exhaled and the ET tube is in the trachea.

  ○ A helpful reminder is that a **y**ellow color change signifies **"yes"**, or **"yes for CO_2."**

  ○ The color may not change until 8 to 10 breaths are given.

  ○ At times, even when intubated, the CO_2 color may not change, *especially* if there is poor cardiac output or a low or no heart rate. Other causes for failure to change color include secretions obstructing the trachea or the lungs not expanding because of tension pneumothoraces.

  ○ If the CO_2 detector color is not changing, troubleshoot the following: a) the ET tube is in the correct location in the trachea (i.e., not too deep or too shallow), b) there is equal chest rise when breaths are given, c) secretions, if any, are suctioned from the tube, d) the possibility of a pneumothorax is considered.

- Exhaled CO_2 is only one parameter that helps confirm the ET tube is in the trachea. Evaluate for the following:

  ○ Vapor condensation in the tube is seen with exhalation.

  ○ Breath sounds are audible in both axillae and are equal when PPV is given.

  ○ There is equal chest rise with PPV.

  ○ Decreased or no sounds are heard over the stomach with PPV.

> *The decision to remove the ET tube, give PPV via mask, and then reintubate the infant should be considered if the heart rate is low and not rising as expected and you are uncertain that the infant is intubated, as evidenced by no change in the CO_2 detector color to yellow and no chest rise when breaths are given (despite increasing the delivered amount of pressure). Follow neonatal resuscitation guidelines for when to initiate chest compressions.[79]*
>
> - *Prior to removing the ET tube, ensure an adequate inspiratory pressure is being given. The PIP may need to be increased to 35 to 40 cmH2O pressure to inflate the lungs.*
>
> - *If confident in the ability to reinsert the laryngoscope to visually inspect whether the tube is in the trachea, hold the tube securely while this procedure is done.[80] Accidental extubation may occur so be prepared to give bag and mask breaths.*

Strategies to Prevent Deep Endotracheal Tube (ET tube) Insertion[63,73,80-82]

Following insertion of the ET tube, the goal is to position the tube tip at approximately T1 to T3, which should position the tip above the carina, as shown on page 154. Inadvertent insertion into the right mainstem bronchus is a common complication that impairs ventilation and increases the risk of pneumothorax. One effective strategy to reduce deep insertion into the bronchus is to decide *before* the tube is placed what the estimated insertion depth at the upper lip should be. Verification of tube depth should occur three more times thereafter: 1) as soon as the tube is inserted and before ventilations are given, 2) prior to securing the ET tube, and 3) after the tube is secured. For ongoing care of the intubated patient, the ET tube location at the upper lip should be recorded at the bedside and verified with nursing and respiratory assessments.

The difficulty with pre-estimating the insertion depth is the potential inaccuracy when using different methods, such as the nasal-tragus length (NTL +1 cm) and the lip-to-tip (weight in kg + 6) rule. Inaccuracy increases with both estimation methods when the infant weighs <1,500 grams. Tables 3.9 and 3.10 review ET tube sizes and insertion depths for orally intubated infants according to weight and gestational age. An online tool for estimating insertion depth for all weight infants can be found at nicutools.org.

Lip-to-Tip Rule *(starting with 1 kilogram [kg])*: Add 6 to the infant's weight in kg.[83]

Weight	Gestational Age (in weeks)	ET Tube Size (mm internal diameter)	Approximate Tube Insertion Depth at the Upper Lip (in centimeters [cm])
<1,000 grams (see Table 3.10 for additional weight categories)	<28	2.5	Varies with weight
1,000 to 2,000 grams (1 to 2 kg)	28 – 34	3.0	7 to 8
>2,000 grams (>2 kg)	>34	3.5	8 to 9

Table 3.9. ET tube sizes and insertion depth for orally intubated infants according to weight and gestational age.[63,80,81] See Table 3.10 for approximate ET tube insertion depths for extremely low-birth-weight infants who weigh <1,000 grams.

The lip-to-tip rule (weight in kg + 6 = the ET tube depth at the upper lip in cm) and the nasal-tragus length (NTL) (distance in cm from the nasal septum to the ear tragus, plus add 1 cm) are used to estimate ET tube insertion depth. However, both measurements can be inaccurate with extremely low birthweight infants and, in particular, overestimate how far to insert the ET tube, which results in a tube on the carina or in the bronchus.

Weight	Gestational Age (in weeks)	ET Tube Size (mm internal diameter)	Approximate Tube Insertion Depth at the Upper Lip (in centimeters [cm])
<500 grams	<23	2.5 (or 2.0)[a]	5 to 5.5
500 to 600 grams	23 – 24	2.5	5.5 to 6
700 to 800 grams	25 – 26	2.5	6
900 to 1,000 grams	27 – 29	2.5	6.5
1,100 to 1,400 grams	30 – 32	3.0	7

Table 3.10. Approximate ET tube sizes and insertion depth for extremely preterm infants according to weight and corrected gestational age. Adapted from Kempley ST, Moreiras JW, Petrone FL. Endotracheal tube length for neonatal resuscitation. *Resuscitation.* 2008;77(3):369-373.[84]

Note:

[a] For extremely small infants, <500 grams, a size 2.0 ET tube may be necessary if a 2.5 ET tube will not fit in the trachea. A 2.0 ET tube has a significantly higher resistance than a 2.5 ET tube, which can impair ventilation and require a higher inspiratory pressure to compensate for the increased resistance.[17]

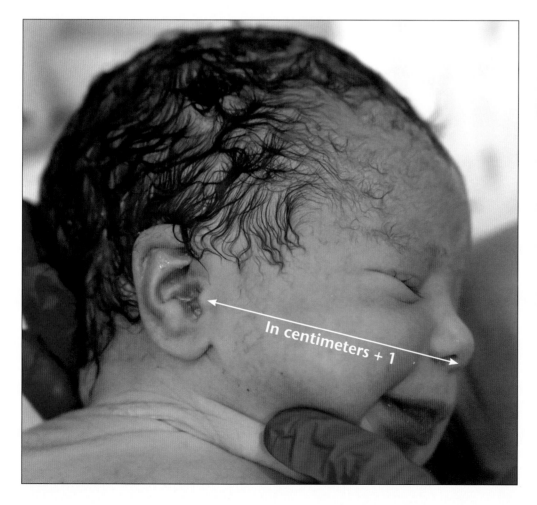

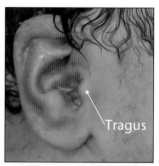

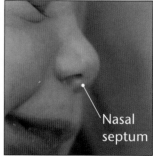

Measure the **nasal-tragus length** from the middle of the nasal septum to the tragus of the ear (in cm); then, add 1 cm.

Location of the Endotracheal Tube on Chest X-ray

Positioning the infant for a chest X-ray[85]

- Position the infant with their shoulders and hips flat and with their arms by their sides or slightly away from the body. The head position, especially if turned far to the right or left, will affect the ET tube tip position. Keep the head midline for every X-ray to allow for comparison. Keep the chin in a neutral position to permit accurate interpretation of the ET tube tip location. If the head is flexed forward (chin down), the ET tube tip will be located deeper in the trachea. If the head is extended backward (chin up), the ET tube tip will move upward in the trachea. A way to remember this is "Head down, tube down. Head up, tube up."

- With proper positioning of the infant, there should be no rotation.

- To optimize comparison of X-rays, position the infant in the same way when repeat X-rays are taken.

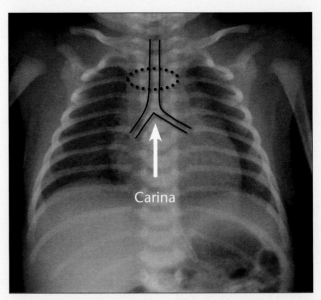

Illustration of the anatomy of the tracheobronchial tree. The dotted area represents the acceptable location for the ET tube tip (mid-trachea).

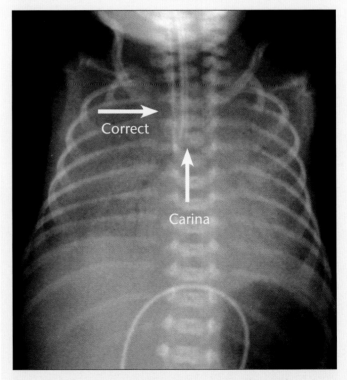

The ET tube tip is at the carina or in the right mainstem bronchus. The arms are along the sides of the head which can cause the head to flex forward (chin down) and advance the tube deeper. The arrow points to the correct ET tube tip location, but the flexed head should be considered since repositioning the head can move the tube into a different location. Both lungs are atelectatic, and air bronchograms are seen in this preterm infant with severe respiratory distress syndrome.

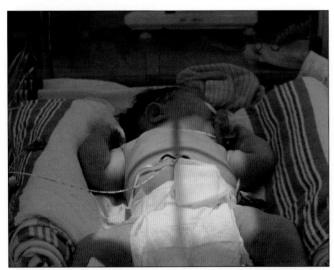

Infant positioned for an X-ray after placement of an umbilical venous catheter.

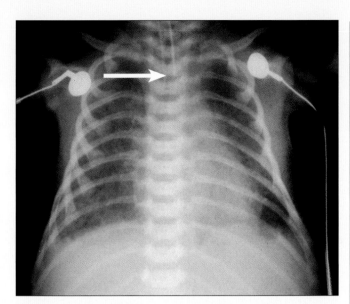

The arrow is pointing to the ET tube, which is in a good position in the mid-trachea.

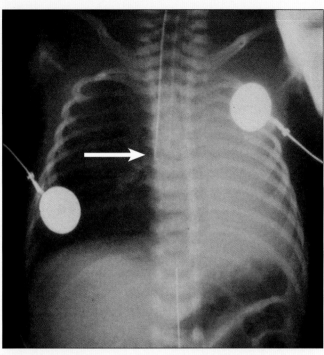

The ET tube is in the right mainstem bronchus, and the left lung is completely atelectatic. Leaving the chest leads on the chest can obscure the lung fields, so they should be removed before the X-ray is taken. The umbilical artery catheter tip is at T-12, which is too low.

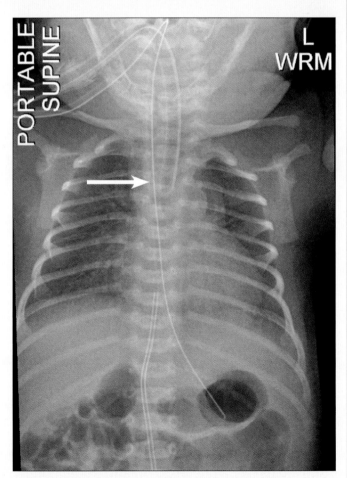

The ET tube is at the carina at T4. The chin is midline, and there is no rotation. The UVC tip is malpositioned and is in the right atrium or through the foramen ovale.

Initial Ventilator Support[9,74]

The infant's history, suspected disease process, response to ventilation, work of breathing, blood gas, and chest X-ray findings are factored in when deciding the level of support to provide and how to deliver that support. Numerous modes of ventilation are in use, such as time-cycled pressure-limited ventilation, assist-control ventilation, pressure support ventilation, volume-targeted ventilation, neurally adjusted ventilatory assist (NAVA), and high-frequency ventilation. Figure 3.5 illustrates the settings that are adjusted when providing positive pressure ventilation (PPV) using a time-cycled pressure-limited mode. The positive end-expiratory pressure (PEEP) provides a continuous distending pressure to the lungs to help maintain functional residual lung volume. The positive inspiratory pressure (PIP), inspiratory time (Ti), and rate are set together. Too long of an inspiratory time, especially with faster rates, shortens the expiratory time necessary for complete exhalation, which can cause gas trapping. The PIP is adjusted to provide an adequate tidal volume to ventilate the infant.

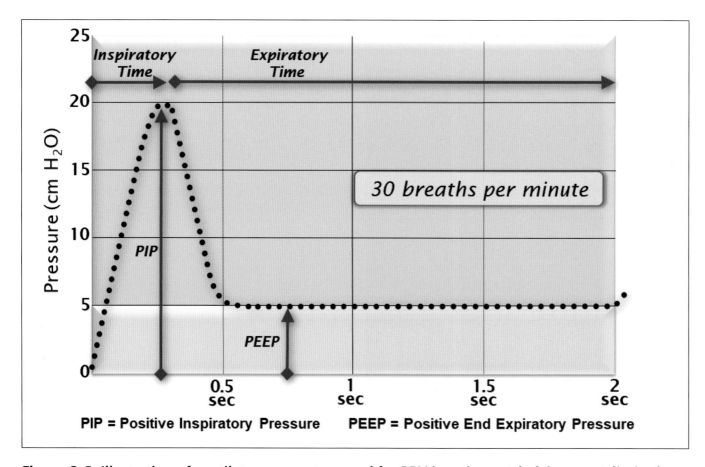

Figure 3.5. Illustration of ventilator parameters used for PPV in a time-cycled /pressure-limited mode. PIP: positive inspiratory pressure, PEEP: positive end-expiratory pressure, inspiratory time, and expiratory time. Note that **time** is shown on the "X" axis, and **pressure** (cmH2O) is shown on the "Y" axis. In this example, each breath is delivered over 2 seconds to deliver a rate of 30 breaths per minute; the inspiratory time is 0.3 seconds, and the expiratory time is 1.7 seconds.

Table 3.11 provides suggestions for the *initial* ventilatory support of infants with varying weights. The goal is to adequately support oxygenation and ventilation while trying to minimize lung injury. **Therefore, it is advised to start with the lowest possible settings** and then increase if necessary. Aim for gentle chest rise, and to reduce lung injury, avoid excessive chest rise. If the infant is not improving on the selected ventilator support, the ventilator settings should be adjusted. For additional information, see the Clinical Tip: *How to approach the ventilated infant who is not oxygenating well* on page 158.

If unsure what level of support to provide or the infant is not responding to the level of support that was chosen, call the tertiary center neonatologist or transport control physician for advice.

Settings	VLBW (< 1.5 kg)	LBW (1.5 to 2.5 kg)	Term (>2.5 kg)
Rate (per minute)	30 to 45	20 to 40	20 to 40
Inspiratory time (in seconds)	0.3 to 0.35	0.3 to 0.35	0.35 to 0.4
Positive inspiratory pressure (PIP) [in cmH2O]	16 to 22	18 to 24	20 to 28
Positive end expiratory pressure (PEEP) [in cmH2O]	5 to 7	5 to 7	5 to 7
Target tidal volume	Approximately 5 mL/kg with an acceptable range of 4-6 mL/kg		

Table 3.11. Initial ventilator support settings for infants of varying weights.[67] VLBW: very low birth weight, LBW: low birth weight. Adjustments in settings are usually required before and after surfactant administration, expecting that the parameters often need to be reduced after surfactant.

If the baby is not responding as expected, assess the patient, obtain an X-ray and blood gas, and seek consultation.

Notes:
- Some programs utilize volume ventilation as a primary mode of support. The suggested starting tidal volume is usually 5 mL/kg and at a rate as above based on patient weight. A chest X-ray can assist in decision-making regarding necessary changes in respiratory support.
- The amount of PEEP selected will be based on the infant's disease process and the goals of therapy.
- Excessive PEEP for the disease process may impair ventilation, lung perfusion, and/or venous return (return of deoxygenated blood to the right side of the heart).
- The amount of pressure required (PIP) will also vary depending on the infant's size, disease state, and response to ventilation. If able, start with pressure at the lower end of the range and adjust up or down as needed based on the infant's response to treatment, chest X-ray, blood gas, and physical exam.
- An inspiratory time greater than 0.5 seconds may result in air trapping and increase the risk of barotrauma and lung injury.

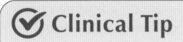 **Clinical Tip** | *How to approach the ventilated infant who is not oxygenating well.[68]*

Several strategies may be used to improve oxygenation. Initially, the easiest thing to do is increase the inspired oxygen. If increasing the oxygen concentration does not improve oxygenation, or if the infant is already on a high percentage of oxygen, then the ventilator settings may be adjusted to increase mean airway pressure (Paw). When increased solely or in combination, three parameters increase the Paw: PEEP, PIP, or inspiratory time. It is helpful to increase just one parameter at a time to see if oxygenation improves: Increase PEEP first, then PIP (which will also affect ventilation), and finally, inspiratory time.

A few reminders regarding changes in ventilator settings:

- Increasing PIP will increase tidal volume, so the PCO_2 may also decrease.

- Increasing PEEP without increasing PIP may decrease tidal volume, so although oxygenation improves, PCO_2 may actually go up.

  o If the PCO_2 is already elevated, then increasing PIP may be a better initial option.

o If the rate is kept the same, increasing inspiratory time will decrease expiratory time; therefore, PCO_2 may increase.

o An increase in inspiratory time reduces exhalation time, but it can be used to increase lung recruitment and Paw.

o If the rate and inspiratory time are increased simultaneously, the expiratory time may be significantly decreased, resulting in insufficient time for expiration and "breath stacking."

Notes:

- These suggestions are for time-cycled pressure-controlled ventilation. Other modes of ventilation, including volume ventilation and high frequency, require adjustments other than mentioned here. In addition, an air leak secondary to pneumothorax or pulmonary interstitial emphysema and other severe forms of lung disease may preclude ventilator changes from being effective.

- If the infant is not responding as desired, repeat the chest X-ray, as new information may help decide the next course of action.

Neonatal Respiratory Illnesses[3,31]

Tachypnea and Low PCO$_2$

Fast breathing (tachypnea) with minimal to no other respiratory distress and a low PCO$_2$ (less than 35) may be secondary to **NON-PULMONARY CAUSES**:

Metabolic acidosis

- Secondary to shock, poor tissue perfusion, and oxygenation

- To compensate for metabolic acidosis, the infant will exhale CO$_2$ via the respiratory system; if the infant does not have concurrent pulmonary disease, then partial or complete compensation is possible

Congenital heart disease

- Tachypnea secondary to shock (left-side obstructive lesions and in response to acidosis) or hypoxemia (right-side obstructive lesions and in response to hypoxemic respiratory stimulation)

- If the lungs are not diseased, or congestive heart failure has not yet developed, the PCO$_2$ may be low

Brain disorders

- Tachypnea secondary to brain irritation from hypoglycemia, hemorrhage, meningitis, or cerebral edema

- Tachypnea secondary to brain injury following perinatal or postnatal hypoxia (is in response to metabolic or mixed acidosis)

Tachypnea and Increased PCO$_2$

Fast breathing (tachypnea) or labored breathing plus an increased PCO$_2$ may be secondary to **PULMONARY CAUSES**:

- Transient tachypnea of the newborn (TTN)

- Respiratory distress syndrome (RDS)

- Pneumonia

- Meconium aspiration syndrome (MAS)

- Persistent pulmonary hypertension of the newborn (PPHN)

- Congenital diaphragmatic hernia (CDH)

- Tracheoesophageal fistula (TEF) / esophageal atresia (EA)

- Airway obstruction

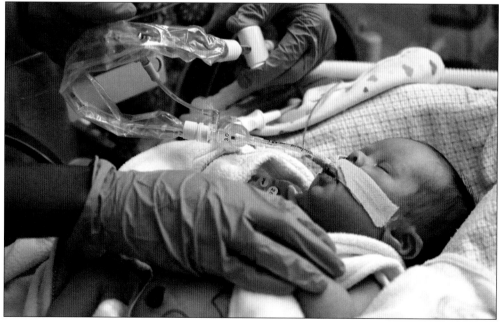

37-week gestation infant who required intubation for MAS.

Airway

As previously discussed, in response to increased CO_2 in the blood, the infant will breathe faster and use accessory muscles of respiration (e.g., will be retracting) to increase minute ventilation. A rising PCO_2 means the infant can no longer compensate despite the increased respiratory rate and work of breathing. Other pulmonary causes of tachypnea with elevated PCO_2 (not included in this module) include chest or lung masses, chest wall deformity, and lung hypoplasia.

The clinical presentation of infants with congenital heart disease (CHD) may be similar to other neonatal illnesses and respiratory conditions, including sepsis, inborn errors of metabolism, persistent pulmonary hypertension of the newborn (PPHN), congenital diaphragmatic hernia, transient tachypnea of the newborn, respiratory distress syndrome, meconium aspiration, pneumonia, or pneumothorax. Infants with severe forms of CHD may also have concurrent respiratory illnesses or conditions. Table 3.12 contrasts key features of pulmonary versus cardiac disease to aid in differential diagnosis.

	Pulmonary	Cardiac
Cyanosis	Yes	Yes or no
Respiratory rate	Usually increased	Usually increased and may be described as "comfortable tachypnea"
Work of breathing (WOB)	Increased WOB; may have nasal flaring, grunting, and/or retractions	Easy effort but increased WOB if CHF has developed
Acid/base balance	Increased PCO_2 Respiratory acidosis or mixed acidosis if in shock	Decreased PCO_2 / metabolic acidosis Hypercarbia if CHF or concurrent pulmonary pathology*
Chest X-ray	May have asymmetric pattern of disease, infiltrates, or other pulmonary pathology	Increased or decreased pulmonary vascular markings; may have pulmonary edema*
Heart size, shape, location	Normal or may have cardiomegaly if there is a history of shock	Normal or may have an abnormal size, shape, or location

*May have infiltrates or other findings consistent with concurrent pulmonary disease.

Table 3.12. Key features of pulmonary versus cardiac disease to aid in differential diagnosis. Infants with CHD may also have concurrent respiratory or other illnesses and exhibit signs of both pulmonary and cardiac disease.[33,42,86-89]

Airway

Transient Tachypnea of the Newborn (TTN)[52,90,91]

- TTN affects term or late preterm infants and is one of the most common causes of respiratory distress in the newborn period.

- TTN is the diagnosis given when there is failure to effectively clear and reabsorb fetal lung fluid into the pulmonary circulation and lymphatics after birth.

- The onset of respiratory distress is usually shortly after birth. The infant may have mild to moderate respiratory distress. CPAP is often used to help clear the pulmonary fluid.

- Other potential etiologies that present with respiratory distress are excluded, such as pneumonia, sepsis, meconium aspiration, respiratory distress syndrome, persistent pulmonary hypertension of the newborn, congenital heart disease, and pneumothorax.

- Risk factors include cesarean delivery without labor, delivery before 39 weeks gestation, preterm delivery, maternal diabetes, and birth asphyxia.

- TTN usually resolves within 24 hours, but in more severe cases, it may not resolve for 72 hours.

- The chest X-ray typically shows evidence of retained fetal lung fluid (i.e., fluid in the fissures), perihilar markings secondary to engorged periarterial lymphatics that assist with clearance of alveolar fluid, hyperaeration, and at times, there may be a small pleural effusion.

Respiratory Distress Syndrome (RDS)[22,52]

- RDS is most commonly seen in preterm infants and occasionally in late preterm infants, particularly males who lag behind females in lung maturity.

- Maternal diabetes increases the risk for RDS (even if the infant is a term gestation) because of the effects of hyperinsulinemia in the fetus, which inhibits the production of surfactant.

- RDS is a disease that is caused by immature lung development and surfactant insufficiency in the alveoli.

- The onset of respiratory distress (tachypnea, retractions, nasal flaring, and grunting) is usually at birth or shortly after birth. Initiating CPAP early after birth to establish and maintain FRV and giving surfactant are mainstays of therapy.

- The chest X-ray typically shows evidence of atelectasis that is described as a 'ground glass' appearance, air bronchograms that are larger airways apparent against the surrounding microatelectasis, and low lung volumes.

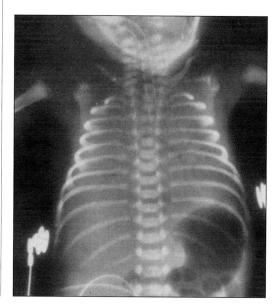

Pneumonia[52,70,92,93]

- Pneumonia affects term or preterm infants.

- The onset of respiratory distress is at birth (congenital pneumonia) or when the lung infection occurs. Congenital pneumonia is usually secondary to ascending infection (vagina/cervix into the amniotic cavity), aspiration of infected amniotic fluid, or transplacental spread from the mother to the fetus.

- Mechanically ventilated infants are at increased risk for acquiring ventilator-associated pneumonia (VAP) because the ET tube serves as a portal of entry for pathogens.

- Differentiate pneumonia from RDS, aspiration, and TTN.

- The chest X-ray is variable and may show unilateral or bilateral diffuse or localized infiltrates (i.e., a shadow seen that may represent pus, blood, or other body fluids in the lungs), hazy or opaque lung fields, or lobar consolidation.

Meconium Aspiration Syndrome (MAS)[19,52,94,95]

- MAS affects term and postterm infants predominantly. Risk factors include small for gestational age, gestation ≥41 weeks, fetal distress, placental insufficiency, cord compression, and other perinatal complications that can compromise placental blood flow.

- Only about 5% of infants born through meconium will develop MAS, and when it occurs, MAS is a common cause of hypoxemic respiratory failure. Severe PPHN is a common complication seen in infants with MAS.

- Respiratory distress can be severe and include cyanosis, tachypnea, retractions, grunting, and nasal flaring. Infants with MAS are at increased risk for developing a pneumothorax.

- MAS is also associated with a several-fold increased risk for bacterial sepsis. *The problem begins in utero:* Impaired placental blood flow and oxygenation causes the anal sphincter to relax and evacuate (pass) meconium. Gasping respirations move amniotic fluid and meconium particles deep into the lungs. After birth, obstruction of the airways leads to both atelectasis and hyperinflation, which increases the risk of pneumothorax, impaired ventilation and oxygenation, surfactant inactivation, and pulmonary hypertension. At times, intrauterine infection is a predisposing factor in the development of MAS. The distressed, gasping fetus can inhale infected fluid deeply into their lungs, which causes pneumonia and sepsis.

- The chest X-ray typically shows coarse, nodular opacities (likely from meconium in the small airways), atelectasis, and over-inflation.

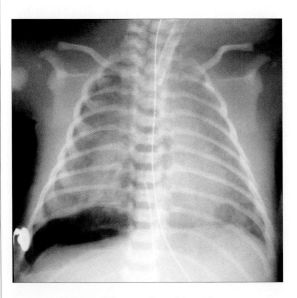

Severe MAS with a subpulmonic pneumothorax on the right side.

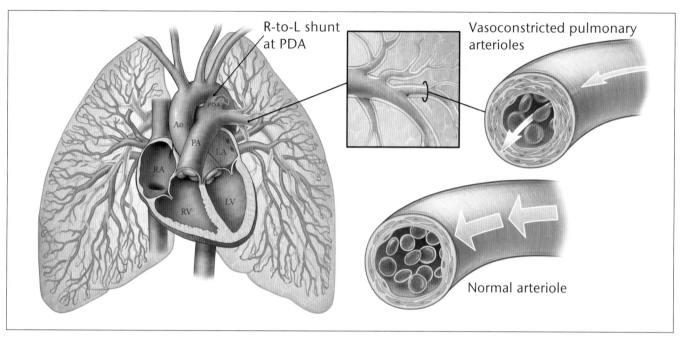

Illustration of a right-to-left shunt through the patent ductus arteriosus (PDA) secondary to vasoconstricted pulmonary arterioles and increased PVR. Because of increased PVR, blood shunts via the pathway of least resistance, right-to-left through the PDA, then into the aorta.

Persistent Pulmonary Hypertension of the Newborn (PPHN)[1,30,52,96,97]

- PPHN affects term infants predominantly but may affect preterm infants at times.

- Elevated pulmonary vascular resistance causes right-to-left shunting of blood across the patent ductus arteriosus (PDA) and/or foramen ovale (FO), which leads to hypoxemia.

- Clinically, the infant may present with respiratory failure and significant hypoxemia within hours of birth, but PPHN may present later when the infant becomes sick with other illnesses, such as sepsis. Treatment involves medications that relax the pulmonary vasculature, including oxygen and cardiorespiratory support that may include mechanical ventilation.

- PPHN may be associated with pulmonary diseases—including meconium aspiration syndrome, pneumonia, respiratory distress syndrome, congenital diaphragmatic hernia, or pulmonary hypoplasia—or cardiovascular abnormalities, including congenital heart disease and heart failure secondary to infection or asphyxia. It may be associated with sepsis and can be idiopathic (underlying cause undetermined).

- Investigate whether the mother took nonsteroidal anti-inflammatory agents (aspirin, ibuprofen, indomethacin) during pregnancy, as these medications are prostaglandin synthetase inhibitors which may constrict the ductus arteriosus and cause structural changes in the pulmonary vasculature, leading to PPHN.

- Prenatal exposure to a selective serotonin reuptake inhibitor, or SSRI, may also increase the risk for idiopathic PPHN. Infants born following SSRI exposure may require extra vigilance during transition and pulse oximetry monitoring to detect hypoxemia.

Congenital Diaphragmatic Hernia (CDH)[52,98-101]

- CDH affects term or preterm infants.

- There is a hole in the diaphragm that allows the stomach and intestine to herniate into the chest.

- The lung on the side with the abdominal contents is compressed and is, therefore, hypoplastic, which makes oxygenation and ventilation very difficult.

- The onset of respiratory distress is at birth or very shortly after. The infant will be cyanotic and have decreased breath sounds on the side with the hernia, which is usually the left. The abdomen may appear sunken (scaphoid) because the stomach and intestine are up in the chest. Bowel sounds may be heard in the chest on the side with the hernia.

- To reduce the amount of air entering the stomach and bowel, proceed with endotracheal intubation or laryngeal mask airway insertion as soon as possible.

- Place a double-lumen gastric tube (such as a 10 Fr Replogle tube) and connect it to low intermittent suction between 30 to 40 mmHg to remove air that enters the stomach. Air that fills the bowel will compress the lung on the opposite side of the hernia and worsen the respiratory distress. If a double-lumen tube is not available, insert an 8 or 10 Fr gastric tube and use a syringe to aspirate air from the stomach every 5 to 10 minutes.

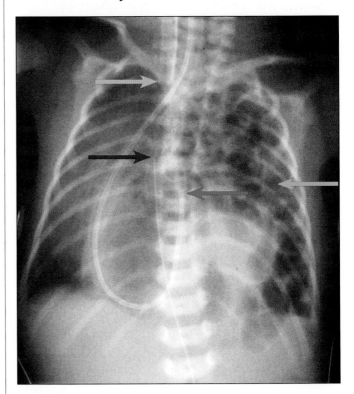

Chest X-ray of an infant with CDH.

- ET tube in the trachea that is shifted to the right.

- UAC tip in the aorta that is shifted to the right.

- Intestine in the chest.

- Gastric tube tip in the stomach that is displaced in the chest.

Term infant with critical COA, hypoplastic aortic arch (unrepaired), and congenital diaphragmatic hernia (post-operative day 10).

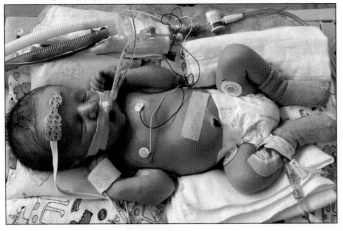

Tracheoesophageal Fistula (TEF) / Esophageal Atresia (EA)[100,102-104]

- TEF and EA affect term or preterm infants.

- In 85% of cases, both TEF and EA are present, most commonly with the atretic proximal esophagus ending in a blind pouch in the lower neck or upper mediastinum and the distal esophagus connecting from the trachea to the stomach (known as Type C). Figure 3.6 shows the different types of TEF and EA.

- Respiratory distress is usually apparent shortly after birth or with the first feeding. Provision of respiratory support can be particularly challenging, especially before the tracheal fistula is ligated. If possible, avoid using positive pressure ventilation since the stomach and intestine fill with air, but there is no way to pass a gastric tube into the stomach to remove the air. If the stomach becomes grossly distended, emergency gastric decompression (needle aspiration) may be necessary.

- Classic signs of TEF/EA are excessive salivation or drooling, choking, coughing, and cyanosis with feeding.

- The goal of stabilization is to prevent aspiration-induced lung injury.

  o Place the infant prone with the head of the bed up 30 degrees to help prevent gastric secretions from refluxing through the fistula into the trachea and lungs.

  o Oral secretions will accumulate rapidly and increase the risk for aspiration, so place a large-bore, double-lumen tube, such as a 10-French Replogle tube, in the esophageal pouch. Connect the tube to low continuous suction between 30 and 40 mmHg.

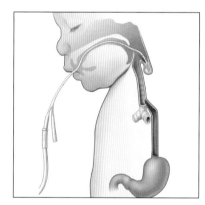

  o If a double-lumen tube is not available, insert a 10-French gastric tube into the esophageal pouch, secure it well, and then use a syringe to aspirate secretions every 5 to 10 minutes or more often as needed.

- Many infants with TEF/EA have other anomalies of the heart, gastrointestinal tract, genitourinary tract, skeletal system, or neurologic system. Investigation for other anomalies within the constellation of the VACTERL association is part of the initial care for these infants. VACTERL stands for **v**ertebral, **a**norectal, **c**ardiac, **t**racheal, **e**sophageal, **r**enal/genitourinary, and **l**imb.

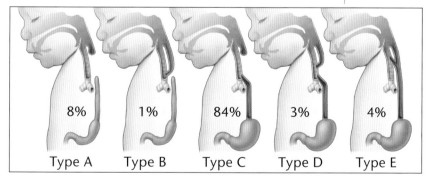

| 8% | 1% | 84% | 3% | 4% |
| Type A | Type B | Type C | Type D | Type E |

Figure 3.6. The five types of TEF and EA. Type A is pure esophageal atresia. Type B has no connection from the trachea to the stomach. With type C (the most common type) and type D (a very rare type), there will be air seen in the stomach and the risk for stomach overdistension is high. In type E, which is called an H-type fistula, there is no esophageal atresia.

Airway Obstruction[23,99,105-107]

Obstruction may occur at the nose, mouth and jaw, larynx, trachea, or bronchi. In addition to respiratory distress (tachypnea, nasal flaring, grunting, retractions), stridor may be heard if the upper airway is narrowed or partially obstructed. Two obstructive airway conditions that present shortly after birth are choanal atresia and Pierre-Robin syndrome.

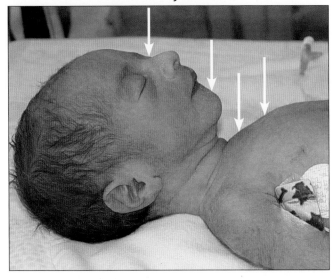

Choanal Atresia

• Choanal atresia affects term or preterm infants and females more than males. The incidence of choanal atresia is approximately 1 in 5,000 to 1 in 9,000 births.

• One or both posterior nasal passages are blocked by a bony septum (more common) or an obstructing membrane. If unilateral, the right nare is obstructed more often.

• If choanal atresia is suspected, try to insert a 6-French feeding tube or suction catheter that is coated with a water-soluble lubricant into each nostril. The inability to pass the tube into the nares mandates further evaluation to rule out choanal atresia.

• Because infants breathe predominantly through their nose and not their mouth, when both nasal passages are blocked, there is **complete airway obstruction and severe hypoxia**. Signs include severe cyanosis while at rest or asleep but "pinking up" with crying as air enters the lungs via the mouth. The O_2 saturation drops again when the infant stops crying.

• Stabilization options to treat airway obstruction and hypoxia include the following:

  o Insert a size 00 oral airway (preterm infants) or size 0 oral airway (term infants).

  o Cut off the end of a feeding nipple or pacifier, insert it into the mouth (called a McGovern Nipple), and secure it with ties around the occiput.[107,108]

  o Intubate the infant (insert an endotracheal tube) and place on mechanical ventilation (CPAP or PPV).

  o In more than half of the cases, there are other associated congenital anomalies, including congenital heart defects.[109]

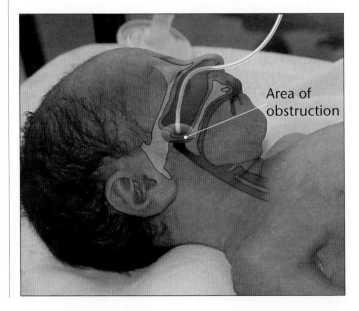

Area of obstruction

Pierre Robin Syndrome (also called Robin Sequence)

- Pierre Robin syndrome affects term or preterm infants.

- Infants with Pierre Robin syndrome have a very small jaw with a normal-sized tongue that obstructs the airway. The lower jaw is set back compared to the upper jaw, and up to half of these infants also have a cleft palate.

- Respiratory distress may be mild to severe.

- To relieve airway obstruction, **turn the infant prone** to help the tongue fall forward by gravity.

- **If the airway is still obstructed**, insert a nasopharyngeal (NP) tube as follows:[107]

  o Coat the tip of a 2.5 mm ET tube with water-soluble gel (do **not** use an oil-based lubricant).

  o Gently pass the lubricated tube through one nostril until the tube is located at the end of the nasal passage and past the base of the tongue but not through the vocal cords.

  o Secure the tube with tape.

  o Once the NP tube is in place, provide CPAP at approximately 6 cm H_2O pressure. PPV may also be necessary to support oxygenation and ventilation.

- Combined with prone positioning, an NP tube is often very effective for opening the airway. However, if the NP tube is not adequate to maintain an open airway, a **laryngeal mask airway** (LMA) is another alternative. Because of the infant's very small jaw, endotracheal intubation may be technically very difficult to perform.

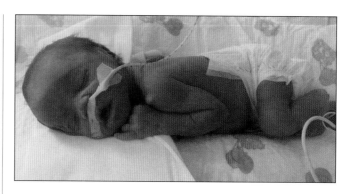

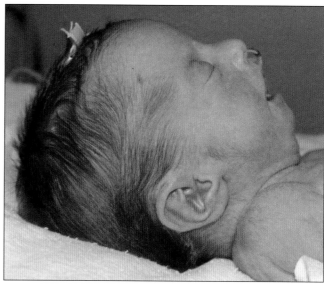

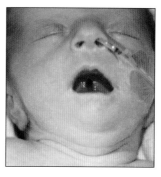

Infant with Pierre Robin syndrome and a cleft palate.

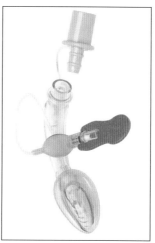

Appendix 3.1 Endotracheal Intubation: Equipment and Securing the ET Tube With Tape

Intubation Supplies and Equipment[63,80,81,110-113]

The supplies and equipment necessary to perform endotracheal intubation should be kept together on a resuscitation cart or intubation tray. Each delivery room, nursery, and emergency department should have a complete set of the items listed below.

- Videolaryngoscope device (if available) with neonatal size blade handle

- Laryngoscope handle with an extra set of batteries and extra bulb
  - Some laryngoscopes are disposable, and the batteries and the bulb cannot be changed (shown in photo below)

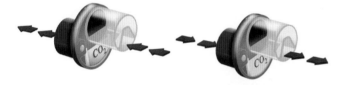

- Blades: Straight rather than curved blades are preferred for optimal visualization
  - No. 1 (term infant)
  - No. 0 (preterm infant)
  - No. 00 (very preterm infant)

- McGill forceps (used for nasotracheal intubation)

- Uncuffed endotracheal (ET) tubes with an internal (inside) diameter of 2.5, 3.0, 3.5, and 4.0 mm
  - A 2.0 ET tube should be available for <500-gram infants in case a 2.5 ET tube won't fit

- Stylet (for optional use and is the appropriate size to fit in the ET tube)

- CO_2 detector (displays a color change when the infant exhales CO_2) or capnography equipment (displays the level of exhaled CO_2)

Mini StatCO2 End Tidal CO_2 Detector (above).

Photo courtesy of Mercury Medical, mercurymed.com

Intubation supplies shown on the tray: Suction catheter, disposable laryngoscope handles and blades, CO_2 detector, ET tubes of varying sizes, and laryngeal mask airway.

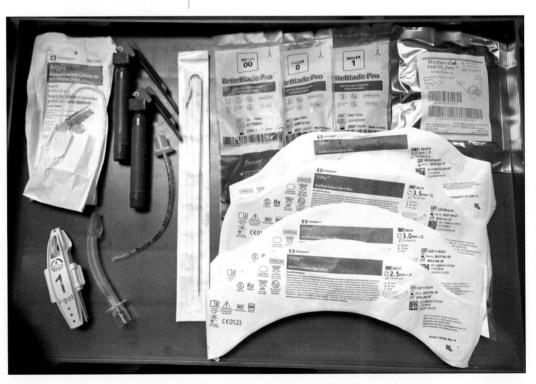

- Suctioning device or suction setup with 8 and 10 Fr suction catheters

  o A size 5 or 6 Fr suction catheter should be available to suction a 2.0 or 2.5 size ET tube

- Shoulder roll

- Adhesive tape (½ or ¾ inch) or endotracheal tube stabilizer for securing the ET tube

- Extra thin hydrocolloid dressing to apply to the cheeks before taping

- Scissors to cut the tape

- Centimeter measuring tape (if the nasal-tragus length is used to determine ET tube insertion depth)

- Oxygen source and blender to permit administration of different O_2 concentrations from 21% to 100%

- Pulse oximeter and probe with cover

- Cardiac monitor and leads (if available)

- PPV bag or T-piece resuscitator (if available) and tubing to attach to the oxygen blender

- Appropriately sized masks for term and preterm infants

- Stethoscope

- Laryngeal mask airway (LMA; size 1) and 5 mL syringe to fill the LMA cuff with air

  o LMA insertion may be selected as the initial advanced airway to insert

  o LMA sizes vary, and newer generation models may become available for smaller infants; follow manufacturer instructions for appropriate size selection

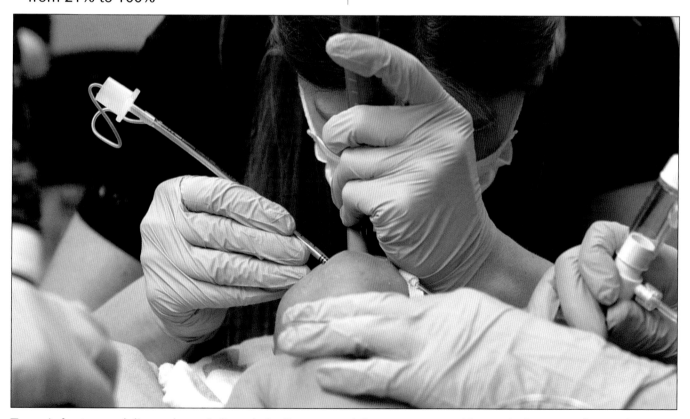

Term infant was delivered precipitously in the car and then transported by ambulance to the tertiary center. The infant required intubation for severe respiratory distress. Cricoid pressure was requested and is being applied.

Securing the ET Tube With Tape—The "X" and "V" Method

1. If the infant is preterm or requires prolonged intubation, protect the cheek skin with a hydrocolloid base layer before applying the tape. Remove secretions from the mouth and upper lip area.

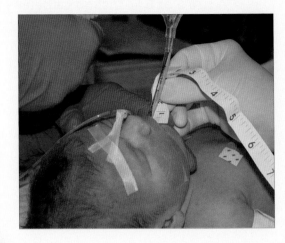

2. Cut adhesive tape into two pieces: a "V" and an "X".

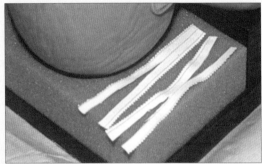

3. Before applying the first piece of tape, re-confirm that the ET tube is at the proper location at the upper lip. An assistant should hold the tube securely at all times. If the tube is being retaped, move it to another place in the mouth so that it is in a different location against the upper gum.

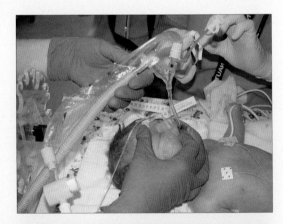

4. The "X" piece is applied firmly to the skin above the upper lip.

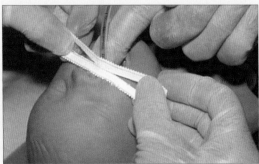

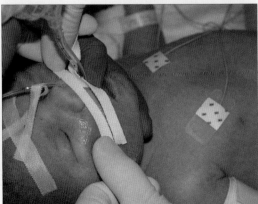

5. One arm of the lower tape is then wrapped around the tube. The other arm is wrapped the opposite way.

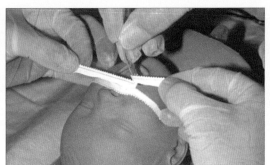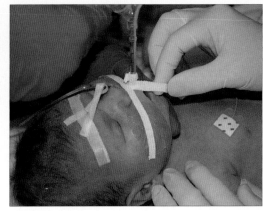

6. Move up slightly on the tube as you wrap, but do not move up so much that the tape puts traction on the tube and pulls it into the mouth. Make a tab at the end of every piece so that it is easier to unwrap the tape if the tube needs to be repositioned. Be sure to check the tube markings at the upper lip throughout the procedure.

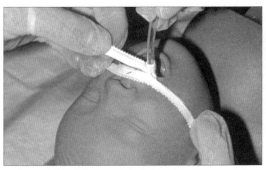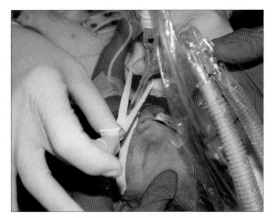

7. Next, apply the "V" shaped piece to help secure the underlying tape. The upper part of the "V" is applied first to the upper lip.

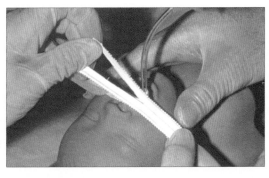

8. The lower piece of the "V" wraps around the tube again. Continue to wrap the tape, moving up slightly until a 1/2 inch of the tape remains.

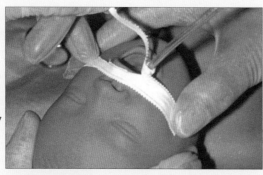

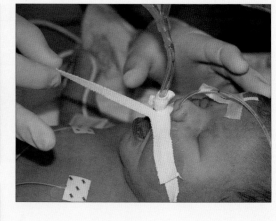

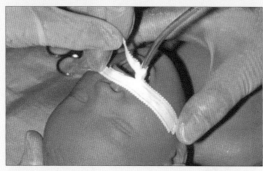

9. Fold the remaining ½ inch of tape to form a tab. The tab allows for easier unfastening of the tape if the tube needs to be repositioned. Check one final time that the tube location at the upper lip is at the desired depth.

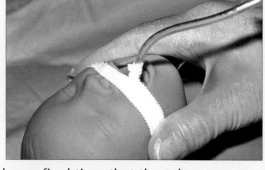

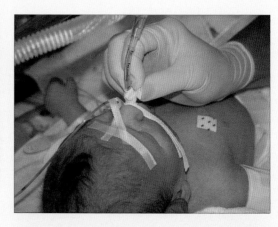

10. Once the ET tube is secure, insert an orogastric or nasogastric tube to decompress the stomach.

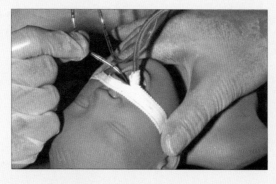

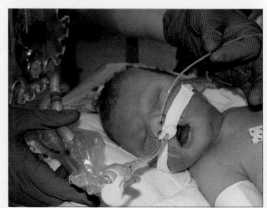

11. Confirm the ET tube location on a chest X-ray.

Blood Pressure Module

Sugar

Temperature

Airway

Blood Pressure

Lab Work

Emotional Support

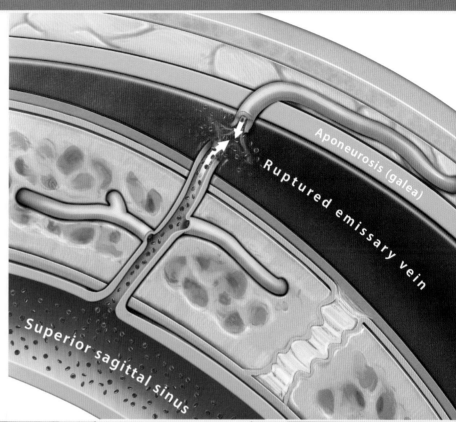

Aponeurosis (galea)

Ruptured emissary vein

superior sagittal sinus

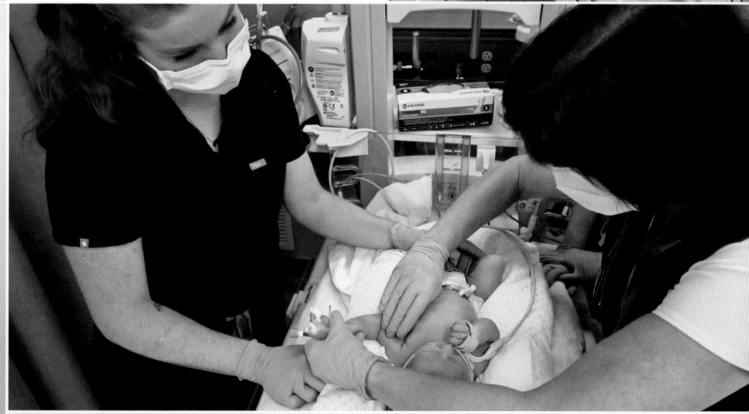

Blood Pressure—Module Objectives

Upon completion of this module, participants will gain an increased understanding of:

1. How inadequate tissue perfusion and oxygenation can lead to shock.

2. The changes in vital signs and physical exam when an infant is in shock.

3. The causes and initial treatment of hypovolemic, obstructive, cardiogenic, and septic/distributive shock.

What Is Shock?

Cells require oxygen to survive and function. Shock occurs when oxygen delivery to vital organs becomes insufficient to meet tissue demands.[1,2] When the oxygen supply is low, the cells will convert from aerobic to anaerobic metabolism to produce energy. Lactic acid will be produced, and lactic acid, combined with low cellular energy, will significantly impair cell function.[3,4]

Three Phases of Shock

Compensated Shock

In **compensated shock**, complex responses, including an increase in systemic vascular resistance (SVR), are activated to maintain blood pressure and preserve blood flow to vital organs (e.g., the brain, heart, and adrenal glands).[1] This response has consequences, however, because blood is diverted from non-vital organs (e.g., the skin, gastrointestinal tract, muscles, liver, lungs, and kidneys) to preferentially perfuse the brain, heart, and adrenal glands.[5,6] If shock is not quickly recognized and reversed, the oxygen debt worsens, lactic acid production increases, and the pH in the blood decreases. As the heart muscle weakens from a lack of oxygen and the effects of acidosis, cardiac output decreases and eventually causes hypotension.

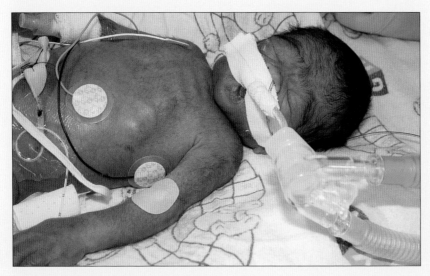

Preterm infant with septic shock.

Uncompensated Shock

Once hypotension develops, the phase of **uncompensated shock** starts. In this phase, perfusion and oxygen delivery to all tissues and organs further decrease. When cellular oxygen content is low, energy is produced by anaerobic metabolism. The large amount of lactic acid produced lowers the pH in the blood and interferes with normal cell function.

Irreversible Shock

Delayed or unsuccessful treatment of shock will lead to the final phase, **irreversible shock**. The infant may rapidly deteriorate and experience complete organ failure. Therapeutic interventions will be unsuccessful, and this phase will end in death.[2,5] Table 4.1 on page 178 and Figure 4.1 on page 180 explain the physical exam to evaluate for shock.

Treatment of shock includes identifying and treating the underlying problem and understanding how to improve and support heart function and appropriate vascular tone.

Hypotension is a late sign of cardiac decompensation. Do not wait for low blood pressure to initiate treatment if there are clinical signs of poor perfusion, which may include a delayed capillary refill time, tachycardia, mottled skin, cool extremities, weak pulses, and declining urine output. Failure to promptly recognize and treat shock may lead to multiple organ failure (brain, heart, liver, kidneys, and gastrointestinal tract) and even death.

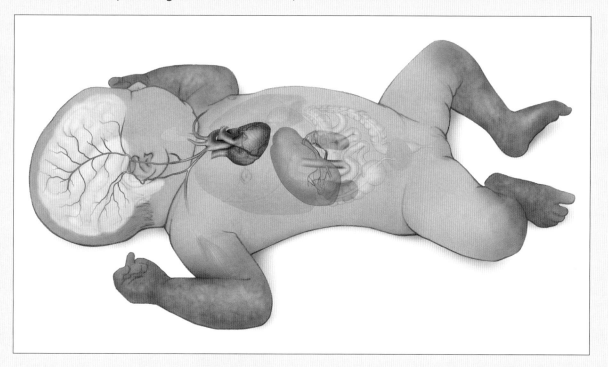

Cardiac Output

The volume of blood ejected from the left ventricle into the aorta with each contraction or heartbeat is called the stroke volume and is measured in liters/beat (L/beat). The heart rate (HR) in beats/minute multiplied by the stroke volume equals the quantity of blood that enters the aorta each minute and is called the *cardiac output*.[4] The formula for cardiac output (CO) is

$$HR_{(beats/min)} \times SV_{(L/beat)} = CO_{(L/min)}$$

The normal blood volume of a neonate ranges between 80 to 100 mL/kg, depending on the gestational age. Therefore, the heart ejects a small fraction of a liter (i.e., milliliters) of blood with each heartbeat. In neonates of varying gestational ages, the normal cardiac output ranges between 150 to 300 mL/kg/minute.[7]

What Can Tachycardia Tell Us About Cardiac Output?

Neonates in shock will try to compensate for a low cardiac output by increasing their heart rate. A sustained heart rate greater than 180 beats per minute is abnormal. Rule out other reasons for *tachycardia,* such as agitation, crying, pain, medications, fever, or an arrhythmia.[4] Although tachycardia is one of the first compensatory mechanisms to help increase cardiac output, a high heart rate may not *effectively* increase cardiac output because the left ventricle has less time to fill.[8] The immature neonatal heart muscle has minimal capacity to stretch to fill more or to squeeze harder to increase the amount of blood ejected with each heartbeat (i.e., SV) unless augmented with a medication and/or intravenous infusion of fluid. **For that reason, tachycardia is the most effective mechanism to increase cardiac output in neonates.**[1,9]

> **A sustained heart rate >180 beats per minute is called tachycardia and is a compensatory mechanism to increase cardiac output.**

The clinical signs seen when an infant is in shock may reflect an attempt to compensate for shock and how well or poorly the patient is doing. For example, tachycardia is the compensatory mechanism to increase cardiac output, whereas a decreased level of consciousness may reflect the effects of brain hypoxia and acidosis.

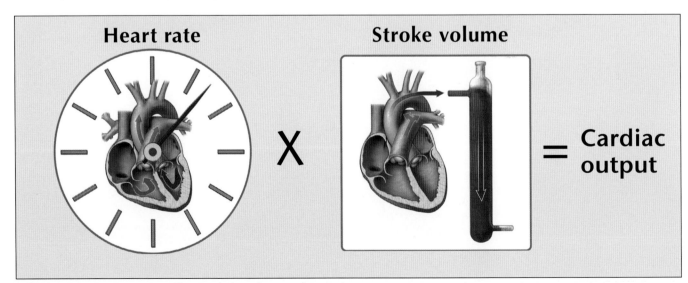

Heart rate X Stroke volume = Cardiac output

Let's Learn More... 3 Factors influencing stroke volume: Preload, afterload, and contractility[10,11]

Understanding the following principles can help guide the treatment of shock:

Preload is the amount of blood in the heart at the end of diastole, just before ventricular contraction begins. The preload, or filling volume, is determined primarily by the amount of blood returning to the heart from the body and lungs.

Impact of decreased preload: If there is a reduced volume of venous blood returning to the heart, the heart has less blood to "pump" with each contraction.

Afterload is the pressure the heart must generate to send blood into the aorta and main pulmonary artery. Afterload increases when there is systemic or pulmonary hypertension or some type of obstruction (e.g., heart valve). Cardiac defects that reduce blood flow through the aorta with closure of the ductus arteriosus (i.e., left-sided obstructive lesions) also increase afterload and stress on the left ventricle.

Impact of increased afterload: The heart works harder to pump blood against arterial resistance and can reduce stroke volume because of incomplete emptying of the ventricles.

Contractility is a measure of how well the heart squeezes with each beat. Factors that can impair contractility include inadequate preload, infections, heart immaturity, and lack of oxygen or glucose to the heart muscle. The metabolic environment is also important, including the amount of lactic acid and electrolytes and minerals (e.g., sodium, potassium, chloride, calcium, and magnesium) in the blood, which affect the function of the heart muscle and the conduction system.

Impact of reduced heart contractility: If the heart squeeze or contraction is poor, less blood is ejected with every heartbeat.

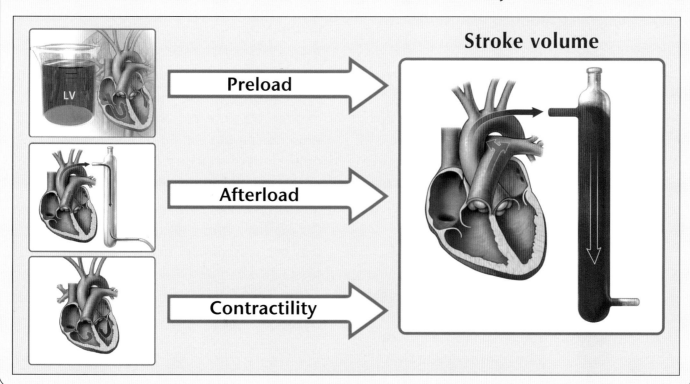

Preload

Afterload

Contractility

Stroke volume

Table 4.1. Physical examination for shock.[3,4,8,12-15]

An infant in shock may exhibit the following signs:

Heart Rate

A normal heart rate is between 120 and 160 beats per minute (bpm) but may range between 80 and 200 bpm, depending upon the infant's activity level (asleep versus active and crying).

Bradycardia (<100 bpm) with Evidence of Poor Perfusion

- Hypoxia and acidosis depress the function of the conduction system and may cause bradycardia. *Bradycardia combined with severe shock is an ominous sign of impending cardiorespiratory arrest.*

- Other causes of bradycardia than shock include hypothermia, increased intracranial pressure, hyperkalemia, hypercalcemia, abdominal distension, hypoglycemia, episodes of apnea (apnea of prematurity), and medications (e.g., beta-blockers and opioids).

- In sinus bradycardia, a p wave precedes each QRS complex. In complete heart block, the p waves are completely unrelated to the QRS complexes. Infants in complete heart block may have a heart rate that is too low to provide adequate cardiac output.

Tachycardia (sustained heart rate >180 bpm at rest)

- Tachycardia is especially concerning if there are signs of poor perfusion and/or congestive heart failure. Other causes of tachycardia than shock include pain, fever, hypoxia, anemia, or medications (i.e., caffeine, dopamine, epinephrine).

- Supraventricular tachycardia (SVT) should be considered if there is an abrupt and sustained heart rate ≥220 bpm, although SVT may be present with a sustained heart rate <220 bpm. Infants in SVT can experience shock.

Pulses

- Pulses should be palpable and feel equal in the upper and lower body. Weak or absent peripheral (radial, dorsalis pedis, posterior tibial) or central (brachial, femoral) pulses are abnormal.

- If central pulses are absent, assess the patient and *initiate cardiopulmonary resuscitation as indicated.*

- If brachial pulses are stronger than femoral pulses, consider coarctation of the aorta or interrupted aortic arch. As the ductus arteriosus closes, blood flow to the lower body decreases. The treatment to reestablish ductal patency is a prostaglandin E1 infusion.

Perfusion

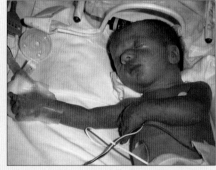

- A capillary refill time (CRT) ≥4 seconds is considered prolonged.

- The hands and/or feet may feel cool secondary to poor perfusion.

- A CRT ≤2 seconds in a sick infant may indicate septic (warm) shock. The hands and feet may also feel warm. Warm shock is not a common presentation but should be considered if other signs of shock are present. Extremely immature infants may also have a short CRT.

- Mottled skin can be a sign of poor perfusion. Differentiate from cutis marmorata, which may occur secondary to altered vasomotor tone when exposed to a cold stressor.[16]

Blood Pressure

- The blood pressure may be within normal range because of vasoconstriction during the period of compensated shock.

- Hypotension is present with uncompensated or irreversible shock.

Skin Color

- Pallor (pale skin color) may indicate severe anemia secondary to significant blood loss, including acute perinatal hemorrhagic events. The skin can appear pale or white secondary to decreased perfusion distal to a thrombus. Neonates with light skin pigmentation can also appear pale.

- A gray color and/or cyanosis of the skin and mucous membranes indicates hypoxemia.

Respiratory Status

- Tachypnea may be a sign of compensation for an acid-base imbalance (i.e., respiratory, metabolic, or mixed acidosis).

- Increased work of breathing may include retractions, grunting, and nasal flaring.

- Apnea can signify worsening cardiorespiratory failure and impending arrest.

- *Gasping* is an ominous sign of impending cardiorespiratory arrest.

Neurologic Status

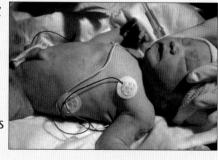

- Monitor for a decline in the level of consciousness and response to stimulation.

- The level of consciousness is altered by sedating medications.

Urine Output

- If the urine output is declining or is less than 1 mL/kg/hour, renal perfusion may be diminished.

- Correlate the urine output with other signs of poor perfusion.

Heart

- A heart murmur is sound caused by turbulent blood flow through the heart or adjacent blood vessels. A murmur may be present for any of the following reasons:

  o Blood forced through a stenotic valve (pulmonary, aortic),

  o Regurgitation of blood through an incompetent valve (aortic, mitral, tricuspid, pulmonary),

  o Blood forced through a narrow area such as a ventricular septal defect (VSD),

  o Blood forced through stenotic arteries (aortic coarctation, branch pulmonary stenosis, peripheral pulmonic stenosis), and

  o Increased blood flow across normal structures (i.e., transient tricuspid regurgitation following birth asphyxia, anemic patients).

- An enlarged heart on chest X-ray (cardiomegaly) correlates with myocardial dysfunction and development of congestive heart failure. Cardiomegaly may also be a sign of underlying congenital heart disease.

- A smaller-than-normal heart on a chest X-ray may reflect low preload or, if on mechanical ventilation, lung hyperinflation and heart compression.

Evaluating the Capillary Refill Time (CRT)[4,17-20]

A prolonged CRT may indicate blood is being shunted away from the skin to preferentially perfuse vital organs. The CRT may vary with gestational or postnatal age, skin and/or ambient temperature, and the duration of pressure applied to blanch the skin. When assessing CRT, concurrently evaluate the strength and quality of the peripheral pulses and the skin temperature in the hands and feet. Follow the same procedure each time CRT is assessed.

- Assess the upper (central) and lower (peripheral) body.

- Press firmly for 2 to 3 seconds, then release.

- Count how many seconds it takes for the skin to refill (e.g., "one-one thousand, two-one thousand, three-one thousand...").

- Compare the upper CRT to the lower body CRT.

Normal CRT

- The CRT should be ≤3 seconds on the upper and/or lower body in a normothermic infant who is in a room with a warm ambient temperature. The hands and feet should also feel warm.

- A CRT ≤2 seconds is normal for healthy older infants and children.

Abnormal CRT

- A CRT >4 seconds may indicate peripheral vasoconstriction in response to shock, especially if the hands and/or feet are cool.

- If the lower body is 2 or more seconds longer than the upper body, this may indicate decreased distal perfusion secondary to a closing ductus arteriosus in a ductal-dependent left heart obstruction congenital heart defect.

- In septic, vasodilated "warm" shock, the CRT is ≤2 seconds, and the hands and feet feel warm.

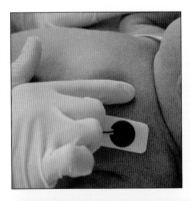 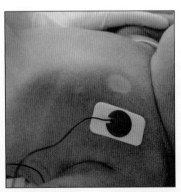 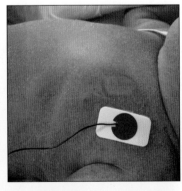 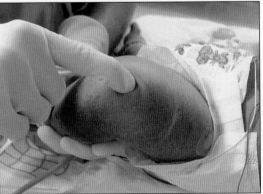 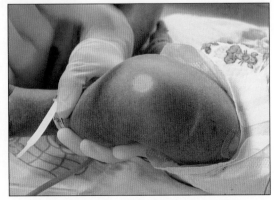

Figure 4.1. Capillary refill time (CRT) is commonly assessed to evaluate perfusion; however, CRT assessment can be subjective and vary between observers.

Blood Pressure (BP)

In newborns and young infants, BP values change with birth weight, gestational age, and postnatal age.[21] A concerning BP should be assessed in combination with heart rate, signs of poor perfusion, and, as indicated, with laboratory tests that may include any of the following: lactate, blood gas, hemoglobin, renal function, liver function, coagulation tests, and electrolytes.[22] See Table 4.3 on page 185 for additional information about laboratory tests to help assess for shock.

Is Assessment of Only the Mean BP Sufficient?

The mean BP alone should not guide therapeutic interventions such as vasopressor or volume administration. Research that supports using a single BP parameter (i.e., mean BP) to assess adequate systemic blood flow, including to the vulnerable brain, is lacking.[5,21,23] Using the mean BP equal to or slightly higher than the infant's gestational age to conclude the BP is 'normal' is not physiologically based and does not correlate with left ventricular output.[23,24] In addition, in sick preterm infants, when the mean BP is <30 mmHg by cuff measurement, the mean is often overestimated compared to the arterial mean BP.[25] Therefore, the risk is that the infant's BP may actually be lower than what is reported by the cuff (oscillometric) measurement.

Assess Systolic, Diastolic, and Mean BP

Systolic, diastolic, and mean BP all provide helpful information, including the numbers needed to calculate pulse pressure as explained in Figure 4.2 on page 184. The systolic, diastolic, and mean BPs spontaneously and steadily increase after birth for all gestational-age infants.[21,24,26-28] If the BP does not rise, or it declines, possible causes should be investigated.[29]

Table 4.2 displays the average systolic, diastolic, and mean BP values and the BP values at the 10th, 50th, and 90th percentile for hemodynamically stable NICU patients (25 to 42 weeks gestational age) who required invasive mechanical ventilation for <24 hours.[30] An interactive tool for reference ranges for non-invasive BP measurement in the first week after birth in healthy preterm and term neonates can be found at www.bloodpressure-neonate.com.

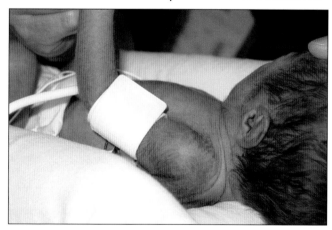

Table 4.2. Average systolic, diastolic, and mean BP values and the BP values at the 10th, 50th, and 90th percentile for hemodynamically stable NICU patients (25 to 42 weeks gestational age) on days 1, 3, and 5 after birth.[30]

Birth Weight (grams)	Blood Pressure Parameter	Day 1				Day 3				Day 5			
%tile = Percentile		Average	10th %tile	50th %tile	90th %tile	Average	10th %tile	50th %tile	90th %tile	Average	10th %tile	50th %tile	90th %tile
≤1000	Systolic	56	40	55	72	60	46	59	77	62	49	62	77
	Diastolic	35	21	36	48	40	27	38	56	39	29	38	51
	Mean	43	27	41	56	48	35	46	64	47	36	47	59
1001–1500	Systolic	56	43	55	71	65	53	65	78	67	54	68	79
	Diastolic	35	24	36	45	42	32	42	53	43	33	43	54
	Mean	43	31	43	56	51	40	51	61	52	41	52	62
1501–2000	Systolic	59	48	58	70	65	54	65	77	68	57	68	81
	Diastolic	35	26	35	44	42	33	41	52	42	32	42	53
	Mean	44	34	44	54	51	42	51	60	52	42	52	64
2001–2500	Systolic	60	50	59	72	68	58	68	79	73	60	73	86
	Diastolic	37	27	36	46	44	35	44	53	45	35	44	57
	Mean	46	36	45	55	53	44	53	62	56	45	55	69
2501–3000	Systolic	67	54	64	82	71	59	71	84	73	63	74	83
	Diastolic	43	30	41	58	45	34	44	56	43	35	42	54
	Mean	52	40	50	68	55	44	54	67	55	45	54	66
3001–3500	Systolic	69	56	69	82	74	62	73	87	75	63	75	88
	Diastolic	42	32	42	52	47	37	46	58	46	37	45	56
	Mean	52	42	52	63	58	46	57	70	57	48	57	68
3501–4000	Systolic	70	59	70	81	75	62	74	86	80	69	80	91
	Diastolic	42	32	41	52	48	37	47	59	48	39	48	59
	Mean	53	43	52	64	58	46	58	70	60	50	60	71
4001–4500	Systolic	71	58	70	88	75	62	75	88	77	61	78	90
	Diastolic	43	35	42	54	47	36	45	59	46	36	44	58
	Mean	53	43	52	66	58	45	58	71	58	45	58	69

Adapted from Kiss JK, Gajda A, Mari J, Nemeth J, Bereczki C. Oscillometric arterial blood pressure in haemodynamically stable neonates in the first 2 weeks of life. Pediatr Nephrol. 2023;38(10):3369-3378.

___

Note:
Patients were excluded from this BP study for any of the following reasons: receiving inotropic medications, postnatal steroids, or invasive mechanical ventilation beyond 24 hours; the presence of an umbilical artery catheter, renal disease, major congenital heart disease, chromosomal anomaly, hypertension, or bronchopulmonary dysplasia; or maternal substance misuse.

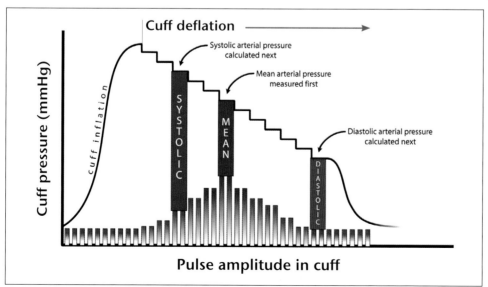

Oscillometric BP Measurement [21,25,31-35]

Noninvasive blood pressure (NIBP) monitoring estimates the systolic, diastolic, and mean arterial BP.

How Does Oscillometric BP Measurement Work?

The cuff inflates to a level above systolic BP. As the cuff slowly deflates, arterial blood flow increases, and pulsatile signals or oscillations are detected in the arterial wall. When the maximum amplitude of the oscillations is reached, the mean arterial BP is measured. The cuff further deflates, and when blood flows smoothly through the artery without further detection of oscillations, the systolic and diastolic BPs are calculated and displayed on the monitor (along with the mean BP). A pressure transducer in the cuff communicates information about the strength of oscillations as the cuff is deflated. This information is analyzed and calculated using device-specific algorithms, which can lead to variability between devices. The illustration shows how the oscillometric method calculates the BP. Correlate findings with patient assessment and report abnormal results to the infant's care team.

Improving the Accuracy of Oscillometric BP Measurement

- Take the BP when the infant is calm because movement interferes with the accuracy of the reading. The BP is usually higher when the infant is awake.

- Keep the arm or leg at the level of the heart. Gently hold the extremity in a straight position distal to the cuff placement.

- Line up the arterial arrow on the cuff with the brachial artery (for an arm BP) or the popliteal artery (for a leg BP). The bladder of the cuff underlies where the tubing is located, and it is the bladder that detects the oscillations in the artery.

- Place the cuff on the arm, thigh, or calf. Taking the BP on the same limb is helpful for comparing results. The right arm is preferred for upper extremity BP measurement because it best reflects the BP in the ascending aorta.

- Use the correct cuff size. Calf and arm BPs correlate closely, providing the proper cuff size is selected for the midarm or calf.

- Using a cuff that is too small will overestimate the BP and may give false reassurance that the BP is normal. Using a cuff that is too large will underestimate the BP and may report a low BP when, in fact, the BP may be normal.

Graph adapted with permission of Bruce Friedman (GE Healthcare).

Pulse Pressure[4,11,36-40]

The pulse pressure is the difference between the systolic and diastolic BP. The difference between these two measurements can be small (narrow) or large (wide). Figure 4.2 shows normal pulse pressures for preterm and term infants and possible causes of a narrow or wide pulse pressure. A narrow or wide pulse pressure should be reported to the infant's medical team.

Gestation	Normal Pulse Pressure (mmHg)
Term	25 to 30
Preterm	15 to 25

Possible Causes of a Narrow or Wide Pulse Pressure	
Narrow Pulse Pressure *Associated with weak pulses*	• Compensation for a low systemic output is to increase systemic vascular resistance that, in turn, raises the diastolic BP and narrows the pulse pressure • Decreased cardiac output is secondary to shock, cardiomyopathy, and myocarditis • Compression on the heart reduces cardiac output • Pneumopericardium, pericardial effusion, tension pneumothorax, lung hyperinflation • Severe aortic valve stenosis • Significant tachycardia Pneumopericardium — Bilateral tension pneumothorax — Lung hyperinflation
Wide Pulse Pressure *Associated with "bounding" pulses*	• Patent ductus arteriosus (PDA), truncus arteriosus, arteriovenous malformation (AVM), aortopulmonary window, aortic regurgitation • Vasodilation secondary to sepsis (warm shock) PDA — Truncus arteriosus — AVM

Figure 4.2. Normal pulse pressure in preterm and term infants and possible causes of a narrow or wide pulse pressure.[41] To calculate the pulse pressure, subtract the diastolic pressure from the systolic pressure.

Laboratory and Other Tests to Evaluate for Shock

In addition to laboratory tests, as outlined in Table 4.3, an echocardiogram will help evaluate heart function and the presence of a structural heart defect that can negatively affect heart function. An electrocardiogram (ECG) will help assess abnormal heart conduction (i.e., an arrhythmia) and evidence of myocardial ischemia. If concerned about an inborn error of metabolism, many of the tests listed in Table 4.3 will be useful, but additional metabolic screening tests may include an ammonia level, plasma amino acids, plasma acylcarnitine profile, and urine organic acids.

Table 4.3. Laboratory evaluation for shock.[14,42-61]

- **Blood gas/acid-base measurement:** Metabolic acidosis may be present. An infant with concurrent respiratory disease or ineffective ventilation will also have an elevated PCO_2 (mixed metabolic and respiratory acidosis).

- **Lactic acid/lactate:** Lactic acid is produced as a by-product of anaerobic metabolism, and as lactic acid accumulates, the pH declines (acidosis/acidemia).

- **Liver function tests (albumin, total protein, and conjugated bilirubin):** These tests may be abnormal after shock. Elevated liver intracellular enzymes can reflect liver injury.

  o Coagulation studies (prothrombin time, partial thromboplastin time, international normalized ratio, fibrinogen) may be abnormal if the liver was injured during a period of shock or the infant has developed disseminated intravascular coagulation (DIC).

- **Complete Blood Count:** Evaluate for sepsis, anemia, polycythemia, and thrombocytopenia.

- **Blood culture:** Evaluate for sepsis.

- **Glucose:** In response to stress and catecholamine release, the glucose may initially be high. Monitor for and prevent hypoglycemia.

- **Electrolytes (hypo or hypernatremia and hypo or hyperkalemia):** If metabolic acidosis is present, calculate the anion gap.

- **Ionized calcium:** Ionized calcium is the measure of 'free calcium' and the physiologically active fraction of calcium in the blood. An adequate ionized calcium concentration optimizes myocardial contractility.

- **Renal function tests (BUN, creatinine, phosphorus):** Evaluate renal injury following shock and adjust medications (i.e., dosing and interval) when they are renally excreted.

- **Cardiac enzymes:** Assess possible myocardial stress or injury.

  o B-type natriuretic peptide (BNP) is synthesized and secreted by the ventricular myocardium in response to increased ventricular pressure overload, volume expansion, and stretching of cardiac myocytes.

  o Troponin is an enzyme released from cardiac myocytes in response to myocardial injury. Troponin levels may be elevated with sepsis, heart failure, tachyarrhythmias, heart block, cardiomyopathies, myocarditis, pericarditis, chest trauma (cardiac contusion), and severe pulmonary hypertension.

The Four Types of Shock: Hypovolemic, Obstructive, Cardiogenic, and Septic

Hypovolemic Shock[4,5,22,62-65]

A low circulating blood volume reduces cardiac output and oxygen delivery to the tissues.

Causes of Hypovolemic Shock

Acute blood loss *during the intrapartum period*

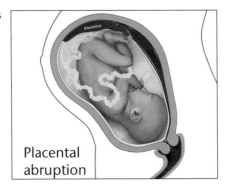
Placental abruption

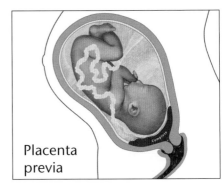
Placenta previa

- Placental abruption or placenta previa (placental separation compromises placental blood flow to the fetus)

- Umbilical cord injury secondary to velamentous cord insertion and/or vasa previa (the umbilical vessels may rupture and lead to an acute hemorrhage)

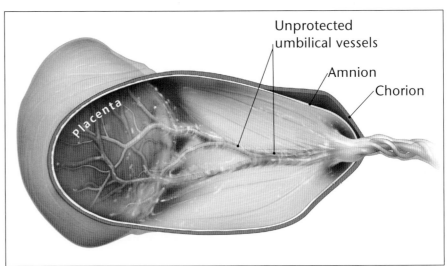
Velamentous Cord Insertion

- Fetal-maternal transfusion (transplacental passage of a large amount of fetal blood into the maternal circulation; severe anemia in the fetus)

- Twin-to-twin transfusion syndrome (acute or chronic hemorrhage); one twin is the donor and may be pale, anemic, hypovolemic, and growth-restricted, and the other twin is the recipient and at risk for hypervolemia, hydrops, and congestive heart failure

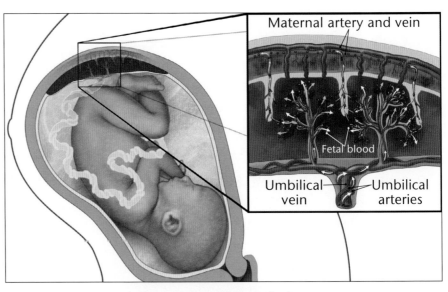
Fetal-Maternal Transfusion

- Organ laceration (liver or spleen) following a difficult delivery or laceration of the placenta during a cesarean delivery

Postnatal hemorrhage

- An intracranial (brain) hemorrhage may occur prenatally, during the intrapartum period, or postnatally

- Blood loss due to disseminated intravascular coagulation (DIC) or other bleeding complications such as hemophilia or vitamin K deficiency

- Subgaleal hemorrhage (see Appendix 4.1 for more information)

- Lung (pulmonary hemorrhage)

- Adrenal gland

Non-hemorrhagic causes of hypovolemic shock

- Severe capillary leak secondary to infection

- Dehydration

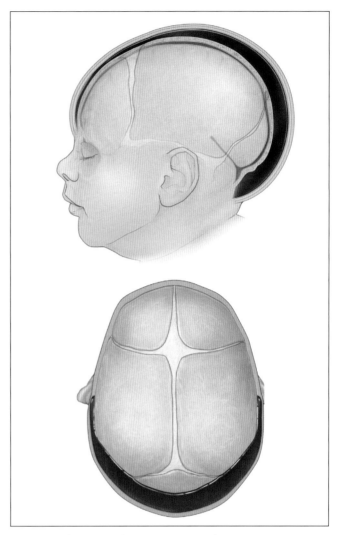

Subgaleal hemorrhage occurs when emissary veins rupture and bleed into the subgaleal space that overlies the periosteum. Because there is nothing to impede blood once it seeps into this space, the infant's entire blood volume (240 to 260 mL) can insidiously bleed into this area.

 In the delivery room, a very pale or 'white' appearing infant may be a sign that the infant is severely anemic. Remember that 3 to 5 grams/dL of hemoglobin needs to be desaturated (not carrying any oxygen) for cyanosis to be visible. If the infant experienced a severe hemorrhage in utero and only has 3 to 5 grams/dL of hemoglobin (which equates to a hematocrit of 9 to 15%), then cyanosis will not be apparent, or it will only become apparent when the O_2 saturation is dangerously low. An emergency blood transfusion of O-negative packed red blood cells (PRBCs) may be lifesaving in this situation.

If the infant has experienced chronic anemia in utero and/or is edematous at birth (hydrops fetalis), take care to give blood or volume infusions slowly. The infant may already be experiencing a degree of heart failure because of the anemia and chronic in-utero hypoxia. Giving blood or volume too quickly may not be tolerated.

Obstructive Shock[4,6,13,22,66]

Low cardiac output because of interruption of blood returning to or leaving the heart is called obstructive shock.

Causes of Obstructive Shock

Perinatal conditions that impede (obstruct) blood flow to the fetus

- Umbilical cord compression secondary to a knot in the cord or a tight nuchal cord

- Cord prolapse

Causes of obstructed blood flow in the veins or arteries leading into or out of the heart

- Tension pneumothorax (compresses the lung(s) and restricts ventilation)

  o As air accumulates, the mediastinum shifts to the opposite side and kinks or compresses the great vessels, which are the large arteries and veins that bring blood into or away from the heart

- Cardiac tamponade:

  o Pneumopericardium (as air collects in the pericardial sac, the heart is compressed and unable to contract effectively)

  o Pericardial effusion (the pericardium is a membrane that encircles the heart; blood or fluid can collect in the pericardial sac and compress the heart, such as occurs when a percutaneously inserted central catheter (PICC) erodes through the sac)

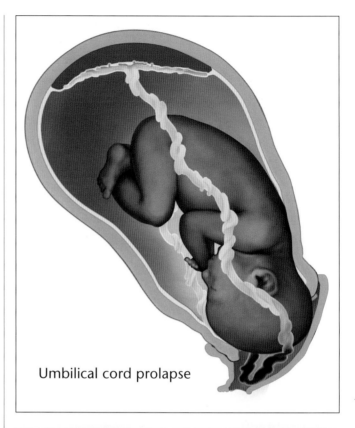

Umbilical cord prolapse

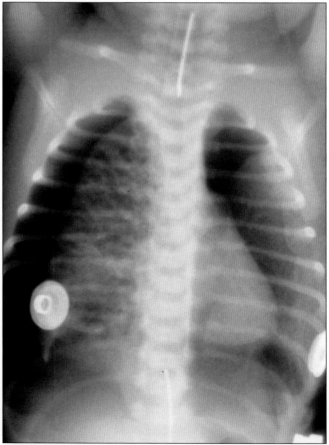

Bilateral tension pneumothorax.

Critical congenital heart defects that can obstruct blood flow

In utero, the ductus arteriosus (DA) is a fetal shunt that allows blood to bypass the non-aerating lungs. Shortly after birth, the DA begins to close. In most term infants, anatomic closure of the DA is by 4 days of age; however, complete closure may take 1 to 2 weeks. With ductal-dependent types of congenital heart disease, as the DA closes, the infant may be in shock (left-side obstructive lesions) or become severely hypoxemic (right-side obstructive lesions). Left-side heart obstruction lesions that can impair cardiac output as the DA closes are shown below.

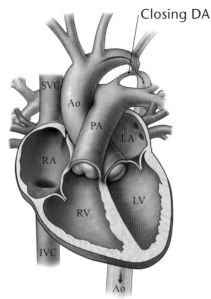

Coarctation of the Aorta—narrowing of the aorta.

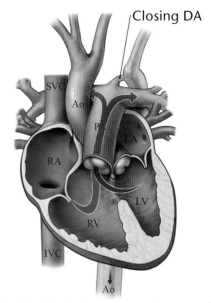

Interrupted Aortic Arch—the most severe form of arch obstruction.

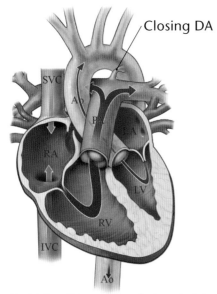

Critical Aortic Valve Stenosis—obstructs blood flow from the left ventricle to the aorta.

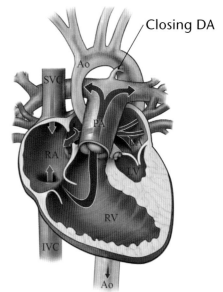

Hypoplastic Left Heart Syndrome—very small left ventricle and aortic hypoplasia secondary to aortic or mitral valve stenosis or atresia.

Cardiogenic Shock[4,67,68]

Impaired heart function or decreased strength of heart contractions leads to a decrease in cardiac output.

Factors That Impair Heart Function

- Intrapartum or postpartum asphyxia (myocardial ischemia)

- Hypoxia and/or metabolic acidosis (heart cell dysfunction)

- Bacterial or viral infection (myocarditis and/or impaired heart contractility)

- Severe hypoglycemia

- An abnormal metabolic environment that may include elevated levels of lactic acid and abnormal electrolytes and minerals (e.g., sodium, potassium, chloride, calcium, and magnesium) may affect the function of both the heart muscle and conduction system

- Arrhythmia

  - Tachycardia secondary to supraventricular tachycardia reduces the time for the ventricles to fill and reduces stroke volume

  - Bradycardia secondary to complete heart block reduces cardiac output and tissue oxygenation

- Congenital heart defects

  - Right-side obstructive lesions impair blood flow to the lungs; hypoxemia may become severe, and poor oxygenation impairs heart function (see illustrations of two severe heart defects on page 191).

  - Left-side obstructive lesions with a closing ductus arteriosus cause obstructive shock; as acidosis worsens, the effects of a low pH on cell function may lead to cardiogenic shock

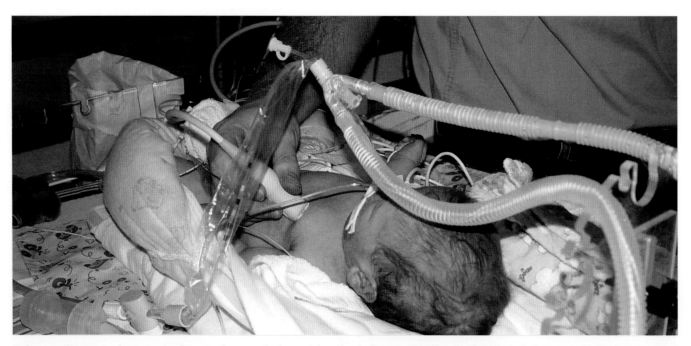

Echocardiogram being performed on a 2-day-old term infant with hypoplastic left heart syndrome.

Septic (Distributive) Shock[4,67,68]

Severe infection may lead to a fourth type of shock known as septic or distributive shock. When some gram-negative bacteria disintegrate, they release a toxic substance that was bound to their cell wall (i.e., endotoxin). Endotoxins trigger a cascade of negative effects, including inappropriate vasodilation and dysfunction of the endothelium. The endothelium is the innermost lining of every blood vessel, and it controls the passage of nutrients and waste products into and out of the vessel. Injury to the endothelium allows capillaries to leak fluid from the intravascular space into the surrounding tissues. Capillary leak reduces venous return (preload) and this, combined with poor heart contractility, leads to a reduced cardiac output and poor delivery of oxygen to the tissues. In addition to fluid resuscitation with a crystalloid solution (normal saline), these infants may also need blood pressure medication to treat hypotension. Infants in septic shock are at high risk for end-organ injury and death.

> **Not infrequently, infants may have a combination of the four types of shock.**

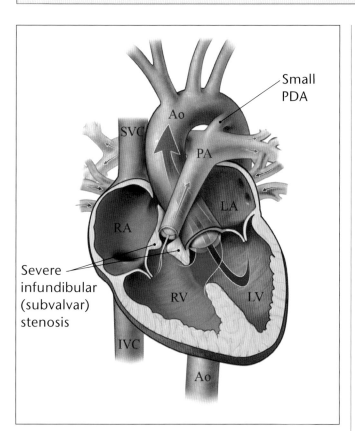

Figure 4.3. Tetralogy of Fallot with severe pulmonary stenosis. The right outflow tract obstruction causes deoxygenated blood to shunt right-to-left through the VSD into the aorta. If the O$_2$ saturation remains less than 75% despite administration of 100% oxygen, then PGE should be considered to establish ductal patency and promote a left-to-right shunt from the aorta to the pulmonary arteries and lungs.

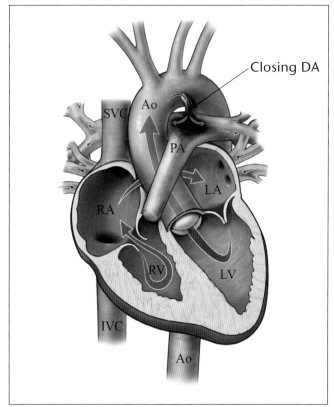

Figure 4.4. Pulmonary atresia with intact ventricular septum with a closing DA. As the DA closes, pulmonary blood flow is significantly decreased. Severe hypoxemia leads to hypoxia and metabolic acidosis. A PGE infusion to maintain open the DA is essential for survival.

Treatment of Shock[8,67,69,70]

The first step in the treatment of shock is to identify the cause and then correct any related or underlying problems that may impair heart function, such as poor cardiac filling because of hypovolemia, anemia, congenital heart disease, tamponade, excessive airway pressure, electrolyte or metabolic disturbances, hypoglycemia, hypoxemia, or arrhythmias. Figure 4.5 illustrates the principles underlying an improvement in the blood pH.

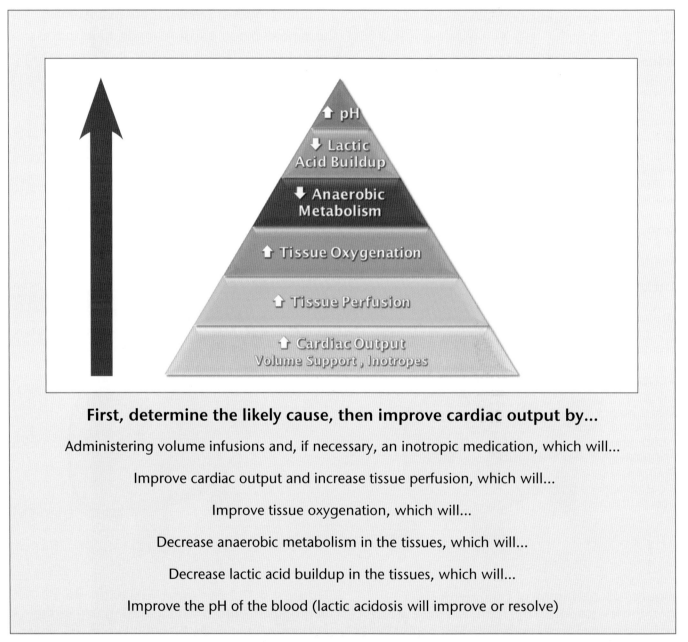

First, determine the likely cause, then improve cardiac output by...

Administering volume infusions and, if necessary, an inotropic medication, which will...

Improve cardiac output and increase tissue perfusion, which will...

Improve tissue oxygenation, which will...

Decrease anaerobic metabolism in the tissues, which will...

Decrease lactic acid buildup in the tissues, which will...

Improve the pH of the blood (lactic acidosis will improve or resolve)

Figure 4.5. Shock treatment goals. Restoring intravascular volume and supporting perfusion, oxygenation, and ventilation is critical when infants are in shock. Oxygen delivery to the tissues must improve to reverse the effects of shock.[1,66]

Treatment of Hypovolemic (Low Blood Volume) Shock[6,66,67,71-73]

The goal of treatment is to improve the circulating blood volume by administering crystalloids, and if there is blood loss, to improve oxygen carrying capacity by administering blood.

If There Is NO Acute Blood Loss

Normal Saline (NS) 0.9% sodium chloride solution

Indications: Volume infusion, to improve preload (circulating blood volume)

Dose: 10 mL per kilogram per dose (10 mL/kg/dose)

Route: IV, UVC, intraosseous

Time interval: Administer over 15 to 30 minutes

Notes:

The administration time is dependent upon the severity of the situation and **may need to be more rapid**.

For treatment of severe shock, it may be necessary to provide two, three, or more volume boluses. Evaluate the infant's response to treatment (changes in heart rate, perfusion, and blood pressure) following each bolus. **Be cautious with giving too much volume** since overdistension of the immature neonatal heart may lead to acute heart failure.

If There IS Acute Blood Loss

Give Normal Saline to begin volume resuscitation while awaiting PRBCs.

Packed Red Blood Cells (PRBCs)

Indications: Treat anemia and improve preload (circulating blood volume)

Dose: 10 mL per kilogram per dose (10 mL/kg/dose)

Route: IV, UVC, intraosseous

Time interval: Administer over 30 minutes to 2 hours (see notes)

Notes:

The administration time is dependent upon the severity of the situation and may need to be as rapid as over 10 to 15 minutes.

If not done already and time allows, obtain the newborn metabolic screen before any blood transfusions, but do not delay giving a transfusion if needed emergently.

 If there is a history of chronic blood loss, some infants in severe shock may not tolerate volume boluses. Consult the tertiary center neonatologist if in doubt about how much and how fast to administer volume.

Example: How to calculate the volume bolus

Desired Dose: 10 mL per kilogram per dose (10 mL/kg/dose)

Weight: 3,100 grams or 3.1 kg

Final Dose: 10 (mL) X 3.1 (kg) = 31 mL

Give 31 mL of volume over 15 to 30 minutes IV, UVC, or intraosseous (IO) route

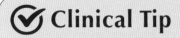 **Clinical Tip**

Emergency transfusion of packed red blood cells (PRBCs) and blood administration in neonates[74-81]

Significant anemia can lead to tissue hypoxia that can be harmful to the infant's organs. During an emergency, Type O-negative PRBCs may be given when time does not allow for crossmatching of blood. **All infants who receive a PRBC transfusion should have blood leukoreduced by filtration before administration.** If an emergency blood transfusion is anticipated (e.g., an emergency cesarean delivery for placental abruption is in progress), it is helpful to notify the blood bank ahead of time to request they prepare a unit of O-negative PRBCs in anticipation the infant may be severely anemic. If a large-volume transfusion is expected, an in-line blood warmer should be used to prevent hypothermia.

Who Should Receive Leukoreduced (Filtered) PRBCs?

All infants who receive a PRBC transfusion should receive filtered PRBCs.

Recommended Staff Assignment

Goal: All staff members will know how to rapidly access PRBCs in an emergency. Knowing how to request and receive blood in an emergency is a patient safety issue. If unsure of the process, call the blood bank and ask the following questions and any additional questions you have:

- Does an order have to be written, or will a verbal order suffice?

- What paperwork, if any, is necessary?

- Who can order the blood (nurses, unit secretary, physician, others)?

- How is the blood sent to the delivery room or nursery/NICU? Does a staff member pick it up?

- How long will it take to receive emergency O-negative PRBCs once requested?

- Is the emergency blood supply available 24 hours per day, 7 days per week?

- Is there a chance that the emergency blood supply can be depleted and then not replenished for 1 or more days?

- Does the blood need to be filtered at the bedside, or does the blood bank filter it? If at the bedside, will the blood be sent with a filter? If not, where are the leukoreduction filters located?

- Are irradiated PRBCs available, and if yes, how long does the irradiation process take?

Clinical Tip ✅

Emergency transfusion of packed red blood cells (PRBCs) and blood administration in neonates[74-81]

Leukoreduction of Red Blood Cells

How blood products are prepared in different countries for administration to infants may vary. In the United States, leukoreduction of red blood cells (i.e., removal of white blood cells) using special filters is a highly efficient method to remove most of the white blood cells from the blood. In the U.S., PRBCs are filtered either soon after collection and before they are stored, after varying periods of storage in the blood bank, or at the bedside using a blood transfusion filter. Leukoreduction performed in the laboratory is subject to quality control, whereas leukoreduction (filtration) at the bedside is not. Filtration with the proper equipment is designed to remove >99.9% of the white blood cells. PRBCs and platelets that are leukoreduced (properly filtered) are considered to be cytomegalovirus (CMV) safe or CMV-reduced risk.

Why is leukocyte reduction important?

CMV infection is especially concerning for very-low-birth weight preterm infants, particularly if the mother is seronegative for CMV because the infant would then lack any immunity to CMV. The risk of acquiring CMV is proportional to the number of WBCs containing CMV virions in the blood product. CMV transmission risk can also be decreased using CMV seronegative donors, but CMV negative blood is not nearly as available as blood that can be leukoreduced by filtration to a safe level for most neonates.

Irradiation of Red Blood Cells in Patients at Risk for Transfusion-Associated Graft Versus Host Disease (TA-GVHD)

Leukoreduction does not remove all the white blood cells (i.e., viable donor lymphocytes) that are capable of replicating and causing transfusion-associated graft versus host disease (TA-GVHD), which can be fatal. Patients at risk for TA-GVHD include but are not limited to preterm infants (<1,200 grams), infants with immunodeficiency such as DiGeorge syndrome, infants with severe combined immunodeficiency, immunosuppression related to chemotherapy or radiation treatment, solid organ transplant recipients, and recipients of intrauterine transfusion. Irradiation prevents lymphocytes from proliferating, thereby reducing the risk that the blood product will cause TA-GVHD. Some facilities also irradiate blood when transfusing directed donor blood into a blood relative, but expert opinion and practice differ in this area. In addition to irradiation, the blood product should also be leukoreduced (filtered) before administering it to the infant.

Treatment of Obstructive Shock[9,13,66,71,82-88]

Pneumothorax

Needle aspiration to remove the air in the pleural cavity may be attempted first and may be all that is necessary to resolve the pneumothorax. If air continually accumulates or the infant fails to improve to a satisfactory level following needle aspiration, a chest tube should be inserted.

Pleural Effusion

Fluid that accumulates in the pleural space can compress the heart and reduce cardiac output. Lung expansion may also be reduced and lead to respiratory failure. Needle aspiration or chest tube drainage may be necessary to remove the fluid.

Cardiac Tamponade

If cardiac tamponade is suspected and the infant is in a *pulseless arrest*, emergently perform needle aspiration of the fluid or air from the pericardial sac. However, if time allows, perform pericardiocentesis guided by echocardiography or ultrasound, including point of care ultrasound (POCUS). Cardiopulmonary resuscitation (CPR) should also be started if clinically indicated.

Congenital Heart Disease (CHD) That Is Ductal-Dependent

If ductal-dependent CHD is suspected, start a continuous intravenous infusion of prostaglandin E1 (PGE) to establish ductal patency. The starting dose varies depending on the infant's age and clinical presentation. Table 4.4 outlines four different clinical situations and the corresponding PGE doses. Figure 4.6 shows the blood flow pattern seen in critical coarctation of the aorta when the DA is closed and then re-opened with a PGE infusion. Detailed information about ductal-dependent congenital heart disease and PGE may be found in the S.T.A.B.L.E. – Cardiac Module manual.[13]

 One serious side effect of PGE is apnea, so continuous cardiorespiratory monitoring is recommended when this medication is used.

Clinical Situation	PGE Dose (micrograms/kg/minute)
Prenatally diagnosed ductal dependent CHD and patient is a newborn (DA is open)	0.01 to 0.03 mcg/kg/minute
CHD was not prenatally diagnosed (DA may not be open or is closing)	Usual starting dose is between 0.05 to 0.1 mcg/kg/minute
Infant is critically ill (severe cyanosis or shock; DA is likely closed or very small)	Reasonable starting dose is 0.1 mcg/kg/minute
NICU management (echocardiogram demonstrates DA is widely open)	Titrate to 0.01 to 0.03 mcg/kg/minute and monitor closely for the desired effect (improved systemic perfusion or improved oxygenation)

Table 4.4. Recommended starting dose of prostaglandin E_1 (PGE) based on four clinical situations.

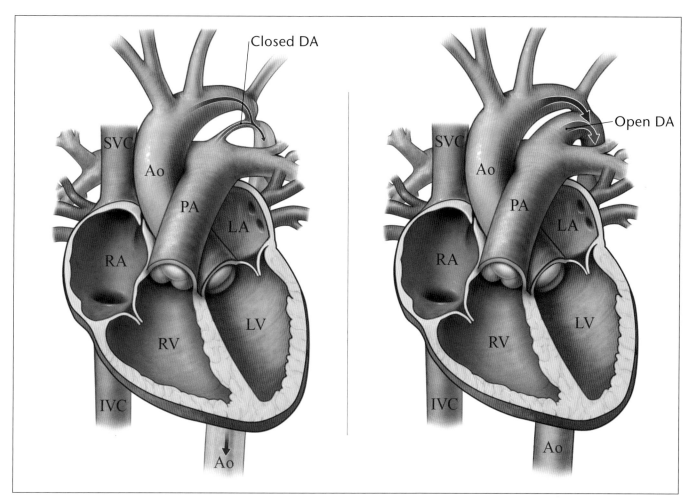

Figure 4.6. Illustrations of coarctation of the aorta (COA) with a closing ductus arteriosus (left side) and a reopened ductus arteriosus (right side). As the ductus arteriosus (DA) closes, the area of coarctation narrows and obstructs blood flow to the systemic circulation.

Reestablishing patency of the DA with a PGE infusion allows blood to flow unobstructed through the aorta as well as shunt right-to-left from the pulmonary artery into the aorta.

Treatment of Cardiogenic (Heart Failure) Shock[6,66,68,71]

Treatment is aimed at correcting the underlying problems that may negatively affect heart function, including the following:

- Hypoxia

- Acidosis

- Hypotension

- Arrhythmias

- Infection

- Electrolyte or mineral imbalances

- Hypoglycemia

- Hypothermia

Pulmonary edema may develop because of poor heart function. Monitor the infant closely during fluid administration to assess whether the patient is tolerating the volume being given. Signs of intolerance may include increased respiratory distress, desaturation, and a worsening of tachycardia.

Treatment of Septic (Distributive) Shock[66,67,69-72,89]

The American College of Critical Care Medicine published clinical practice parameters for hemodynamic support of pediatric and neonatal septic shock.[70] They stressed the importance of rapid recognition of septic shock by using a "*recognition bundle*" and utilizing a best practice "*resuscitation and stabilization bundle.*" In addition to providing respiratory support and hemodynamic monitoring, the resuscitation bundle includes the following:

- Rapid establishment of intravenous access

- Prompt fluid resuscitation with a crystalloid solution (10 mL/kg/dose)

- Prompt administration of antibiotics

- Provision of a blood pressure medication (inotrope)

Infants with septic shock usually require repeated administration of isotonic intravenous normal saline to support their blood pressure. PRBCs are given to treat anemia and improve oxygen delivery to the tissues. Fresh frozen plasma can be given if clotting studies are abnormal or there is active bleeding. Inotropic medicatons used to treat septic shock may include dopamine (in combination with dobutamine at times), epinephrine, or norepinephrine. Adrenal insufficiency is treated with hydrocortisone. Table 4.5 provides additional information about dopamine administration, and page 201 describes how to mix dopamine for continuous infusion if a pharmacist is unavailable to prepare it.

Persistent pulmonary hypertension of the newborn (PPHN) and respiratory failure often complicate the care of infants with septic shock. An inborn error of metabolism may present very similarly to septic shock and, therefore, should be considered in the initial diagnostic workup.

Medications Used to Treat Cardiogenic and Septic Shock

Normal Saline (NS) 0.9% sodium chloride solution

Indications: Volume infusion to improve preload (circulating blood volume)

Dose: The dose recommendations are the same as for hypovolemic shock: 10 mL/kg per dose

Route: IV, UVC, Intraosseous

Dopamine Hydrochloride[1,66,67,71,90]

Indications: Poor cardiac contractility

Dose: 5 to 20 micrograms per kg per minute (mcg/kg/minute)

Route: IV continuous infusion (IV pump)

Additional inotropes used to treat shock may include milrinone, dobutamine, epinephrine, or norepinephrine.

Table 4.5. Dopamine dose and effect.

Dose	Receptors Stimulated	Effect
Low: 1 to 4 mcg/kg/min	Dopaminergic receptors	Renal, coronary, mesenteric vasodilation
Intermediate: 5 to 15 mcg/kg/min	Dopaminergic and beta$_1$-adrenergic receptors	Increase in cardiac contractility and output, blood pressure, and heart rate
High: >15 mcg/kg/min	Alpha-adrenergic receptors	Systemic vasoconstriction and increase in blood pressure; pulmonary vasoconstriction

✓ Clinical Tip — *What is the difference between crystalloids and colloids?[66]*

Crystalloid solutions, such as normal saline and lactated Ringer's, are isotonic and contain water and electrolytes. Crystalloids pass easily through semi-permeable membranes and stay in the intravascular (circulating) compartment for shorter periods of time than colloids. The advantages of crystalloid solutions are that they are inexpensive, readily available for the immediate treatment of shock, and require no special compatibility testing. Colloid solutions, such as 5% albumin and fresh frozen plasma (FFP), have a large molecular weight and do not pass easily through semi-permeable membranes. Consequently, they stay in the intravascular (circulating) compartment longer than crystalloids. Albumin is sometimes administered when there is a low albumin concentration in the blood. The disadvantages of colloids include a longer preparation time, higher cost, and the possibility of sensitivity reactions (FFP) and necessary compatibility testing (FFP) before they can be administered.

Rules for Dopamine Infusion

1 Provide normal saline volume boluses before determining dopamine (or another inotrope) is necessary. In addition, inotropic medications will be more effective if hypovolemia is treated first.[91]

2 Dopamine is usually started at 5 mcg/kg/minute and can be titrated up or down by 1 mcg/kg/minute increments to achieve the desired effect. A maximum dose of 20 mcg/kg/minute is usually recommended, but some care teams may not exceed 15 mcg/kg/minute. See page 202 for a simplified infusion graph when the dopamine is mixed to yield a concentration of 800 mcg/mL of IV fluid.

3 If an arterial line is present, monitor the BP continuously. If an arterial line is not present, monitor the BP by cuff measurement every 1 to 2 minutes for 15 minutes, then every 2 to 5 minutes, depending upon the response to the medication. The BP monitoring interval can be lengthened as clinically able. Continuously monitor heart rate and oxygen saturation and notify the infant's care team if the infant shows signs of deterioration.

4 Never infuse dopamine or any inotropic medication through any arterial site (umbilical artery catheter, peripheral arterial line).

5 Infuse dopamine on an infusion pump and use "smart pump" technology whenever possible to increase safely.

6 **Do not flush** dopamine or lines containing dopamine, as this will cause the blood pressure to surge and the heart rate to abruptly slow.

7 Since IV infiltration may lead to tissue sloughing and necrosis, it is recommended that dopamine be administered through a central venous line (UVC or PICC).

- If no central venous access is available, infuse dopamine through a peripheral IV.
- If infused through a peripheral IV, monitor the infusion site closely. If infiltration occurs, and there is concern that dermal necrosis may develop, phentolamine can be administered to counteract the vasoactive effect of dopamine.

Do not give dopamine via any arterial route (umbilical or peripheral artery) or through an endotracheal tube.

Dopamine Hydrochloride—How to Calculate a Final Standardized Concentration of 800 Micrograms per mL IV Fluid

In some settings, a pharmacist is not available to prepare and dispense high-risk medications, such as dopamine. Therefore, the following information is provided for situations where a pharmacist may not be available and where nurses and physicians may be inexperienced with administering dopamine. In recognition of this clinical challenge, The S.T.A.B.L.E. Program recommends the use of a final dopamine infusion concentration that is relatively diluted (i.e., 800 mcg/mL IV fluid). In NICUs where dopamine is used more frequently, a more concentrated solution is usually prepared, and the rate of increase (or decrease) is usually limited to 1 mcg/kg/minute each time the rate is changed.

Step 1. Select the pre-mixed dopamine solution as described in Option One or mix the solution as described in Option Two.

Option One

Use this option when a commercially-prepared pre-mixed dopamine drip solution with a final concentration of 800 micrograms (mcg) per milliliter (mL) in D_5W **IS** available.

- Please note that this solution is mixed in D_5W. Monitor the infant's blood glucose closely and adjust the maintenance dextrose infusion (concentration and/or rate) as necessary to maintain a normal blood sugar.

- To determine the appropriate rate, go to Step 2 on page 202.

- Always administer dopamine using an infusion pump.

Option Two

Use this option when a commercially prepared pre-mixed dopamine solution IS NOT available. Mix the dopamine drip as follows:

1. Select a dopamine vial containing dopamine 40 milligrams (mg) per mL.

2. From this vial, draw up 5 mL (equals 200 mg) of dopamine.

3. Add this amount (5 mL or 200 mg of dopamine) to a 250 mL bag of $D_{10}W$.

4. This amount of dopamine will provide a dopamine concentration of 800 mcg per mL of IV fluid (or 200 mg per 250 mL IV fluid).

5. Label the IV bag with the following: This 250 mL bag of $D_{10}W$ contains 800 mcg dopamine per mL IV fluid.

6. Always administer dopamine using an infusion pump.

If a pre-mixed dopamine solution is not available, place the following items in a plastic bag or container and keep with emergency medications:

- 250 mL bag of $D_{10}W$

- A 5 mL syringe

- Dopamine hydrochloride 40 mg/mL solution (5 ml vial = 200 mg)

- This instructional information

Ordered Dose (mcg/kg/min) Using a dopamine solution containing 800 mcg per mL of IV fluid							
Weight in kg	5 mcg/kg/min	7.5 mcg/kg/min	10 mcg/kg/min	12.5 mcg/kg/min	15 mcg/kg/min	17.5 mcg/kg/min	20 mcg/kg/min
0.5 kg	0.2 mL/hr	0.3 mL/hr	0.4 mL/hr	0.5 mL/hr	0.6 mL/hr	0.7 mL/hr	0.8 mL/hr
1 kg	0.4 mL/hr	0.6 mL/hr	0.8 mL/hr	1 mL/hr	1.1 mL/hr	1.3 mL/hr	1.5 mL/hr
1.5 kg	0.6 mL/hr	0.8 mL/hr	1.1 mL/hr	1.4 mL/hr	1.7 mL/hr	2 mL/hr	2.3 mL/hr
2 kg	0.8 mL/hr	1.1 mL/hr	1.5 mL/hr	1.9 mL/hr	2.3 mL/hr	2.6 mL/hr	3 mL/hr
2.5 kg	1 mL/hr	1.4 mL/hr	1.9 mL/hr	2.3 mL/hr	2.8 mL/hr	3.3 mL/hr	3.8 mL/hr
3 kg	1.1 mL/hr	1.7 mL/hr	2.3 mL/hr	2.8 mL/hr	3.4 mL/hr	3.9 mL/hr	4.5 mL/hr
3.5 kg	1.3 mL/hr	2 mL/hr	2.6 mL/hr	3.3 mL/hr	3.9 mL/hr	4.6 mL/hr	5.3 mL/hr
4 kg	1.5 mL/hr	2.3 mL/hr	3 mL/hr	3.8 mL/hr	4.5 mL/hr	5.3 mL/hr	6 mL/hr
4.5 kg	1.7 mL/hr	2.5 mL/hr	3.4 mL/hr	4.2 mL/hr	5.1 mL/hr	5.9 mL/hr	6.8 mL/hr
5 kg	1.9 mL/hr	2.8 mL/hr	3.8 mL/hr	4.7 mL/hr	5.6 mL/hr	6.6 mL/hr	7.5 mL/hr

Note:
Some rounding has occurred to simplify the infusion rate.

Step 2. Using the table, select the infusion rate.

1. Find the **patient's weight** in the first column marked **Weight in kg**. Round up or down as needed if the weight is in between the 0.5 kilogram increments.

2. Read across the row to the ordered infusion dose in mcg/kg/min.

3. The result is the infusion pump setting in **mL/hr**.

4. Double-check all calculations and reconstitution with another nurse or physician before administering dopamine to the infant.

Practice session: Dopamine rate

A dopamine standardized concentration of 800 mcg per mL IV fluid has been prepared.

Using the infusion graph above, answer the following questions:

1. A dose of 10 mcg/kg/minute of dopamine is ordered for a 3.8 kg infant. What continuous infusion rate will this infant require? _____mL/hour

2. A dose of 5 mcg/kg/minute of dopamine is ordered for a 1.4 kg infant. What infusion rate will this infant require? _____mL/hour

Check your answers below.

Answers
1. 3 mL/hour   2. 0.6 mL/hour

Appendix 4.1 Scalp Swellings: Caput Succedaneum, Cephalohematoma, and Subgaleal Hemorrhage[63,92-101]

Scalp swelling is a common finding in newborn infants. Three types of extracranial swelling can occur: caput succedaneum, cephalohematoma, and subgaleal hemorrhage.

Normal Scalp Anatomy

The word "scalp" is an acronym; from outer to inner, the scalp consists of the skin, connective tissue, aponeurosis (galea), loose connective tissue (subgaleal), and periosteum.

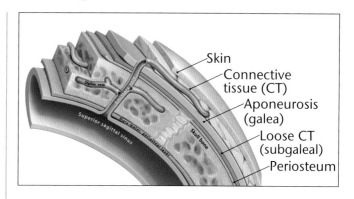

Skin
Connective tissue (CT)
Aponeurosis (galea)
Loose CT (subgaleal)
Periosteum

Caput Succedaneum

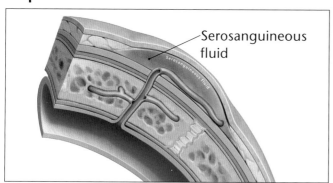

Serosanguineous fluid

Soft tissue edema of the scalp develops due to the pressure of the head against the slowly dilating cervix during labor contractions. The swelling is superficial and is composed of serosanguineous fluid that is usually limited to the part of the scalp that was the presenting part. The edema may cross suture lines and shift with changes in the infant's position. Bruising may also be present. The edema may be significant enough to obscure the sutures and fontanel. The caput is usually largest just after birth, then recedes over time, and disappears within a few days. If the edema does not recede by 72 hours or there is a decline in the level of consciousness, further investigation, including skull imaging, may be necessary.

Cephalohematoma

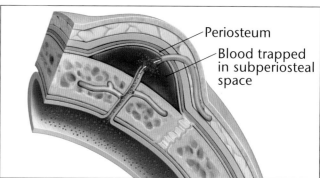

Periosteum
Blood trapped in subperiosteal space

The shearing forces of labor and delivery can rupture the diploic or emissary blood vessels and lead to bleeding beneath the periosteum, which is a fibrous membrane that lines the skull bones. A cephalohematoma occurs more frequently in primiparous mothers and/or when there has been a difficult or prolonged labor or when delivery was assisted by vacuum or forceps. Bleeding is unilateral in 85% of cases and is usually over the parietal bone, but it can also be over the occipital bone. Bleeding beneath the periosteum may be slow, and the cephalohematoma may not appear for several hours or days after birth. Because the periosteum limits the extension of bleeding, the swelling does not cross suture lines, making it easier to diagnose. Initially, the swelling may feel fluctuant and then slowly become firmer. There is an occasional association of a linear (nondepressed) skull fracture; therefore, additional imaging (skull X-ray and/or CT scan) may be indicated. In rare cases, the bleeding can be severe enough to cause anemia. The infant should be monitored for hyperbilirubinemia. Although rare, bacterial infection of the cephalohematoma may occur, usually in association with septicemia and meningitis. Calcification that requires neurosurgical removal is another complication. A cephalohematoma usually resolves within 2 to 12 weeks but may take as long as 6 months to resolve completely.

Subgaleal Hemorrhage

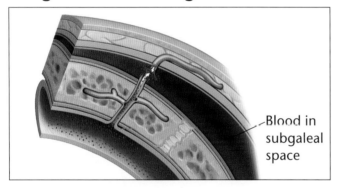

Blood in subgaleal space

Emissary veins drain blood from the scalp to the heart. Subgaleal hemorrhage (SGH) occurs when the emissary veins rupture and bleed into the subgaleal space (aponeurosis galea) that overlies the periosteum. Because there is nothing to impede blood once it seeps into this space, the infant's entire blood volume (240 to 260 mL) can bleed into the subgaleal space. The bleeding can be slow and insidious with a characteristic diffuse, fluctuant accumulation (i.e., a fluid wave) that is felt when palpating the scalp. A study that used magnetic resonance imaging (MRI) to evaluate study patients with SGH found that serous fluid also collects in this space, which explains why some infants can have SGH without significant cardiovascular compromise while others may have significant blood loss and develop severe hypovolemic shock and require blood product transfusions.

When the neonate has signs of encephalopathy, then SGH is associated with an adverse neurological outcome.

The subgaleal space extends from the orbits of the eyes to the nape of the neck. One characteristic finding of subgaleal hemorrhage is the lateral spreading of edema toward the ears, which may displace the ears anteriorly (shown in the photo on page 205). Swelling around the eyes is also present in some cases.

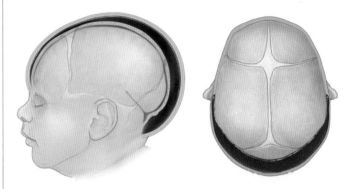

SGH can occur following spontaneous and cesarean delivery, although, with cesarean delivery, the incidence of SGH is not increased unless the patient is in labor first.[102] When delivery is assisted by vacuum or forceps (i.e., an operative vaginal delivery), the risk for SGH increases. There are specific maternal and fetal indications for operative vaginal delivery and guidelines for when it is safe to apply the vacuum or forceps, how to perform the procedure correctly, how many pop-offs should be permitted (understanding that no safe number has been established), how many minutes the procedure should be allowed to continue, and importantly, when to abandon the attempt.[94] Following operative vaginal delivery, bleeding may also occur in the subdural, subarachnoid, intraparenchymal, and intraventricular regions.

Risk Factors Associated With the Development of SGH

- Nulliparity

- Prolonged second stage of labor

- Vacuum suction applied for >20 minutes

- Sequential use of vacuum and forceps (increases the risk for both infant and maternal injury and should be avoided)[103]

- Vacuum-assisted delivery with two or more pop-offs (although no safe number has been established)

Pop-offs are usually related to an improperly placed cup. After a vacuum-assisted delivery, inspect the scalp for where the cup mark is located, as improper cup placement may be a clue that scalp injury has occurred.

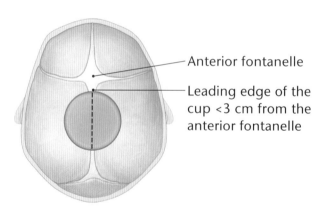

Anterior fontanelle

Leading edge of the cup <3 cm from the anterior fontanelle

Deflexing cup application

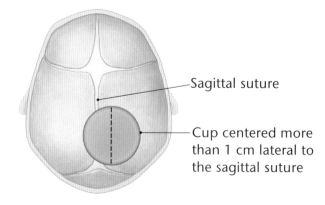

Sagittal suture

Cup centered more than 1 cm lateral to the sagittal suture

Paramedian cup application

If there was a difficult delivery, such as a prolonged second stage, or if vacuum assistance was required, then neonatal caregivers should be made aware so they may assess the infant and monitor for complications. S.T.A.B.L.E. recommends hourly monitoring of the following for at least 8 hours:

- Any concerning change in the level of consciousness

- Vital signs and oxygen saturation

- A change in skin color, such as the appearance of pallor

- Increase in head circumference

- Location and characteristics of scalp swelling

Treatment of subgaleal hemorrhage may include any or all of the following to treat anemia, stop the bleeding, and restore the blood pressure:

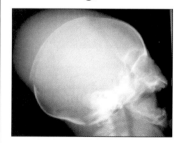

PRBCs, fresh frozen plasma, platelets, cryoprecipitate, normal saline volume infusions, and dopamine.

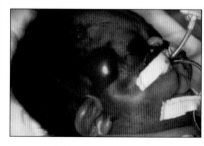

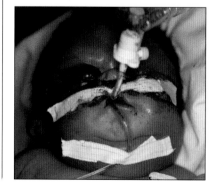

Top image is a skull X-ray of this infant with a severe subgaleal hemorrhage. This infant required numerous blood product transfusions to stabilize. The infant's outcome is unknown.

Lab Work Module

Sugar

Temperature

Airway

Blood Pressure

Lab Work

Emotional Support

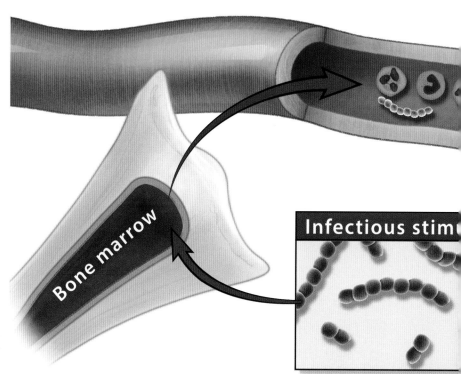

Bone marrow

Infectious stim

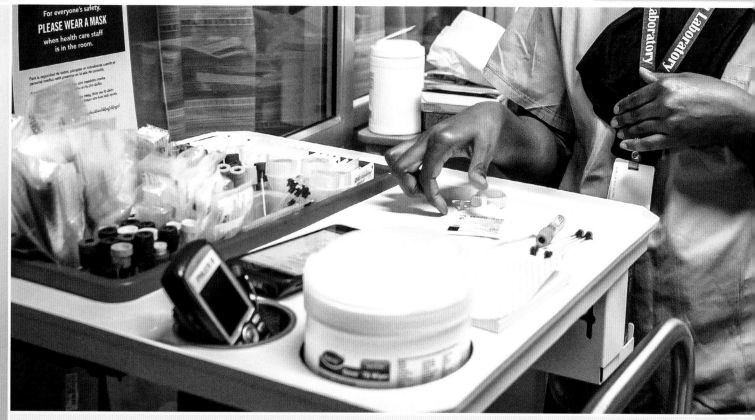

For everyone's safety,
PLEASE WEAR A MASK
when health care staff
is in the room.

Lab Work—Module Objectives

Upon completion of this module, participants will gain an increased understanding of:

1. Why neonates are more vulnerable to infection than older infants and children.

2. The clinical signs of neonatal sepsis.

3. Bacterial and viral organisms that may cause infection.

4. Perinatal and postnatal risk factors that predispose neonates to infection.

5. Initial laboratory tests to obtain in the pre-transport / post-resuscitation period.

6. White blood cell (WBC) development and how neutrophils respond to an infection.

7. The initial antibiotic treatment for neonates with suspected sepsis.

The term sepsis is used interchangeably with infection in this module.

Key Concepts

1 The Immature Neonatal Immune System Increases the Risk for Infection

Exposure to an infectious agent activates a complex series of responses to identify, neutralize, and eliminate the invading organism. Neonates have an immature immune system and an impaired ability to effectively eliminate invading organisms.[1-3] Preterm infants are at an even greater disadvantage than term infants.* The younger the gestation, the higher the risk for infection and adverse outcome.[4-7] Neonatal sepsis may lead to significant long-term morbidity, including central nervous system injury, developmental delays, visual impairment, and in severe cases, death.[6] For these important reasons, evaluation for and treatment of suspected sepsis is a top priority in the pre-transport / post-resuscitation period.[8]

2 Signs of Sepsis May Mimic Other Noninfectious Conditions

One challenge encountered when trying to diagnose neonatal sepsis is that infected infants often present with nonspecific signs that are commonly seen with noninfectious conditions, such as transient tachypnea of the newborn (TTN) and respiratory distress syndrome (RDS), congenital heart disease, or inborn errors of metabolism.[9-11] Compared with TTN or RDS, neonatal sepsis is rare. Yet, the infant's initial presentation may be so similar to a respiratory or other illness that clinicians often err on the side of caution because of the devastating effects of delayed treatment of infection.[1,12]

*The term "infant" is used interchangeably with "neonate" in this module.

Respiratory Distress

- Apnea
- Tachypnea, retractions, nasal flaring, grunting
- Cyanosis
- Development of an oxygen requirement or an increase in oxygen requirement and/or ventilator support

 Abnormal Temperature

- Hypothermia (more common) and hyperthermia (less common)
- Persistent fever (especially concerning as a presenting sign for neonatal sepsis, including viral infection)

 Gastrointestinal Signs

- Poor feeding, disinterest in feeding, or weak suck
- Vomiting
- Abdominal distension
- Diarrhea

 Cardiovascular Signs

- Tachycardia, bradycardia
- Hypotension
- Poor perfusion, prolonged capillary refill time, skin mottling
- Pale or gray skin color

 Abnormal Neurologic Status

- Irritability
- Increased sleepiness
- Lethargy
- Hypotonia
- Seizures

 Abnormal Skin Findings or Bleeding Problems

- Vesicles (skin or mucous membranes)
- Oozing from puncture sites, unexplained bruising, petechiae
- Purpura (viral infection, sepsis, coagulation defect)
- Omphalitis (periumbilical erythema)
- Cellulitis
- Soft tissue swelling and/or redness

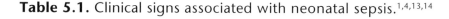

Table 5.1. Clinical signs associated with neonatal sepsis.[1,4,13,14]

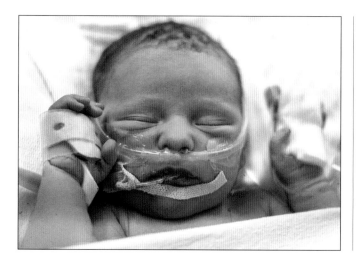

Early-Onset and Late-Onset Sepsis

An infection acquired before 72 hours of age is called *early-onset sepsis (EOS),* and an infection acquired after 72 hours is called *late-onset sepsis (LOS).*[1,5] Most infants with EOS have signs of infection within the first 24 to 48 hours after birth.[11,12] Poor feeding or disinterest in feeding and lethargy may be early signs of sepsis.[1] Table 5.1 summarizes signs that may be seen when an infant has an infection.

Pathogens

Infants can become infected with bacteria, viruses, fungi, or other pathogens. Group B Streptococcus (a Gram-positive organism) and Escherichia coli (a Gram-negative organism) are the two most common organisms that cause early-onset bacterial infection.[4,13,15,16] In the U.S., a large study of more than 200,000 babies reported the bacterial organisms that caused EOS. These organisms are listed in Table 5.2.

Table 5.2. Bacterial organisms that cause EOS in preterm and term infants, from higher to lower frequency of the infecting bacteria.[7]

Gram-Positive Organisms	Gram-Negative Organisms
Group B Streptococcus (GBS)	Escherichia coli
Enterococcus species	Haemophilus species
Group A Streptococcus	Klebsiella species
Viridans streptococci	Morganella morganii
Streptococcus bovis	Citrobacter species
Streptococcus species	Enterobacter species
Streptococcus pneumoniae	Flavobacterium species
Coagulase-negative staphylococci	Proteus species
Listeria monocytogenes	Pseudomonas species
Staphylococcus aureus	

 Let's Learn More... **What does Gram-positive and Gram-negative mean?**[17]

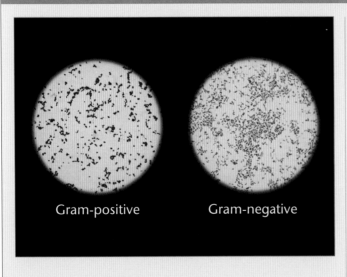

Gram-positive   Gram-negative

Gram staining refers to a bacterial staining procedure that was developed by a Danish bacteriologist, Hans Christian Gram, in 1883. Gram staining is the first step in identifying an organism. The procedure allows differentiation of bacteria into one of two categories—positive or negative. The determination is based on color change. Organisms that stain a blue/purple color (because they retain the stain applied to them) are Gram-positive bacteria. Organisms that stain a pink/reddish color (because they lose their color when the destaining step is performed) are Gram-negative bacteria.

Viral Infection[13,18,19]

Viral infection may occur anytime during pregnancy or after delivery. Viruses that cause infection in the fetus or newborn include but are not limited to **herpes simplex virus (HSV), human immunodeficiency virus (HIV), cytomegalovirus (CMV), varicella, adenovirus, enterovirus, Zika virus, coronavirus, hepatitis, human parvovirus B19, and rubella.**

Infection during the first trimester may severely impact fetal growth and organ development. In addition to significantly increased risk for intrauterine growth restriction, the neonate may also have visual, hearing, brain, cardiac, and/ or liver damage. Late pregnancy, intrapartum, or postpartum viral exposure may result from maternal or family illness that presents with diarrhea, vomiting, and/or respiratory symptoms. It is important when taking the maternal medical history to ask about early gestation viral exposure, as well as recent viral illness in siblings, other family members, and the mother.

 When an infant is unwell, attention is commonly directed at bacterial infection as the cause. It is important to also consider viral infection by carefully evaluating the maternal history for viral exposure during any of the trimesters.

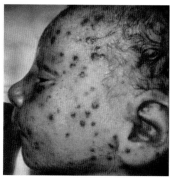

Photo courtesy Dr. David A. Clark

"Blueberry muffin" lesions secondary to extramedullary hematopoiesis in an infant with congenital CMV. These lesions may also be observed with congenital rubella syndrome and other viral infections.

Herpes Viral Infection

Herpes simplex virus (HSV) type 1 or 2 may be present in the maternal genital tract without the pregnant person knowing they have an infection. A negative history of HSV exposure is not uncommon, since asymptomatic viral shedding is possible.[18,20-22] Globally, neonatal HSV infection is estimated to occur in 1 in 10,000 live births, with the highest rates in Africa.[23] In the United States, HSV infection occurs in approximately 1 in 2,000 to 1 in 3,000 live births.[18,21]

 Infants exposed to HSV may develop clinical signs at any time between birth and 6 weeks of age, with most presenting within the first month after birth.[18,22]

Risk of transmitting HSV to the infant[18,21,22,24]

- If the pregnant person acquires a first-episode, primary genital infection near the time of delivery, the risk of transmitting the infection to the infant is estimated between 25 to 60%.

- If the pregnant person has recurrent HSV or if they acquired HSV in the first half of their pregnancy and the infection is reactivated, the risk of transmitting HSV to the infant is approximately 2% because of protective maternal antibodies.

Both type 1 and type 2 HSV infection can present in newborns in one of three ways:[21,22,24]

1) Disease limited to the skin, eyes, and/or mouth (SEM)—occurs in approximately 45% of cases.

2) Central nervous system (CNS) disease (encephalitis), although the skin, eyes, and/ or mouth may also be involved—occurs in approximately 30% of cases.

3) Disseminated disease involving multiple organs, including the liver, adrenal glands, and lungs—occurs in approximately 25% of cases. Skin vesicles may be absent in up to 40 to 50% of these infants. The CNS is involved in about 60 to 70% of cases. Infants with disseminated disease are critically ill with shock, extensive liver and lung involvement, and disseminated intravascular coagulation (DIC). **The risk of dying is highest in these infants.**

Signs of HSV infection[19,21,22,24]

Signs may include skin vesicles; however, some infants with HSV infection never develop skin lesions. Other signs may include fever, poor feeding, lethargy, irritability, or seizures. Fever, especially in the first 4 weeks after birth, should raise suspicion for HSV infection. If the history and/or presentation suggests HSV infection, treatment with an antiviral medication such as Acyclovir should be started while awaiting culture and/or polymerase chain reaction (PCR) testing. If HSV infection is diagnosed, antiviral therapy is usually given for 2 to 3 weeks, but in some cases, treatment may need to be longer.[21,24]

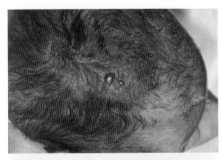

Herpes vesicles on the scalp.

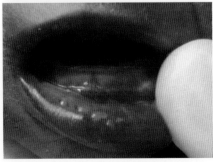

Herpes vesicles in the mouth.

Photos courtesy Dr. David A. Clark

Risk Factors for Sepsis

Infection can begin prior to birth (*intrauterine infection*), during the birth process (*intrapartum infection*), or after birth from various causes, including from the mother, the hospital environment, hospital personnel, or post-birth procedures.[13] Perinatal risk factors for neonatal infection are summarized in Table 5.3.

Microorganisms can enter the amniotic cavity and infect the fetus in several ways.

Ascending Infection[25]

As shown in Figure 5.1, the most common route for fetal infection is when microorganisms ascend from the vagina and cervix into the intrauterine cavity and eventually pass through the amnion into the amniotic fluid. Ascending infection can occur even if the membranes are not ruptured. Presence of bacteria in the amniotic fluid (stage 3) may lead to infection of the fetus by several ports of entry: the oropharynx (where it is swallowed), ears, eyes, lungs, and umbilical cord. If the fetus is distressed in utero and gasps, infected fluid can be inhaled deeply into the lungs and cause pneumonia, bacteremia, and sepsis.[4,26]

Transplacental Infection

Another route of infection is from the maternal bloodstream to the placenta, then on to the fetus. Bacterial infection may present with severe sepsis at birth. Viral infection in early gestation increases the risk for miscarriage, stillbirth, and congenital malformations.

Invasive Procedures

Infection may occur by accidental introduction of bacteria during invasive procedures, such as amniocentesis, chorionic villus sampling, or percutaneous fetal blood sampling.[27]

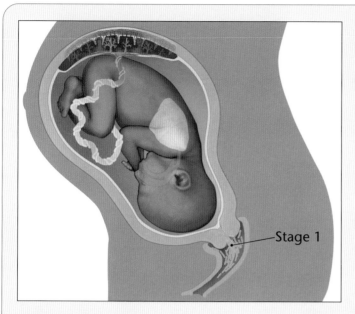

Stage 1: Pathologic bacteria ascends from the vagina to the cervix.

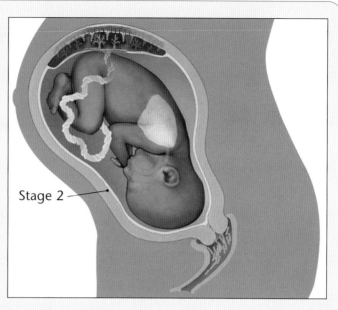

Stage 2: The bacteria gains access to the intrauterine cavity and may be located in the chorioamniotic membranes.

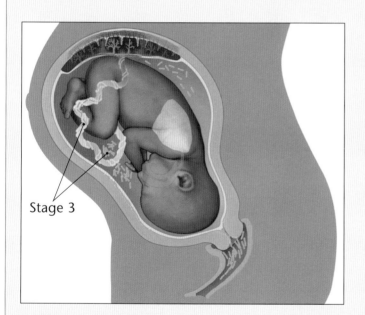

Stage 3: The bacteria invade the fetal vessels and/or penetrate through the amnion into the amniotic fluid.

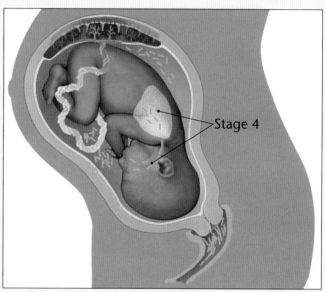

Stage 4: Fetal infection may occur by several ports of entry: oropharynx, ears, eyes, lungs, and umbilical cord.

Note: The green color in the illustrations represent bacteria.

Figure 5.1. Ascending infection from the vagina into the amniotic cavity, leading to an intraamniotic infection. Premature rupture of membranes and preterm labor are commonly associated with intraamniotic infection. Fetal infection can occur by several ports of entry: the oropharynx, ears, eyes, lungs, and umbilical cord.

Table 5.3. Perinatal risk factors for neonatal infection.[1,4,8,13,15,26,28-30]

- Prematurity and low birth weight.
- Preterm labor.
- Preterm premature rupture of membranes (Preterm PROM; before labor begins).
- Prolonged rupture of membranes (ROM) >18 hours.
- Maternal GBS colonization.
- Intraamniotic infection* (also referred to as chorioamnionitis):[25,30,31]
  - Markedly elevated maternal intrapartum temperature ≥39°C (102.2°F).
  - Maternal temperature 38 to 38.9°C (100.4°F to 102°F) **and** one or more of the following: fetal tachycardia >160 BPM for ≥10 minutes, elevated maternal WBC count, purulent discharge from the cervical os, or evidence of microbial invasion of the amniotic cavity (biochemical or microbiologic fluid results).
- Recent maternal infection or illness.
- Maternal genitourinary tract infection, including urinary tract infection and sexually transmitted diseases.

- Intrapartum fetal distress:
  - Fetal tachycardia, meconium-stained amniotic fluid, and severe depression at birth may indicate the infant has acquired an infection in utero and/or is at increased risk for EOS.
  - If the fetus gasps in-utero, infected amniotic fluid may be inhaled into the lungs and cause pneumonia, bacteremia, and sepsis.[4,26]

Procedures

- **Prior to delivery**—accidental introduction of bacteria into the amniotic cavity during invasive procedures, such as amniocentesis and chorionic villous sampling.
- **Instrumentation at delivery**—vacuum assist, placement of a fetal scalp electrode.
- **After delivery**—intravenous and central lines, endotracheal intubation, mechanical ventilation, needle thoracentesis, and other invasive procedures.

* For more infomation, see page 216: *Let's Learn More...Will "Triple I" replace the term chrorioamnionitis?*

✅ Clinical Tip | *Why is blood culture volume so important?*

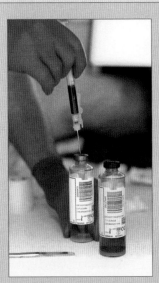

The blood culture is the gold standard for detecting bacteria in the bloodstream. As many as one-quarter of all infants with sepsis have a very small number of bacteria in their blood (≤4 colony-forming units [CFU]/mL).[8] The chance that bacteria will grow in the sample increases *significantly* when at least 1 mL of blood is placed in the culture bottle(s).[15,32-34]

Modern microbiology labs incubate blood culture bottles in automated machines that continuously monitor for bacterial growth. The culture media that the blood is placed in has special ingredients to help neutralize any antibiotics that may have been given, as well as to break up the WBCs to release any bacteria that may have been engulfed. These machines can detect growth of even very small amounts of bacteria, providing the inoculum (blood volume added to culture) is sufficient.[4,15] To avoid contamination of the culture, prepare the infant's skin with an antibacterial solution, then follow your hospital's protocol for preparing the culture bottle and transferring the blood.

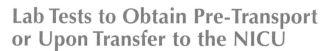

Lab Tests to Obtain Pre-Transport or Upon Transfer to the NICU

The following four laboratory tests may help guide initial care. See Appendices 5.1 and 5.2 for additional laboratory tests that may be ordered post-transport/transfer.

Complete Blood Count (CBC)[35]

- A CBC is one of the most commonly obtained tests in newborns to assess the white blood cell (WBC) count and differential, hemoglobin, hematocrit, erythrocyte indices, and platelet count.

- A CBC may provide helpful information to assess the infants' response to an infection and identify other treatable causes of deterioration, such as severe anemia, polycythemia, or thrombocytopenia.

Blood Culture[1,4,32,33]

- Obtain **at least 1 mL of blood** per culture bottle. This culture volume is critically important, as it improves the chance that bacteria will grow in the sample.

- For EOS evaluation, if only able to obtain 1 mL of blood, then request approval from the infant's care team to place the full 1 mL in the aerobic bottle only.[34] Ensure the care team approves not obtaining blood for the anaerobic culture bottle.

- Blood cultures are usually monitored for 5 days, although longer times are sometimes requested.

- Use sterile technique when drawing the culture and transferring the blood into the culture bottle.

- Obtain the culture before starting antibiotics.

 If having difficulty obtaining a blood culture, contact the infant's care team to report the situation and request assistance.

Blood Glucose (Sugar)

- Sick infants are at increased risk for abnormal glucose levels (both high and low) secondary to various causes, including poor feeding, respiratory distress, genetic disorders, infection, and/or shock.

- Achieve glucose stability, as able, between 50 mg/dL (2.8 mmol/L) and 100 mg/dL (5.6 mmol/L).

Blood Gas

- Infants with an infection often have some respiratory distress and a supplemental oxygen requirement.

- Infants with an advanced infection may be in shock. In combination with an exam and consideration of the suspected disease process, a blood gas will help guide cardiovascular and respiratory support.

- Assess the pH, PCO_2, bicarbonate, and base deficit to determine if the blood gas is abnormal from respiratory, metabolic, or both causes. If the blood gas is a capillary or venous sample, utilize pulse oximetry to evaluate oxygenation status.

When concerned about LOS, or an infection that occurs >72 hours after birth, other sources of infection can include the urine or cerebrospinal fluid. Obtaining cultures from these sites, in addition to the blood, is important to aid in the identification of the invading microorganism and to help select the appropriate antimicrobial medication and duration of therapy. Lastly, it is important to recognize that cultures may not be as helpful, although they are obtained as part of a sepsis work-up, when an infection is in the lung (pneumonia), bone (osteomyelitis), or intestine (necrotizing enterocolitis). Regional differences exist regarding other screening labs to help assess for infection. These labs include a CBC, C-reactive protein (CRP), procalcitonin, and interleukin-6 (IL-6).[36-38]

Let's Learn More... Will "Triple I" replace the term chorioamnionitis?

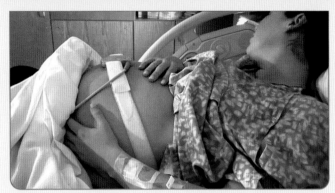

This information is provided to acquaint perinatal caregivers with terminology that might be encountered when providing care to obstetric and neonatal patients.

The terms intraamniotic infection and chorioamnionitis are often used interchangeably; however, this is a complicated topic because not all chorioamnionitis is caused by infection.[39] The American College of Obstetricians and Gynecologists (ACOG) describe intraamniotic infection as infection that results in inflammation of any combination of the amniotic fluid, placenta, fetus, fetal membranes, or decidua.[30] Most infections occur by bacteria that ascend from the vagina into the amniotic cavity. In rare circumstances, infection may occur via the maternal bloodstream if there is a systemic infection or following invasive procedures such as amniocentesis or chorionic villus sampling. One to 3% of infants will develop neonatal sepsis. Preterm birth is a common outcome and contributes heavily to the morbidity associated with chorioamnionitis: increased risk for bronchopulmonary dysplasia, retinopathy of prematurity, and cerebral palsy.[29] Maternal consequences of intraamniotic infection include dysfunctional labor that may need additional intervention, postpartum hemorrhage secondary to uterine atony, postpartum infection (endometritis, peritonitis, urinary tract infection, pyelonephritis, perineal and wound infection, sepsis), readmission, adult respiratory distress syndrome, and in rare circumstances, death.[40,41]

In 2015, a panel of U.S. maternal and neonatal experts were assembled by the National Institute of Child Health and Human Development (NICHD) to discuss the topic of chorioamnionitis. This expert panel suggested replacing the word chorioamnionitis with a descriptive term: "intrauterine inflammation or infection or both," abbreviated "Triple I."[42]

The rationale for the recommendation to change to "Triple I" included the following:

1) The term "chorioamnionitis" is outdated and implies infection is present. "Chorioamnionitis" triggers investigations and management decisions in the pregnant patient and infant without probable cause or clinical findings.

2) The diagnostic work-up and/or the neonatal or obstetric management to treat chorioamnionitis lack agreement, often resulting in many well-appearing infants being empirically treated with antibiotics. Concurrent with antibiotic treatment are the additional lab tests and very often, admission to a neonatal intensive care unit (NICU). In addition to the significant financial costs related to NICU admission, the emotional burden includes separation from the family and the potential to interfere with successful breastfeeding. Unnecessary antibiotic exposure may also negatively alter the infant's microbiome.

The NICHD expert panel explained that the term *chorioamnionitis* includes inflammation as well as infection, where inflammation leads to tissue edema, swelling, and irritation, and infection includes inflammation and invasion of bacteria, viruses, fungi, or other infectious agents.[42] Further, the term chorioamnionitis is used even when the only sign is a maternal fever.

Let's Learn More... Will "Triple I" replace the term chorioamnionitis?

Lab Work

L

Recognizing that **maternal fever** can occur from noninfectious etiologies (epidural anesthesia during labor, dehydration, elevated room temperature, hyperthyroidism, use of pyrogens, including prostaglandin E2 for induction of labor), it is inappropriate to proceed with a 'rule out chorioamnionitis' or 'presumptive chorioamnionitis', as this results in overtreatment of the pregnant patient and the baby. However, if there is an isolated maternal fever during labor, but unknown GBS status at ≥37 weeks gestation, the panel recommended following the Centers for Disease Control and Prevention (CDC) guidelines to give intrapartum antibiotic prophylaxis.

To guide clinicians through this complicated conundrum, the panel proposed an evaluation and management algorithm that differentiates what to do when there is an isolated maternal fever versus fever *WITH* one or more of the following:

- Fetal tachycardia, >160 beats per minute for 10 minutes or longer
- Maternal white blood cell (WBC) count >15,000 per mm³ in the absence of corticosteroids
- Purulent fluid coming from the cervical os (cloudy or yellowish thick discharge seen by speculum exam)
- Evidence of microbial invasion of the amniotic cavity (biochemical or microbiologic fluid results)

In summary, three categories of cases were proposed by the NICHD expert panel:

1. **Isolated maternal fever (not Triple I)**
2. **Suspected Triple I**
3. **Confirmed Triple I**

Retrospective confirmation would follow laboratory findings of infection in the amniotic fluid or histopathological evidence of infection or inflammation or both in the placenta, fetal membranes, or umbilical vessels.

The American College of Obstetricians and Gynecologists (ACOG) Committee on Obstetric Practice[30] differs from the NICHD expert panel in that they recommend a diagnosis of *intraamniotic infection* includes the following:

- When the maternal temperature is markedly elevated, ≥39°C (102.2°F), or
- When the maternal temperature is 38°C to 38.9°C (100.4 to 102°F), **_and_** there is one additional clinical risk factor present

A diagnosis of ***isolated maternal fever*** is reserved for any maternal temperature between 38°C to 38.9°C **without** additional clinical criteria indicating intraamniotic infection and with or without persistent temperature elevation.

An important distinction between the NICHD expert panel and ACOG is that ACOG asserts that absent an obvious cause for a fever, a markedly elevated temperature ≥39°C is a clinically important sign that is most likely due to an infection.

 To optimize appropriate assessment, monitoring, and care of the newborn, the neonatal team should be informed of any intrapartum maternal fever.

Note:
Further research may determine whether the treatment algorithm recommended by the NICHD expert panel is sufficient to protect both mothers and their infants from the significant and, at times, devastating effects of intrauterine infection. The research question is whether isolated maternal fever without other signs of infection is as benign as envisioned by the NICHD expert panel, and if assigning a 'not Triple I' diagnosis in the setting of an isolated maternal fever potentially delays treatment of clinically relevant infection.[43]

Understanding the Complete Blood Count (CBC)

The CBC[a] assesses the WBC count and differential, hemoglobin, hematocrit, erythrocyte indices, and platelet count. WBCs are involved in protection against infective organisms and foreign substances and are produced in the bone marrow along with red blood cells and platelets. On the first day of age, in noninfected infants, the WBC count ranges between 5,300 (5th percentile) and 28,200 (95th percentile)/mm^3.[44]

What WBC Count Number Is Concerning?

For all gestational ages, a WBC count below 5,000 may correlate with neonatal sepsis, especially if the infant is clinically unwell. The lower the number, the more concerning the finding. However, a WBC count within a normal range for age may be observed even in infants with a positive blood culture. Clinicians should utilize all available laboratory and clinical data and not rely solely on the WBC count as an indicator of sepsis.[44,45]

A neonate with sepsis may have a normal CBC in the early phase of illness.[46] The time between the onset of infection and the first change in the CBC may be as long as 4 to 6 hours.

It's important to remember that an infection may be present even if the CBC results are normal.

Conversely, abnormal CBC results do not always mean that an infant has an infection.[46,47] Infants with Trisomy 13, 18, and 21 may also have abnormal WBC counts but not necessarily sepsis.[48,49]

Because the CBC can change with time, it is very important to repeat the CBC and trend the results.

Neutrophils

Neutrophils are the WBCs primarily responsible for killing and digesting bacteria.[6,50] The other WBC types are explained in the *Let's Learn More: The WBC differential—A review* on page 220. In response to an infection, neutrophils are released from the bone marrow into the circulation to travel to the site of infection where they phagocytize (ingest) bacteria.[51] However, this response is impaired in term and especially preterm infants because of several factors:[2,50,52]

- Slow movement of neutrophils to the site of infection (chemotaxis). *Impact*: neutrophils don't reach the site of infection as quickly as needed.

- Stiffer neutrophil cell membrane. *Impact*: neutrophils have difficulty migrating into the tissue where the infection is located.

- Impaired *phagocytosis* (engulfing and ingestion of pathogens). *Impact*: ineffective elimination of bacteria or other foreign substances.

- Impaired or slow 'tagging' (opsonization) of the microorganism for phagocytosis. *Impact*: impaired phagocytic activity of neutrophils.

- Impaired ability to make *neutrophil extracellular traps* (NETs) that capture and destroy microbes without phagocytosis. *Impact*: ineffective elimination of bacteria.

There are other factors that impair the neonatal immune response, but those factors are beyond the scope of this program.

Note:
[a]In some nations, the CBC is called a full blood count (FBC).

As shown in Figure 5.2, neutrophils mature in the bone marrow, from the myeloblast, to the promyelocyte, to the myelocyte, to the metamyelocyte, to the band neutrophil, and finally to the mature **segmented neutrophil**. This process of maturation takes approximately 2 weeks. In the bone marrow, the metamyelocytes, band neutrophils, and segmented neutrophils comprise the *neutrophil storage pool (NSP)*.[35,50] In neonates, the NSP is significantly smaller per kilogram of body weight than in adults. Depletion of the NSP may occur with severe bacterial infection, placing the infant at a significantly increased risk of complications and even death.[2]

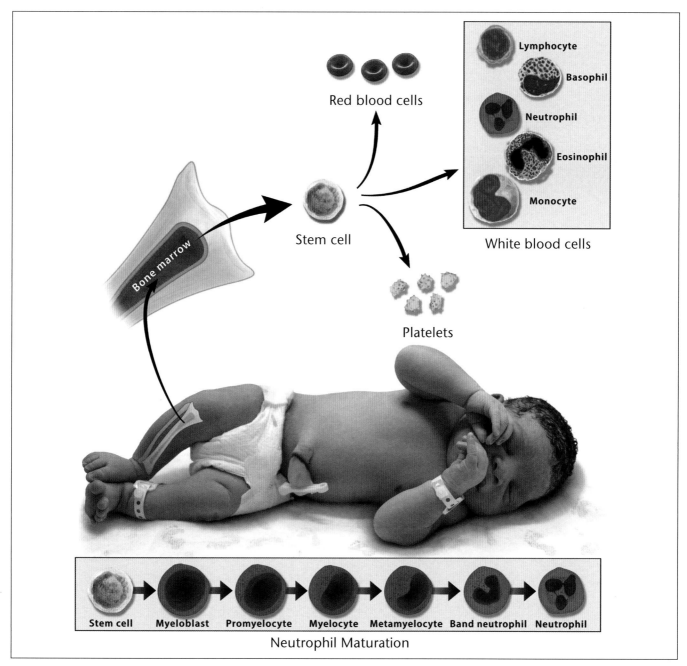

Figure 5.2. Blood cell development—from the bone marrow to the bloodstream. The stem cell differentiates into red blood cells, platelets, neutrophils, lymphocytes, monocytes, basophils, and eosinophils.

Let's Learn More...The white blood cell differential—A review[6,52-55]

The differential count reports the proportions of the five types of WBCs: neutrophils, eosinophils, basophils, lymphocytes, and monocytes. When all proportions (or percentages) are added together, they equal 100%. A normal differential count for a healthy, term infant is found below.

 Neutrophils generally account for the highest proportion of the WBCs. Neutrophils are primarily responsible for killing and digesting bacteria. They travel to the site of infection and destroy microorganisms by phagocytosis. They also release enzymes that kill the microorganisms.

 Eosinophils account for a very small proportion of the WBCs. Eosinophils are a type of immune cell that can collect in tissues where allergic reactions occur, such as the skin following an allergic skin reaction and the lung in patients with asthma. Their role in responding to an allergic reaction is to detoxify some of the inflammation-inducing substances released during an allergic reaction. Neonates may have an elevated eosinophil count (mild, moderate, or severe eosinophilia) associated with infection (Candida species and bacteria), necrotizing enterocolitis, and following transfusion of packed red blood cells.[5,56] Infants with allergic colitis or eosinophilic proctocolitis secondary to a cow milk or soy protein allergy may also have eosinophlia.[57]

 Basophils account for a very small proportion of the WBCs. Basophils have numerous functions that assist with the immune response. Basophils help protect against microbial pathogens, viruses, and parasites. They also release histamine during an allergic reaction and enzymes to help prevent blood clots.

 Lymphocytes account for the second highest proportion of the WBCs after neutrophils. Lymphocytes are a type of immune cell found in the blood and in lymph tissue. Along with drainage of lymph from the lymph nodes and other lymphoid tissue, lymphocytes enter the circulation continually. Lymphocytes have a lifespan of weeks or months, depending upon the body's need for them. There are two main types of lymphocytes: B lymphocytes that make antibodies and T lymphocytes that help kill tumor cells and control immune responses.

 Monocytes are a type of phagocyte and account for a small proportion of the WBCs. Monocytes travel from the blood into the tissues, where they differentiate into either a macrophage or a dendritic cell. Macrophages have numerous functions: surround and kill microorganisms, ingest foreign material, remove dead cells, and boost immune responses. Dendritic cells process antigens to help initiate an immune response, and they also help develop immunologic memory of the antigen.

Percentage (%) of the total WBCs in the blood of a healthy, term newborn (shortly after birth)[58]

Neutrophils*	61%
Lymphocytes	31%
Monocytes	6%
Eosinophils	2%
Basophils	0%

Shortly after birth, the differential proportions change; however, under noninfected conditions, the neutrophils and lymphocytes remain the highest proportions in the blood.[59]

*Includes myelocytes, metamyelocytes, band neutrophils, and mature, segmented neutrophils.

Note:
Reference intervals in neonatal hematology, from birth through various gestational ages may be found in this textbook: Christensen RD. Reference intervals in neonatal hematology. In: De Alarcon PA, Werner EJ, Christensen RD, Sola-Visner MC, eds. *Neonatal Hematology: Pathogenesis, Diagnosis, and Management of Hematologic Problems.* 3rd ed. Cambridge University Press; 2021:440-469.[59]

Figure 5.3. Bone marrow response to bacterial infection. In response to bacterial infection, the NSP releases immature and segmented neutrophils into the blood. Notice the increased numbers of band neutrophils and metamyelocytes in the bloodstream. Group B streptococcus bacteria is shown in the illustration.

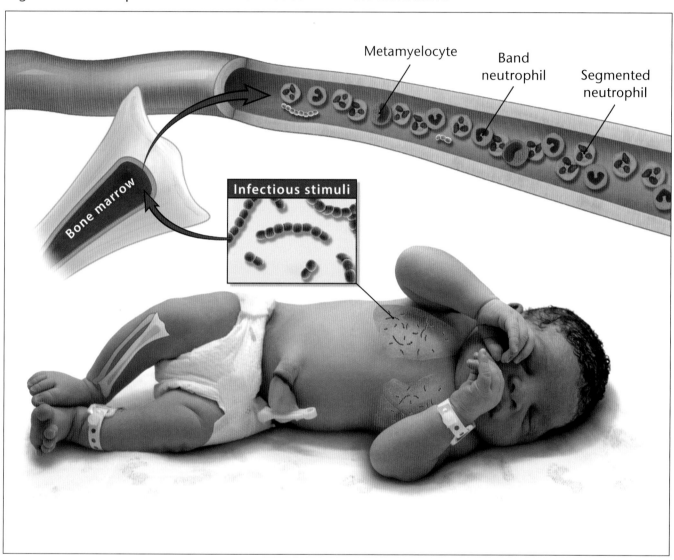

Under normal, non-infected, non-stressed circumstances, mature segmented neutrophils are released from the NSP into the bloodstream where they circulate for a short period (6 to 8 hours), and then they migrate into the tissue where they live for approximately 24 hours.[50]

In the presence of infection, immature forms of neutrophils—*bands and metamyelocytes* (and sometimes even more immature neutrophils such as myelocytes and promyelocytes)—are also released from the bone marrow into the bloodstream to maximize the number of circulating neutrophils (illustrated in Figure 5.3). The ability of immature neutrophils to neutralize a bacterial infection is significantly impaired. The term **left shift** refers to the appearance of immature neutrophils in the blood.

The Immature to Total (I/T) Ratio

The immature to total ratio (I/T ratio) calculation provides information about the proportion of immature to mature neutrophils in the blood. The I/T ratio is the most sensitive of the calculations for estimating the risk that infection may be present.[44]

Why is it helpful to calculate the I/T ratio?

The majority of neutrophils that appear in the bloodstream should be mature cells, or *segmented neutrophils*. When more than 20 to 25% of the neutrophils in the blood are immature neutrophils, suspicion should increase that the infant is responding to a bacterial infection.[2,44,60]

Making sense of the I/T ratio calculation

- Two normal I/T ratios obtained 8 to 12 hours apart and a negative blood culture at 24 hours *most likely* indicate the infant is not infected.[61]

- An I/T ratio >0.20 raises the index of suspicion for infection. The higher the I/T ratio, the more likely the infant may have EOS.[44,[a]]

- An I/T ratio >0.8 correlates with a higher risk of death from sepsis.[62]

Directions to calculate the I/T ratio

1) Identify the immature neutrophils (metamyelocytes and band neutrophils) and add them together. Do not include neutrophils that are more immature than metamyelocytes. This number equals the **I**mmature neutrophil count. Place this number as the numerator.

2) Add together the mature (segmented neutrophils) and immature neutrophils (metamyelocytes and band neutrophils). This number equals the **T**otal neutrophil count. Place this number as the denominator.

3) Divide the **I**mmature by the **T**otal neutrophil count as shown in the example on page 223.

> ⚠ *The decision to treat with antibiotics is based upon the clinical history, risk factors for infection, the patient condition and signs. Do not withhold antibiotic treatment in an ill neonate on the sole basis that the CBC is normal.*

Note:

[a]The data was derived from 166,092 infants who had a blood culture obtained within 3 days of birth and who were born in 293 NICUs between 1996 and 2009. Contaminated blood cultures were excluded.

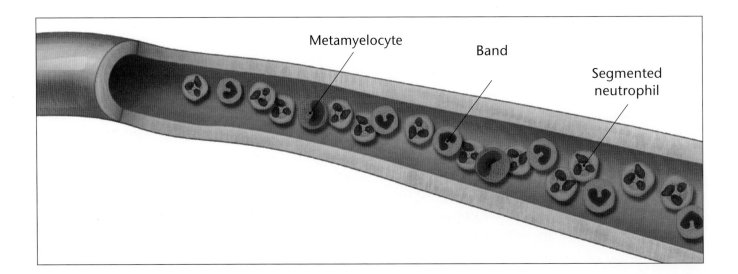

Metamyelocyte   Band   Segmented neutrophil

Example I/T Ratio Calculation

Case: A term infant was delivered after an uncomplicated pregnancy, except for rupture of membranes for 24 hours. At 4 hours old, the infant developed respiratory distress (tachypnea, cyanosis, retractions) and was hypothermic (36.1°C; 97°F). Oxygen and pulse oximetry were started, and the infant's doctor was notified. A complete physical exam was completed. A CBC, blood culture, capillary blood gas, blood glucose, and chest X-ray were obtained when the infant was 5 hours old.

CBC Results at 5 Hours of Age

	White Blood Cell (WBC) Count	6,200 (reported as 6.2 x 10³/µL)
WBC Differential	Segmented neutrophils (segs)	42 (%)
	Band neutrophils (bands)	20 (%)
	Metamyelocytes (metas)	2 (%)
	Lymphocytes	36 (%)
	Eosinophils*	0 (%)
	Basophils*	0 (%)

1) 20 bands + 2 metas = 22 (%) of the neutrophils are immature

2) 20 bands + 2 metas + 42 segs = 64 (%) of the WBCs

3) 22 (immature neutrophils) divided by 64 (total neutrophils) 22 / 64 = 0.34
   The I/T ratio is 0.34

Interpretation: **34%** of the neutrophil types are the **immature forms**. This elevated I/T ratio should raise concern that the bone marrow is responding to a bacterial infection by sending immature forms into the bloodstream before they have had time to fully mature.

*These values may be 0%—that is, they are not present in the differential count for that CBC. Lymphocytes, eosinophils, basophils, and neutrophils more immature than metamyelocytes are not included in the I/T ratio calculation.

The Absolute Neutrophil Count (ANC)[2,3,45,48,63-67]

When evaluating the CBC for possible bacterial infection, it is useful to know the concentration of neutrophils in the blood. The ANC calculation will provide this information. Normally, the WBC and neutrophil counts rise for the first day after birth. Therefore, a *low white blood cell count* and *declining total neutrophil count*, rather than the expected physiologic rise in count, should raise concern that the infant may be responding to an infection. Repeating the CBC at an interval relevant to the infant's clinical condition (i.e., 12, 24, or 48 hours) may be useful since the initial CBC may be normal and subsequent CBC results abnormal. See Appendix 5.3 on page 237 for more information about the ANC, including reference ranges based on gestational age.

Platelet Count and Thrombocytopenia[4,68-72]

A low platelet count is called thrombocytopenia. Thrombocytopenia may result from either decreased platelet production or increased platelet destruction (or utilization). Conditions that may cause thrombocytopenia include the following:

- **Infectious etiology:** bacterial (especially if Gram-negative), fungal, viral (e.g., CMV, HIV, rubella, herpes), or parasitic (toxoplasma)

- **Maternal medical conditions:** gestational hypertension, preeclampsia, etc.

- **Maternal auto- or isoimmunization:** alloimmune or autoimmune thrombocytopenia (idiopathic thrombocytopenic purpura, systemic lupus erythematosus)

- **Genetic etiology:** chromosomal (trisomy 13, 18, 21, Turner syndrome), familial thrombocytopenias, or specific mutations in the genes MPL, RUNX1, or PTPN11

- **Other etiologies:** necrotizing enterocolitis, hyperviscosity, disseminated intravascular coagulation following perinatal asphyxia, metabolic (propionic methylmalonic, isovaleric acidemias)

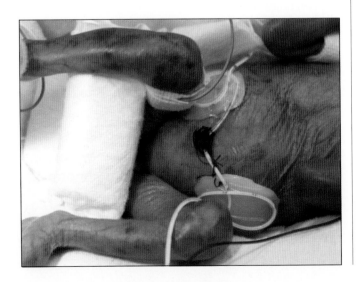

What Platelet Count Numbers Are Concerning?[59,70,73-75]

The platelet count increases with increasing gestational age. The 5th percentile for infants <32 weeks gestation is 104,200/µL and for late preterm and term infants, 123,000/µL.

- **Mild** thrombocytopenia is defined as a platelet count in the range 100,000/µL to 149,000/µL.

- **Moderate** thrombocytopenia is between 50,000 and 100,000/µL.

- **Severe** thrombocytopenia is when the platelet count is less than 50,000/µL.

A platelet count less than 100,000/µL is abnormal and needs to be re-evaluated, especially if there is a downward trend. In addition, the infant should be examined for signs of bleeding (oozing from puncture sites, bruising, petechiae, GI bleeding, etc.). Consult the tertiary center if any of these signs are present.

A platelet count less than 50,000/µL is termed "severe" thrombocytopenia and indicates that the risk of bleeding is increased.[68] If the platelet count is <50,000 in a neonate who has no petechiae and no signs of bleeding, consider repeating the count to make sure it is accurate (i.e., there is no platelet clumping). As mentioned above, evaluate for signs of bleeding and consult the tertiary center if any signs of bleeding are present.

Platelet counts less than 25,000/µL can be dangerously low. Consult the tertiary center for assistance with diagnosing the cause and treating this problem. As mentioned above, evaluate for signs of bleeding and be prepared to administer a platelet transfusion if instructed to do so.

Initial Antibiotic Therapy for Sick Infants

When Should Antibiotics Be Started?

In years past, antibiotics were frequently started in newborns even if they only had subtle signs of infection. With the emergence of antibiotic-resistant organisms and increased knowledge of the adverse effects, including long-term impacts of antibiotic overtreatment, the decision to start antibiotics should be based on careful evaluation of risk factors for infection and the infant's clinical condition.

Antibiotic Regimens May Vary From Hospital to Hospital and Region to Region

In the United States, early-onset sepsis (EOS) is commonly treated with Ampicillin and Gentamicin to provide coverage against both Gram-negative and Gram-positive organisms.[1,47] It is important to monitor resistance to both Ampicillin and Gentamicin and adjust the antibiotic regimen as indicated. **Before starting antibiotics, obtain an adequate volume blood culture.**

How long does it take for a blood culture to turn positive?

In infants at risk for EOS, one large study in the U.S. evaluated the time it took for a blood culture to become positive (grow bacteria or other pathogens). Thirty-seven percent of the blood cultures grew pathogenic bacteria, and 63% were contaminants. Blood cultures were positive by 36 hours in 94% of cases and by 48 hours in 97% of cases, even if the patient received maternal intrapartum antibiotic prophylaxis.[76]

With late-onset sepsis (LOS), microorganisms may grow more slowly. In a large Canadian study, most blood cultures were positive by 36 to 48 hours of incubation.[77]

When Should Antibiotics Be Stopped?

Once antibiotics are started, the goal should be to stop antibiotics as soon as possible. For infants at risk for EOS, consider stopping antibiotics if:[4,76-78]

- The blood culture remains negative after 36 hours.

- The infant is clinically well-appearing, and laboratory tests do not suggest that an infection is present.

- Other screening cultures (urine and cerebrospinal fluid), if obtained, are negative.

- Clinical suspicion for sepsis is low.

The Neonatal Early-Onset Sepsis Calculator is a tool used to help guide administration of empirical antibiotics in newborns ≥34 weeks gestation.[47,79-84] This tool has assisted national and international goals to reduce antibiotic use in newborns by synthesizing clinical correlates with neonatal exam findings.[85-87] For more information, see the Clinical Tip: *What is the Neonatal Early-Onset Sepsis Calculator?* on page 228.

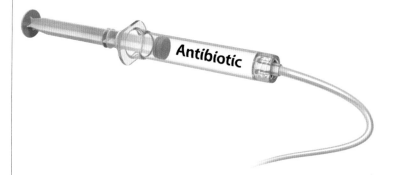

 Any delay in obtaining the blood culture or carrying out the order for administering antibiotics should be reported promptly to the infant's care team.

Ampicillin

Ampicillin dosing may vary depending on the reference utilized. This information is from the Lexidrug® reference.[88] The dose is adjusted based on gestational age, postnatal age, and the indication for use.[13] Ampicillin is used in combination with Gentamicin for broad-spectrum coverage to treat suspected or confirmed EOS.

Gestational Age	Postnatal Age	Dose (when meningitis / CNS involvement **IS NOT** suspected)
≤34 Weeks	≤7 days	50 mg/kg/dose every 12 hours
	8 to 28 days	75 mg/kg/dose every 12 hours
>34 Weeks	≤28 days	50 mg/kg/dose every 8 hours

Gestational Age	Postnatal Age	Dose (when meningitis / CNS involvement **IS** suspected)
≤34 Weeks	≤7 days	100 mg/kg/dose every 8 hours
	8 to 28 days	75 mg/kg/dose every 6 hours
>34 Weeks	≤7 days	100 mg/kg/dose every 8 hours
	8 to 28 days	75 mg/kg/dose every 6 hours

Route of Administration

Intravascular (IV)—preferred route

- Use sterile water or normal saline to reconstitute the Ampicillin medication.

- For IV infusion, maximum concentration is 100 mg/mL.

- Administer over 3 to 5 minutes (not faster than 100 mg per minute).

- If feasible, avoid infusing at the same time as Gentamicin.

- To avoid loss of potency, use reconstituted solutions within 1 hour of mixing.

- If there is reduced kidney function (renal impairment), consult your neonatal pharmacist or neonatal expert for guidance on dosing adjustments.

Intramuscular (IM)

- If having difficulty establishing IV access, consider giving Ampicillin IM for a few doses. Once IV access is established, change to IV administration.

- In the neonate, IM injections should be given in the anterolateral aspect of the thigh muscle (vastus lateralis).

- In small infants, the maximum volume per injection is 0.5 mL; therefore, more than one injection may be necessary to administer the full dose.[89]

- For IM injection, mix to a final concentration of 250 mg/mL.

One serious side-effect of Ampicillin is that it prolongs bleeding time because of its impact on platelet function. In 33- to 41-week gestation infants receiving between 50 to 100 mg/kg every 12 hours, bleeding times started to become more prolonged following the third or fourth dose.[90] In very-low-birth-weight infants, bleeding time was prolonged an average of 2 minutes when these infants received more than 10 doses of 50 mg/kg every 12 hours.[91]

Prolongation of the bleeding time may have implications for intracranial (including intraventricular) hemorrhage or pulmonary hemorrhage in vulnerable, sick infants. Therefore, Ampicillin given over many days and/or in higher doses should be based on clinical indications and with caution because of the potential effect on prolonged bleeding times.

Gentamicin

Higher dose, longer interval Gentamicin administration is usually administered. Doses and intervals should be adjusted based on the goals of therapy, renal function, and tolerance of the doses administered. This information is from the Lexidrug® reference.[92]

Gestational Age	Postnatal Age	Dose
<30 Weeks	≤14 days	5 mg/kg/dose every 48 hours
	≥15 days	5 mg/kg/dose every 36 hours
30 to 34 Weeks	≤10 days	5 mg/kg/dose every 36 hours
	11 to 60 days	5 mg/kg/dose every 24 hours
≥35 Weeks	≤7 days	4 mg/kg/dose every 24 hours
	8 to 60 days	5 mg/kg/dose every 24 hours

Route of Administration

Intravascular (IV)—preferred route

- Administer via an infusion pump over 30 minutes.

Intramuscular (IM)

- If having difficulty establishing IV access, Gentamicin may be given IM for a few doses. Absorption may be variable; IV administration is the preferred route.

If there is reduced kidney function (renal impairment), consider giving a single dose of Gentamicin with careful monitoring of serum concentration to decide when the next dose of Gentamicin can be safely administered.

To avoid toxicity, neonatal pharmacists can help with dosing pharmacokinetics and when to monitor serum concentrations and dosing intervals. Consult the tertiary referral center for guidance as needed.

Neonatal care recommendations and drug therapies are constantly evolving. Please consult current medication references and expert neonatal pharmacists as necessary since dosing regimens may change as new evidence becomes available.

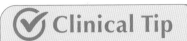

Clinical Tip — *What is the Neonatal Early-Onset Sepsis Calculator?*[47,79-84,87,93]

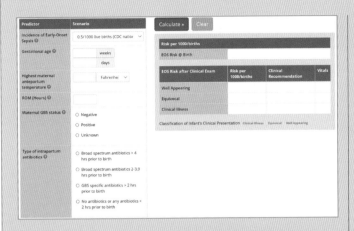

The **Neonatal Early-Onset Sepsis (EOS) Calculator** is an open source tool that was developed to guide clinical recommendations for determining the frequency of vital signs and antibiotic administration in newborns ≥34 weeks gestation.[a] To use the tool, the clinician first selects the incidence of early-onset sepsis in their region. The Centers for Disease Control (CDC) national incidence can also be used as necessary. Next, gestational age, the highest maternal antepartum temperature, and duration of rupture of membranes are entered. An important predictor in the model is the maximum maternal temperature. The final entries are for Group B Streptococcus status and any intrapartum antibiotic administration. Most importantly, the calculator includes the clinical presentation after birth. The product that the calculator computes is the risk of early-onset sepsis per 1,000 births.

Only half of the infants with EOS will be clinically ill after birth, so it is important to monitor the infant for deterioration through the first 24 hours of age. If the infant's clinical status changes over the first 24 hours, recalculate the EOS risk and follow the recommendation for that illness category.

[a] The EOS calculator tool may be accessed at this site: https://neonatalsepsiscalculator.kaiserpermanente.org/InfectionProbabilityCalculator.aspx.

[b] See EOS Calculator, Frequently Asked Questions for additional information about maternal fever, antibiotic prophylaxis, and other questions and clarifications from the study authors: https://neonatalsepsiscalculator.kaiserpermanente.org/GenFAQ.aspx

Classification of the Infant's Clinical Presentation

Clinical Exam	Description	
Well Appearing	No persistent physiologic abnormalities	
Equivocal (Note: abnormality can be intermittent)	1. Persistent physiologic abnormality ≥4 hours • Tachycardia (HR ≥160) • Tachypnea (RR ≥60) • Temperature instability (≥100.4°F or <97.5°F) • Respiratory distress (grunting, flaring, or retracting) not requiring supplemental O_2	2. Two or more physiologic abnormalities lasting for ≥2 hours • Tachycardia (HR ≥160) • Tachypnea (RR ≥60) • Temperature instability (≥100.4°F or <97.5°F) • Respiratory distress (grunting, flaring, or retracting) not requiring supplemental O_2
Clinical Illness	1. Persistent need for NCPAP / HFNC / mechanical ventilation (outside of the delivery room) 2. Hemodynamic instability requiring vasoactive drugs NCPAP: nasal continuous positive airway pressure HFNC: high flow nasal cannula	3. Neonatal encephalopathy / Perinatal depression • Seizure • Apgar Score @ 5 minutes <5 4. Need for supplemental O_2 ≥2 hours to maintain oxygen saturations >90% (outside of the delivery room)

Lab Work—**Key Points**

- Review the maternal and neonatal history for risk factors for infection.

- Infected infants often present with nonspecific signs that are commonly seen with other noninfectious conditions; be suspicious of subtle signs of infection.

- A neonate with sepsis can have a completely normal CBC early in the illness. Trend the CBC results and don't withhold antibiotic treatment in an ill neonate who has risk factors for infection solely on the basis that the CBC is normal.

- Draw at least 1 mL of blood for blood culture to increase the opportunity to grow even small amounts of bacteria that may be present in the blood.

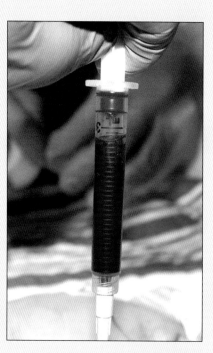

- Initiate antibiotics promptly if concerned for sepsis.

- Base the decision to discontinue antibiotics on the following:

  ○ Perinatal history and risk factors for infection

  ○ Clinical course

  ○ Blood culture results

  ○ Other culture and screening results (urine, cerebrospinal fluid, PCR test, if obtained)

  ○ Laboratory data (CBC, CRP, other biomarkers)

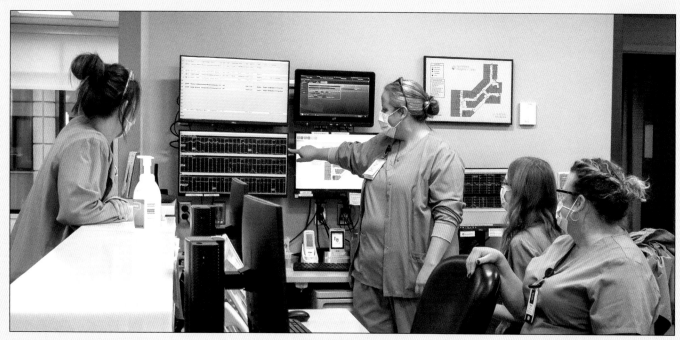

Appendix 5.1 Laboratory Tests That May Be Evaluated in the Post-Transport/Transfer Period

Depending upon the infant's history, risk factors, and clinical presentation, additional laboratory tests may be indicated as part of the neonatal intensive care unit (tertiary center) evaluation. These tests are **usually not necessary prior to transport** unless directed by the transport control or tertiary center physician.

Bilirubin[94,95]

Bilirubin is an end-product of hemoglobin metabolism that occurs when a red blood cell is hemolyzed. Jaundice is the term used to describe the identifiable yellow color seen when bilirubin is deposited in the skin and mucous membranes. Two forms of bilirubin are measured: direct (conjugated) and indirect (unconjugated). Almost all newborns have an elevated unconjugated bilirubin level initially that declines over the days and weeks after birth, providing there is no hemolysis or other pathologic process. An imbalance between bilirubin production and elimination can cause an increase in jaundice and hyperbilirubinemia.

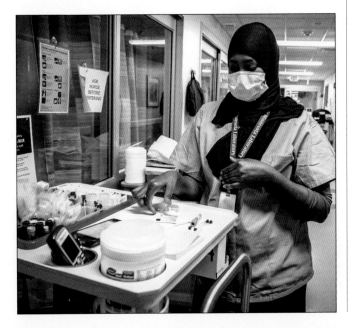

Electrolytes[96,97]

- An elevated potassium level, or **hyperkalemia,** can cause life-threatening cardiac arrhythmias. ECG signs of hyperkalemia include peaked T waves, a widened QRS, bradycardia or tachycardia, supraventricular tachycardia, and ventricular tachycardia or fibrillation. Acidosis may cause the potassium to acutely rise.

- A low potassium level, or **hypokalemia,** may occur because of diuretic administration, renal dysfunction, diarrhea, or gastric losses.

- An elevated sodium level, or **hypernatremia,** may occur secondary to increased insensible water or urinary losses, excessive sodium administration, or inadequate water intake.

- A low sodium level, or **hyponatremia,** may occur for various reasons, including retention of free water before kidney function normalizes and urinary sodium losses.

Renal Function Tests (Creatinine and Blood Urea Nitrogen)[96,98,99]

- Infants with acute kidney injury (AKI) secondary to perinatal asphyxia or shock often have oliguria, elevated **creatinine** levels (reflecting changes in kidney function), and electrolyte abnormalities. In the first few days of life, the serum creatinine reflects maternal values. After an insult, serum creatinine may not rise for 48 to 72 hours, so trending this test provides helpful information.

- An elevated **blood urea nitrogen (BUN)** may be observed when the kidneys are not effectively filtering urea, which is a waste product of protein breakdown. The BUN may be elevated because of acute kidney injury, heart failure, dehydration, or a diet high in protein.

Ionized Calcium[100-104]

The most abundant mineral in the body is calcium, with the majority of calcium accumulating during the last trimester. Ionized calcium is the measure of 'free calcium' and is the physiologically active fraction of calcium in the blood. By 24 to 36 hours of age, ionized calcium stabilizes at approximately 1.2 mmol/L (4.9 mg/dL). Calcium plays an important part in the excitation-contraction coupling and generation of impulses in myocardial cells and is also a major factor in vascular smooth muscle tone. An adequate ionized calcium concentration optimizes myocardial contractility. Normal serum concentrations of total and ionized calcium in term infants are summarized in the table. By 1 week of age, in healthy, term infants, the serum calcium concentration rises to equal levels found throughout childhood.

Term Infant, Age	Normal Serum Concentrations of Total and Ionized Calcium From Birth Through 24 Hours in Term Infants		
	Total Calcium	Ionized Calcium	
	mg/dL	mg/dL	mmol/L
Birth (Cord Blood)	10.2 (9.0–11.4)	5.82 (5.22–6.42)	1.45 (1.3–1.6)
2 Hours Old	9.7 (8.5–10.9)	5.34 (4.84–5.84)	1.33 (1.21–1.46)
24 Hours Old	9.0 (7.8–10.2)	4.92 (4.40–5.44)	1.23 (1.1–1.36)

Adapted from Loughead (1988)[101] and Namgung (2020).[103]

Magnesium[102,104-106]

A magnesium level may be indicated if the patient received magnesium during labor or if there are concerns for congenital heart disease, including arrhythmias. Magnesium is an essential mineral that has many important roles in physiologic functions. Magnesium is the second most abundant intracellular cation, influencing membrane integrity, neuromuscular excitability, nervous tissue conduction, protein synthesis, muscle contractility, and hormone secretion.

Hypermagnesemia in neonates is usually a result of maternal administration of magnesium sulfate. Hypermagnesemia may cause hypotonia, respiratory depression, decreased gastrointestinal motility, and meconium plug syndrome.

Signs of **hypomagnesemia** are similar to signs of hypocalcemia—tremors, irritability, and seizures. When hypocalcemia is present, then assessment for hypomagnesemia should follow since the two are closely associated. Causes of hypomagnesemia (usually considered less than 1.6 mg/dL) may include the following:

- Insulin-dependent and gestational maternal diabetes
- Intrauterine growth restriction
- Neonatal hypoparathyroidism
- Maternal hyperparathyroidism
- Defect of intestinal magnesium transport: primary hypomagnesemia with hypocalcemia
- Infantile isolated renal magnesium wasting
- Hypomagnesemia with hypercalciuria and nephrocalcinosis

Liver Function Tests (LFTs)[107-111]

- LFTs are useful to assess and monitor the degree of liver damage that may have occurred during periods of shock or damage to the liver from other etiologies, such as hepatitis or other viral infections.

- Infants with critical congenital heart disease (e.g., coarctation of the aorta, interrupted aortic arch, critical aortic valve stenosis, and hypoplastic left heart syndrome) are especially vulnerable to end-organ damage, including the liver if the ductus arteriosus closed.

Liver Enzymes

- When liver cells are damaged or diseased, the following liver enzymes might be increased:

  - Alanine aminotransferase (ALT), also called alanine transaminase

  - Aspartate aminotransferase (AST), also called serum glutamic-oxaloacetic transaminase (SGOT)

  - Gamma-glutamyl transpeptidase (GGT)

  - Alkaline phosphatase (liver fraction portion)

In addition to enzymes, liver function testing evaluates levels of proteins made in the liver (albumin and total protein) and bilirubin that is processed in the liver. An elevated conjugated (direct) bilirubin can be seen with liver injury or extrahepatic etiologies. Ammonia is processed by the liver into urea, then excreted in the urine. An elevated ammonia level may be observed with liver and/or kidney failure, some inborn errors of metabolism, or other genetic conditions.

Coagulation Tests

These laboratory tests are usually obtained if bleeding is observed, if there is a family history of bleeding disorders, or if there is a history of shock or liver injury.

- **Prothrombin time** (PT) measures how long it takes for a clot to form after adding thromboplastin to a patient's sample. It tests the integrity of the extrinsic clotting pathway. Prothrombin itself is a protein made by the liver, which is involved in blood clotting. A prolonged PT may also indicate a vitamin K deficiency or disseminated intravascular coagulation (DIC).

- **Partial thromboplastin time** (PTT) measures how long it takes for a blood clot to form. It tests the integrity of the intrinsic clotting pathway. Calcium and other substances are added to the patient's plasma sample and the number of seconds it takes for the clot to form is measured.

- **International normalized ratio** (INR) is a method used to standardize the value of a patient's PT. The INR is calculated by dividing the patient's PT by a control PT value obtained using a reference reagent developed by the World Health Organization (WHO).

- **Fibrinogen** is a protein made by the liver. Low levels can be due to hypoproduction, as in liver dysfunction, or excessive consumption, as in DIC.

Urine Culture[1,112]

- For EOS, a urine culture is not recommended as part of the sepsis work-up. However, for LOS, a urine culture is helpful since urinary tract infections may occur secondary to renal seeding during bacteremia.

Cerebrospinal Fluid (CSF) Culture and Analysis[1,18]

- CSF is usually obtained when there is a concern for CNS involvement, including meningitis

- Gram stain and culture

- WBC count with differential

- Glucose and protein concentration

- PCR testing for bacterial pathogen panels

- PCR testing for herpes virus (if concerned about herpes infection) or other viruses, such as enterovirus

Blood Gas[113,114]

This test is usually ordered when the infant is experiencing respiratory distress or there is a history of shock. Arterial samples are the gold standard to assess oxygenation, ventilation, and acid/base status: pH, PCO_2, PO_2, and bicarbonate. Capillary samples obtained from a well-warmed heel (to arterialize the capillary sample) provide a good estimation of ventilation and acid/base status (pH, PCO_2, and bicarbonate) but not oxygenation. If a venous blood gas is obtained, the pH value will be lower than an arterial sample by approximately 0.02 to 0.04, and the venous PCO_2 level will be higher than an arterial sample by approximately 5 to 8 mmHg.[115,116] For both capillary and venous blood gases, oxygenation should be evaluated by pulse oximetry.

Lactate[113,115,117-120]

Cells require adequate amounts of oxygen for survival. When tissue perfusion and oxygen delivery to the cells is inadequate, cells rely on anaerobic metabolism to produce energy. Lactic acid is produced as a by-product of anaerobic metabolism, and as lactic acid accumulates, pH declines (acidosis/acidemia). A normal blood lactate concentration is between 0.5 to 1 mmol/L. A persistently elevated lactate greater than 2 mmol/L is concerning. In combination with metabolic acidosis, the higher the number, the more dire the situation. Sampling error can account for some causes of a falsely elevated lactate level. In particular, the test should be promptly analyzed after being drawn, whenever possible, from a free-flowing sample such as an umbilical venous catheter (UVC) or arterial site. If the feet are cool or poorly perfused, a capillary lactate level may be more elevated than a sample drawn from a free-flowing vessel.

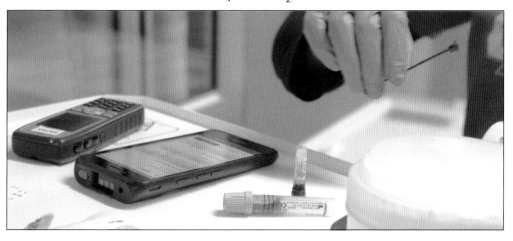

Appendix 5.2 Biomarkers: Laboratory Tests to Help Evaluate for Neonatal Infection

A biomarker is a 'biological marker' that can be measured accurately and reproducibly. Examples of biomarkers include heart rate and blood pressure, basic blood chemistries, and more complex laboratory tests or tissue analyses.

Biomarkers reflect normal and pathologic biologic processes and pharmacologic response to therapeutic intervention(s).[121,122] The search for a sensitive and accurate biomarker or combinations of biomarkers to confirm the diagnosis of neonatal sepsis has been a research topic for many years.[45,123-141]

An ideal biomarker to evaluate for neonatal sepsis would have the following characteristics:[142,143]

- Able to identify the cause of sepsis (bacterial, viral, fungal)

- Ability to detect sepsis close to 100% of the time when sepsis is present (high sensitivity)

- Ability to rule out sepsis (prevent false-positive tests) when sepsis is absent (high specificity)

- Accurately predicts the presence or absence of sepsis close to 100% of the time (high predictive value)

- Rapid results to allow early diagnosis of sepsis

- Low cost technology readily available

- Only requires a small sample of blood

To date, no biomarker has proven sensitive and specific enough to guide when it is safe to withhold administration of empiric antibiotics to treat suspected early-onset sepsis.[12] The blood culture is the gold standard for diagnosing neonatal sepsis. Analysis and culture of cerebrospinal fluid is also done when there are concerns for bacterial or viral meningitis. With EOS, blood cultures can take 24 to 36 hours to yield results, with most cases of positive blood cultures reported by 36 hours.[76,77,144] At times, however, the blood culture fails to reveal the bacteria or pathogen causing illness. In combination with a physical exam, clinicians frequently order various laboratory tests to help decide if an infant is infected.[34] Stopping antibiotics as soon as possible is an international goal in neonatology to reduce emergence of antibiotic-resistant microorganisms and to reduce hospital stays, costs, and morbidity associated with treatment.[77,145] To assist with this goal, researchers have studied combining blood culture results with other lab tests, including C-reactive protein (CRP) and procalcitonin (PCT).[144-146]

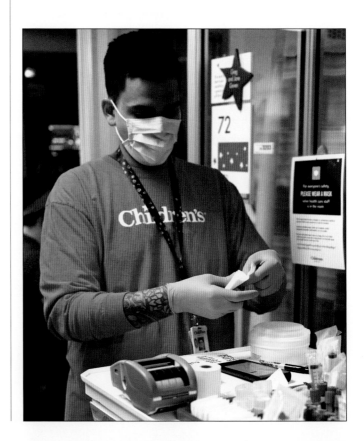

Lab Work

C-Reactive Protein (CRP)[1,4,34,45,50,137,142,147,148]

CRP is a protein produced by the liver in response to inflammatory stimuli, including infection, trauma, or tissue necrosis. Because of this property, CRP is considered an "acute-phase reactant."

- Some laboratories report CRP concentrations as mg/L and others report as mg/dL.[148] Verify the reference range and unit of measurement used for CRP in your hospital laboratory.

  - A normal value for CRP is <1.6 mg/dL for the first 2 days after birth and then 1 mg/dL or less thereafter.[50]

- Since CRP does not cross the placenta, results reflect the infant's level.

- Elevation of CRP can be nonspecific and multifactorial.

  - CRP levels are higher following vaginal birth than cesarean birth.

  - In addition to bacterial infection, CRP levels can increase with respiratory illnesses (meconium aspiration syndrome, respiratory distress syndrome), perinatal asphyxia, surgery, traumatic or ischemic tissue injury, following vacuum-assisted or forceps delivery, with prolonged active labor, following antenatal steroid administration, with hemolysis, and after immunization. One study of 22 healthy babies who received hepatitis B vaccination (HBV) demonstrated a significant rise in CRP 24 hours after vaccination. Therefore, exposure to HBV should be considered when evaluating the CRP as part of a sepsis evaluation.[149]

- CRP changes following the onset of infection:

  - Within 10 to 12 hours of the onset of infection, the CRP usually begins to rise. CRP peaks between 24 and 48 hours. Because of this delay in elevation, *CRP is not reliable for the early diagnosis of neonatal sepsis.*

  - Bacteria and some fungi express an antigen that is recognized by CRP. CRP binds to the antigen and activates the complement system. The organism is then opsonized (tagged for elimination), then cleared through phagocytosis by neutrophils, monocytes, and macrophages.[50]

  - CRP declines rapidly in response to antimicrobial therapy; therefore, serial evaluation of CRP is useful to evaluate response to treatment.

- CRP is not always elevated (even with proven sepsis), so other parameters, including changes in the CBC, clinical status, and blood or other culture results, should be evaluated when deciding whether to treat or not treat for sepsis.[1,50]

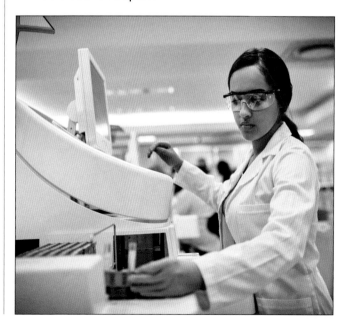

Procalcitonin (PCT)

- Another inflammatory biomarker to aid in the evaluation for neonatal sepsis is *procalcitonin (PCT)*.

- PCT is produced predominantly by monocytes and hepatocytes.

- When exposed to a bacterial endotoxin, PCT levels rise within 3 to 4 hours and usually peak by 6 to 8 hours.[1]

- A normal physiologic rise also occurs within 24 hours of birth, and a normal PCT level can be seen even when there is severe sepsis.

- Serial evaluation of CRP and PCT is necessary since a single measurement is of little clinical value.[45,150] The decision to stop antibiotics as soon as possible can be assisted by serial CRP and/or PCT evaluation. One study found that PCT and CRP levels stopped rising within 36 hours of starting antibiotics and that antibiotics could be safely stopped if, within 36 hours after starting antibiotics, the CRP or PCT remained below thresholds of 16 mg/L (equals 1.6 mg/dL) and 2.8 ng/L, respectively.[145]

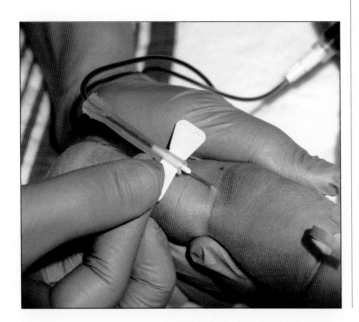

The Future of Biomarker Research

Early and accurate diagnosis of sepsis can improve clinical outcomes, and antibiotic overuse can be minimized. In association with clinical data, it is expected that the search for biomarkers to assist rapid and reliable diagnosis of early- and late-onset sepsis will continue for years.[45] A recent analysis in Sweden assessed 15 biomarkers, and *serum amyloid A (SAA)*, an acute-phase reactant that is produced in the liver similar to CRP, was the most favorable for diagnosing neonatal sepsis.[130] In another study, SAA levels in infected infants were much higher than in healthy infants at all time points evaluated (birth, 8 and 24 hours of age).[45,151] Mean platelet volume (MPV) as a predictive marker for neonatal sepsis has also been studied. In a meta-analysis, MPV was significantly higher in septic infants than in healthy control infants.[152] Clinical correlation, assessment of risk factors for sepsis, culture, and biomarker lab results are all integral aspects of the decision-making process.

A promising technology to rapidly identify microbes that grow in blood culture is peptide nucleic acid (PNA) fluorescent in situ hybridization (PNA-FISH). Another test increasingly used to diagnose infection and guide antimicrobial selection is the polymerase chain reaction (PCR) assay. PCR testing can detect the most common Gram-positive and Gram-negative bacteria found in blood and cerebrospinal fluid cultures. Some Candida (yeast) species and *aspergillus fumigatus* are also detected by PCR. However, since PCR testing fails to identify all pathogens, a blood culture must still be obtained.[140]

Appendix 5.3 The Absolute Neutrophil Count (ANC)—What It Means, How to Calculate the ANC, and Reference Ranges for Gestational Age[2,35,44,50,51,58,62,66,153,154]

Understanding the ANC

The total WBC count is comprised of neutrophils, eosinophils, basophils, lymphocytes, and monocytes.

A segmented neutrophil percentage of "38" means 38% of the WBCs are segmented neutrophils (the most mature form).

A band percentage of "12" means 12% of the WBCs are band neutrophils. Thus, 50% of the WBCs in this scenario (38% segmented neutrophils plus 12% band neutrophils) are those primarily responsible for phagocytizing and killing bacteria.

The remaining 50% of the WBCs are a combination of eosinophils, basophils, lymphocytes, and monocytes and are involved with other functions of the immune system.

The WBC count and the mature, segmented neutrophils and band neutrophils are included in the ANC calculation. Neutrophils more immature than bands (metamyelocytes, myelocytes, promyelocytes) and the other types of WBCs are **not** included in the calculation. As a reminder, when calculating the I/T ratio, the bands and metamyelocytes *are* included for the "immature" numerator as described on page 222.

Neutrophil counts vary with age as shown in the graphs on pages 239 to 240. Preterm infants have a lower ANC than term infants because their WBC count and circulating neutrophil concentration are lower prior to term gestation.

Neutropenia

- An ANC less than 1,000/µL (per microliter) or 1,000/mm³, twice sequentially, is considered neutropenia.

- An ANC less than 500/µL (per microliter) or 500/mm³, twice sequentially, is considered severe neutropenia.

When the ANC falls into the neutropenic range for gestational age and postnatal age, it is possible the infant has a congenital neutropenia versus neutropenia associated with sepsis. If the infant is well-appearing, then congenital neutropenia should be considered. A maternal history of hypertension is important to consider when evaluating ANC results. Infants born to mothers with hypertension may have a low ANC compared with infants whose mothers are not hypertensive.

 Most concerning are infants who have a low ANC for their postnatal age because this may mean there are not enough neutrophils to fight a bacterial infection. Neonates who deplete their neutrophil reserves while fighting infection are at the highest risk of dying from sepsis.

Causes of Neutropenia	
Infection	Premature birth
Severe preeclampsia	Birth depression
Small for gestational age size	Hemolytic disease
Neonatal Alloimmune Neutropenia	Neonatal Autoimmune Neutropenia
Severe Congenital Neutropenia	Syndromes that Include neutropenia (i.e., Barth's, Fanconi, glycogen storage disease 1B, Chediak-Higashi)

Practice Calculating the ANC

Case scenario: A 38-week gestation infant is delivered to a mother who is Group B Streptococcus positive and who did not receive any intrapartum antibiotics. The highest intrapartum maternal temperature was 38°C. Spontaneous rupture of membranes (SROM) was 12 hours before delivery, and the fluid was clear. At 2 hours of age, the infant developed respiratory distress (tachypnea, cyanosis, and retractions). The infant's temperature was normal. Oxygen and pulse oximetry were started, and the infant's doctor was notified. A complete physical exam was completed. A CBC, blood culture, glucose, capillary blood gas, and chest X-ray were obtained at 3 hours of age.

White Blood Cell (WBC) Count	5,300 (reported as 5.3 x 10³/µL)
Segmented neutrophils (segs)	38 (%)
Band neutrophils (bands)	12 (%)
Metamyelocytes (metas)	2 (%)
Lymphocytes	48 (%)

Add the segmented neutrophils and bands together (do not include metamyelocytes). Multiply this number by the total white blood cell count.

1) 38 segs + 12 bands = 50 (percent)

2) 5,300 multiplied by 0.5 = 2,650 (= the ANC)

3) Plot this number (2,650) for a 3-hour-old infant on the >36 weeks gestation chart

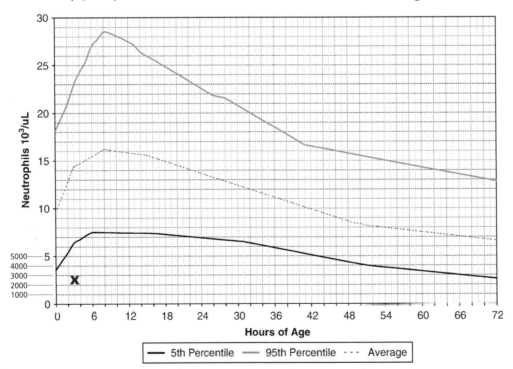

Interpretation: For a 3-hour-old term infant, this ANC is low. Repeating the CBC at an interval appropriate to the infant's clinical condition would be helpful to follow the trend in the WBC count, ANC, and I/T ratio. In this example, the I/T ratio is 0.27 (14 / 52 = 0.27).

Graphs showing the normal range for the absolute neutrophil count (ANC) in infants based on gestational age in the first 72 hours of life[48]

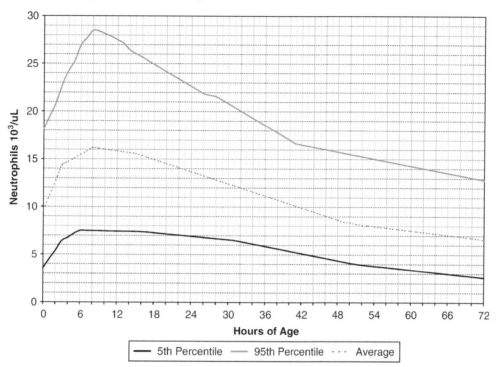

Neonates greater than 36 weeks gestation

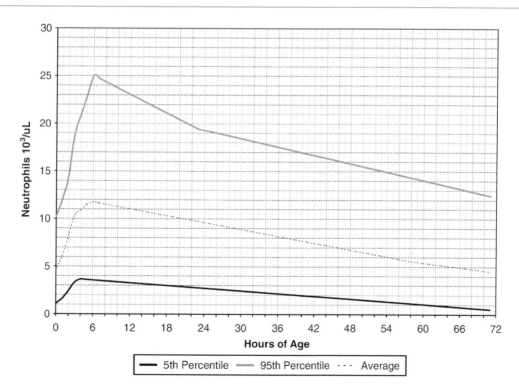

Neonates between 28 to 36 weeks gestation

Graph showing the normal range for the absolute neutrophil count (ANC) in infants based on gestational age in the first 72 hours of life[48]

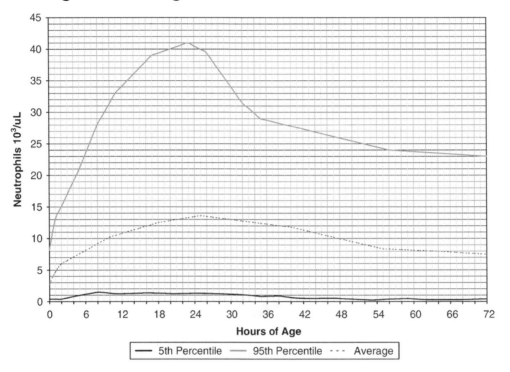

Neonates less than 28 weeks gestation

Note that the 5th percentile is very low and remains low through 72 hours of age.

Optional activity:

a) Enter the data from the case scenario into the EOS calculator: https://neonatalsepsiscalculator.kaiserpermanente.org.

b) Calculate the **EOS Risk at Birth**.

c) Discuss the **Clinical Recommendation and Vitals** output results with your study group.

Notes:

1) Infants were excluded from this study by Schmutz, Henry, Jopling, and Christensen if they had early-onset bacterial sepsis, congenital neutropenia, abnormally low or high neutrophil concentrations, trisomy 13, 18, or 21, or the mother had pregnancy-induced hypertension.

2) All CBCs were analyzed using modern automated blood cell counting instrumentation.

3) The upper limits of ANC in infants born at altitude[48,155] were higher than studies performed on infants born at sea level.[63,67] This finding is attributed to either different methodology used to count the neutrophils versus the effect of the higher altitude of the Intermountain Region study hospitals (average 4,800 feet or 1,463 meters above sea level), compared to Manroe's study, which was conducted in Dallas, Texas (500 feet or 152 meters above sea level).

Graphs reprinted with permission from Macmillan Publishers Ltd: Journal of Perinatology, Schmutz N, Henry E, Jopling J, Christensen RD. Expected ranges for blood neutrophil concentrations of neonates: the Manroe and Mouzinho charts revisited; Figures 1, 2, and 3. 28:275-81, © 2008.

Emotional Support Module (E)

S ugar

T emperature

A irway

B lood Pressure

L ab Work

E motional Support

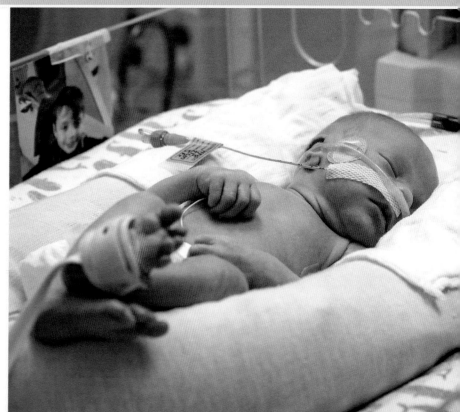

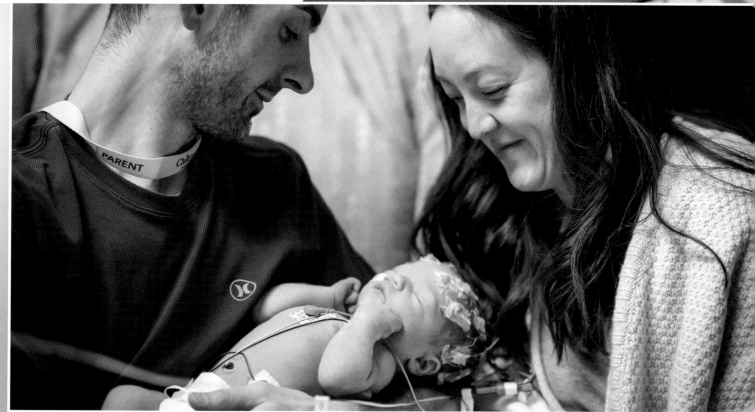

Emotional Support—Module Objectives

Upon completion of this module, participants will gain an increased understanding of:

1. The crisis families experience when an infant requires transport to or care in a neonatal intensive care unit (NICU).

2. Ways healthcare providers can support parents of sick infants.

3. Methods neonatal healthcare providers can use to help reduce parental stress and facilitate parenting in the NICU.

Introduction

When an infant is born preterm or sick, parents experience a complicated crisis.

Perinatal caregivers should recognize that each family brings a unique, potentially complicated history, and diverse cultural background to each childbirth experience. Parental reactions are sometimes hard to interpret, and coping styles vary, as do responses seen from the parents of the same baby. It is important that caregivers engage in reflective practice, being aware of how their own experiences, intentions, desires, and feelings may impact their care. Caregivers should approach all families in a curious, compassionate, and nonjudgmental manner and activate support systems as necessary.

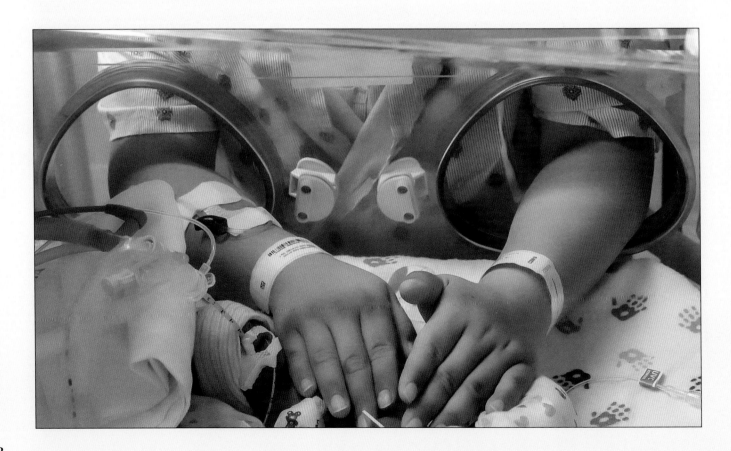

Parents may experience many emotions when their infant is sick and/or preterm. These emotions include guilt, anger, disbelief, sadness, a sense of failure, powerlessness, fear, blame, uncertainty, depression, grief, and importantly, hope. Guilt and a sense of responsibility for the situation are often the first and strongest emotions experienced by mothers. Parents may initially appear "numb" and in shock as they try to understand the situation and explanations provided to them. With the crisis of a NICU admission, parents may not function to the best of their ability. They may not know what questions to ask or what to do in a situation they did not expect or for which they were unprepared. Provide support and assistance to help the family cope with this crisis and their grief by normalizing and validating their emotional responses. Explain the infant's medical situation and involve the family in decision-making.

See Appendices 6.1 and 6.2 for more information about relationship-based care and parental trauma and grief, respectively. Appendix 6.3 offers an enlightened perspective on providing emotional support to healthy and sick infants.

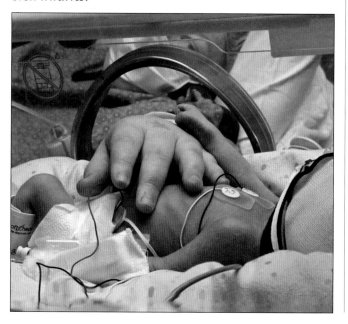

When the Infant Requires Transport to Another Facility

Initial Stabilization Period

In the community hospital, nurses are in an ideal position to offer emotional support to the family. The following are suggestions to guide this initial care:

- If the mother is alone, inquire about their support system and encourage them to call or allow you to help call those they identify as significant others, family members, friends, and/or clergy. In the case of U.S. military families, the active-duty member's ombudsman* may be a supportive resource.

- If the mother's medical condition permits, take them to the nursery to be with the infant before the transport team arrives. Encourage them to talk to and touch their baby. If their medical condition does not allow them to be at the bedside, the transport team, in most cases, will take the baby to the parent's room for a brief visit before their departure. It is helpful for at least one of the postpartum caregivers to accompany the transport team to the mother's room so they can hear explanations provided to the parent(s). When the team has departed, the caregiver can answer any additional questions and help the parent(s) understand the situation and what may happen next.

*Note:
The ombudsman is the liaison between the Command structure and the family members. They can be an enlisted person or, for example, the wife of a senior ranking officer. The ombudsman ensures that the Command knows and can respond to the needs of the family members. Also, if a spouse/significant other is deployed, the Red Cross can send an emergency message to that person's Command. It is never guaranteed that the active duty member will be returned to the U.S., but it at least provides the Command with updated information about what is happening with the active duty member's family.

Emotional Support

- Within hospital protocol, allow and encourage photos and videotaping of the infant, as these may be a source of support after the baby is transported. Once transported, encourage the family to take frequent photos to document their infant's progress.

- Although analgesics are important for maternal care post-delivery, they may also interfere with the mother's ability to remember their time with the infant. Therefore, if you explain this fact to the mother and give them a choice, they may agree that receiving an analgesic after spending time with their infant is best.

- A small cloth can be given to the mother soon after birth to wear in their bra/shirt or be placed on their chest. It can then be included in the transport incubator near the baby to carry the mother's familiar scent to the new hospital. The mother may find comfort in doing something very tangible for their preterm or sick infant.

- Ask the parent(s) if the infant has been given a name and, if yes, call the infant by name.

- In some cultures, name selection and the timing of naming the baby varies; parents may not give a name in the immediate post-birth period. Understanding and respecting the parent's choice about when to name their baby will demonstrate cultural sensitivity.

- Referring to the infant as "your son," "your daughter," or "your baby" will help the parent(s) to identify as the parent(s) of this infant. Particularly for infants in the NICU for extended periods, it is important not to misgender the infant, as doing so may be distressing and diminish their confidence in the healthcare provider. Using the baby's name is a helpful way to avoid the mistake of misgendering the baby and reassures parents that you know who their child is.

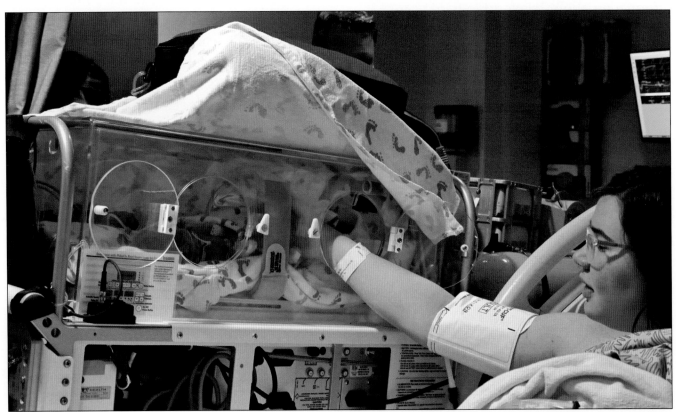

When the Transport Team Arrives

- Accompany the transport team to the mother's room and listen to explanations of the infant's condition and likely medical treatments.

- This situation is often overwhelming for parents. Because of the large amount of information they hear, parents may have difficulty remembering what was explained to them. Help parents understand information: ask them what questions they have, be prepared to repeat explanations, and be aware that explanations are easily misinterpreted or misunderstood.

- Recommend to parents that they write down questions as they arise. It is often difficult for them to remember questions and information when talking with the infant's healthcare providers.

- Most parents have limited backgrounds in healthcare, and many have no prior experience with sick newborns. Keep explanations simple but accurate. Provide illustrations and written materials when possible.

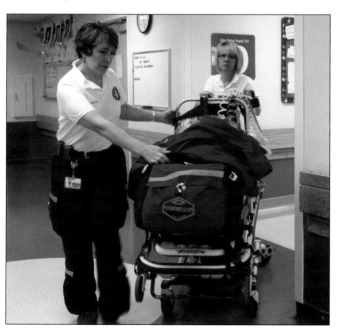

- Be aware of reading limitations. If this problem is identified, appropriate alternative resources should be provided.

- If there is a language barrier, avoid using family or friends to interpret. Instead, use medical interpreters, online video, or over-the-phone interpretation/translation services.

- When grandparents are present, they are often overlooked. They should also receive acknowledgment of the birth of their grandchild and support as warranted. Grandparents may be feeling anxious, fearful, and grieving not only for their new grandchild but also for their own child. When possible, discuss feelings and concerns with parents and grandparents, recognizing that the parents must always receive medical information about their baby first.

- Observe privacy laws at all times and ask the parent(s) for permission to discuss the infant's medical condition in front of other family members.

- Given the difficult circumstances, some parents report having a hard time hearing "congratulations" that their baby has been born. This feeling does not mean you should not say "congratulations," as different families are receptive to different information. Perinatal caregivers can enhance attachment to the infant by highlighting specific things to celebrate or be encouraged by. Regardless of the outcome, the infant's birth (day) will be a significant moment in this family's life.

- If you are the postpartum nurse, try to go to the nursery to see the infant before transfer. Ask the parent(s) if they have a photo of their baby, and if not, facilitate taking a photo before the transport team departs. Parents may also appreciate being in a photo with their baby, even if the baby is in the transport incubator.

- Often, the transport team will provide specific information regarding how to locate the hospital and NICU where the infant will be transported. When possible, they will also describe the caregivers (neonatology, cardiology, surgery, etc.) who will be responsible for the infant's care. This information is instrumental for parents because they, especially mothers, often fear the unknown and separation from their infant. If there is a whiteboard in the mother's room, put the name of the hospital and NICU phone number on that board.

- Notify the mother's care providers of the neonatal transport and explore feasibility to have the mother transported to the receiving hospital or options for early discharge if the mother's condition allows.

Care of the Family After the Infant Is Transported

In the Community Hospital

- If the infant is in very critical condition, and if possible, call the NICU nurse who is caring for the infant to request that you or the infant's birth physician or midwife be notified if "bad news" is given to the family so that you can activate increased levels of support. If it appears the mother will be alone after the infant is transported, encourage a family member or friend to remain with them. This support will be especially helpful if distressing news is provided from the NICU.

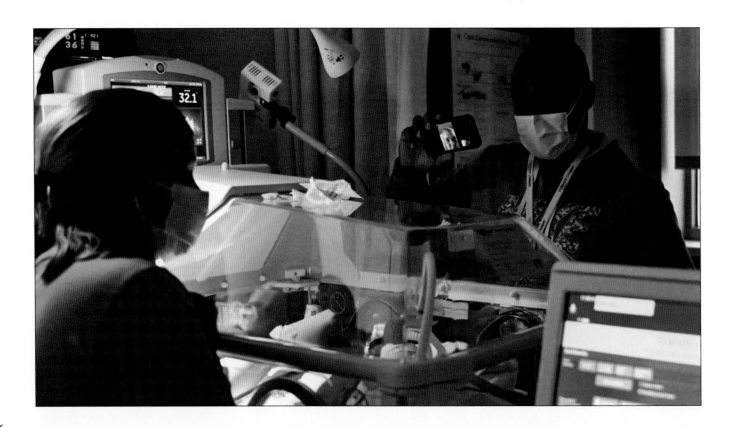

- If parents express overwhelming fear or anxiety, provide reassurance that you can help activate resources, such as the hospital social worker, to help.

- If parents seem to be in denial or unusually calm, don't be surprised. Sometimes, reality sinks in slowly, and every family member has their own approach to coping and dealing with a crisis. It may be that the family had no warning that their infant would be anything but healthy, and it will take time for them to work through their complex emotions. For more information on common expressions of traumatic stress in parents, see Appendix 6.2.

- Ask the mother about their plan to offer breastmilk. Normalize feelings of conflict around pumping during this unexpected crisis. While it is important to respect mothers' wishes, in most cases, it is best to encourage the mother to proceed with hand expression and pumping rather than wait to start. Early initiation of pumping and continued support with an electric pump will help to establish the milk supply. Also, realize that many mothers feel that providing their milk for the infant is a significant and unique contribution to the infant's care, which is reassuring to them.

- Parents may need assistance calling the NICU to check on the baby's status. Facilitate communication with the infant's nursing and/or medical staff as needed.

- If the parent(s) have multiples whose medical conditions are very different from each other (in the case of twins, one is doing well and staying while the other is being transferred or has died), support them in their ambivalence in being happy about the baby who is doing well and anxious or sad about the baby who is not. Provide professional support if needed.

In the Neonatal Intensive Care Unit

- Remember, adults are accustomed to having control over events in their lives. This situation takes their control away. They are not able to "parent" their baby the way they had dreamed of. Depending upon the infant's state of health, the parent(s) may not be able to do much or any of the normal "parenting" activities without asking permission; for example, to hold or feed their baby or change their diaper. By being aware of these feelings, healthcare providers will be better able to empathize with what the family is experiencing, especially if they seem angry toward healthcare providers or the situation.

- Facilitate parenting in the NICU by involving the parent(s) in the infant's care and medical decision-making. Help the family become aware of the many support groups available within the NICU, such as parent and sibling, breastfeeding, social worker, clergy, and, if necessary, grief support groups.

- Recognize that within a couple, parents may cope and respond very differently to stress and the hospital experience. Social expectations and responsibilities may influence how they react and choose to cope. Financial stress, limited childcare and transportation resources, and the fear of losing jobs because of missed work all factor into the complexity of family care in the NICU.

- Fathers or significant others may struggle to balance the stress of caring for the mother, spending time with the baby, caring for other children at home, and work obligations. Mothers may have similar challenges with work obligations, the needs of their other children, and their own physical and emotional needs. The family may live a significant distance from the hospital and have limited transportation resources. It is important not to make assumptions nor make them feel guilty about why they may not be present in the NICU. Ask supportive questions to help them establish a routine that allows them to participate in caring for their baby and facilitate video visits with the baby using available technology.

- Often, family and friends flock to the mother's side, while the father or significant other is left somewhat alone and unsupported; they may not verbalize or express their thoughts and feelings as openly as the mother. Unintentionally, even healthcare givers can be more responsive to mothers' needs than fathers or significant others. Maternal and paternal depression may occur. Know how to activate appropriate resources and screening as necessary.

- Differences in stress management and coping among partners can often place additional strain on parents. Encourage them to communicate with each other about their stress, their feelings, and their infant.

- This is **their** infant, not ours. When healthcare givers refer to an infant as "my baby," we mean "my patient;" however, parents may not understand that is our intent. Rather, refer to the infant as "your baby" or by name if a name has been given.

- As mentioned earlier, if there is a language barrier, use medical interpreters, online video, or over-the-phone interpretation/translation services. Inquire if there are cultural/religious customs that they wish to include or provide for the infant.

- It is essential to collaborate with other healthcare team members on the plan of care and encourage the family to speak up if they hear conflicting information. Often, parents complain that "everyone is telling me something different" and "no one seems to agree with the plan of care." Encourage parents to participate in patient rounds so they may hear the discussions that take place, including interval changes that occurred and/or the rationale for necessary alterations in the previous plan of care. As necessary, provide telephone or telehealth options for parents to attend rounds. Periodically, ask parents for their understanding of their infant's condition and care plan and identify opportunities to clarify. Provide simple, clear explanations (and illustrations when needed) to explain their infant's condition.

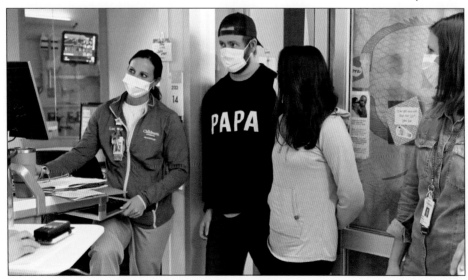

- Parents may not know it is possible to hold their infant skin-to-skin or may be afraid to ask. Facilitate early, frequent, and prolonged skin-to-skin contact when it is most appropriate for the baby's medical condition and the parents' availability.

Caring for Parents in the NICU

Contributed by Rhonda Reed, NICU nurse and Director of Programs for the family support group, Hand to Hold.

As NICU professionals, it is increasingly difficult to care medically for the infant and emotionally for the parent. It often feels like there are just not enough hours in the shift. Engaging parents and viewing them as a valuable part of the healthcare team can lead to better outcomes for the infant and the family, as well as establish a collaborative relationship between the parents and the healthcare team.

When working with families through our parent support organization Hand to Hold (handtohold.org), parents often tell us they don't feel like parents or are afraid they will not bond with their infant. Even the smallest task, like changing a diaper or taking a temperature, can reassure them that they are a parent. Not involving parents as valued members of the care team can lead to stress and anxiety, which can contribute to the development of post-traumatic stress disorder (PTSD) and perinatal mood and anxiety disorders (PMADS).

Working with and supporting families faced with end-of-life decisions can be difficult. From a medical professional perspective, we may encounter families who appear reluctant to hear or discuss information about a devastating prognosis. Regardless of what they are told, the family acts unwilling to transition to palliative care. Instead, they seem to hold onto hope that a miracle will happen, believing that their child will survive. But they do "get it." They do hear you. They just may not be ready. In fact, I had this very experience when I was a bedside nurse caring for an infant who was not expected to survive. I heard multiple comments in rounds: "This mom is just not getting it" and "The parents are not accepting the inevitable." When the parents visited that day, I asked them what they understood regarding their infant. The mom said, "I completely understand it all, but I just can't walk in here every day and only hear and talk about the negative. I have to see something positive each day." Eventually, this family reached a decision to transition their infant to palliative care, and the mother expressed to me that she was at peace with the most difficult decision she would ever make in her life. She also said she would forever cherish every moment she had with her baby. Personally, this experience enriched my perspective as a NICU nurse. As medical professionals, our best approach is acknowledging the gravity and complexity of parents' decisions and supporting families while they process this very difficult decision in their own time. For more resources to support NICU families, scan the QR code.

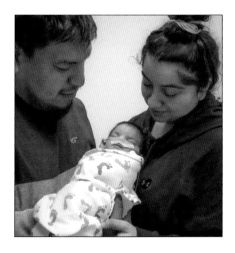

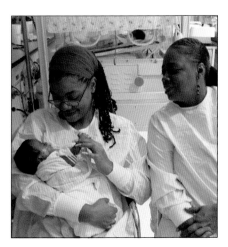

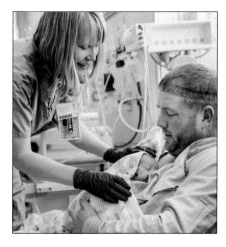

Appendix 6.1 Providing Relationship-Based Care to Babies and Their Parents

Contributed by Deborah L. Davis, Ph.D., and Mara Tesler Stein, Psy.D., PMH-C

In the NICU, relationship-based care is a philosophy of care that recognizes the healing power of sensitive, responsive, and supportive relationships. This healing power is found in the therapeutic relationships that medical professionals form with babies and parents, and particularly in the nurturing relationships parents form with their babies. Relationship-based care is neuroprotective, as attentive relationships protect infants from the physical and emotional stress and trauma associated with intensive care. It is also neuroessential, as it prioritizes keeping the baby and parents in close contact, fostering parental attunement, which helps the baby develop and thrive. Parents who are integrated into their baby's care also thrive because they feel valued, respected, and competent rather than dismissed and inept. Relationship-based care is foundational to holistic, individualized, and developmentally supportive care, as outlined by the Newborn Individualized Developmental Care and Assessment Program (NIDCAP). It is also the core concept of family-integrated care, which prioritizes kangaroo care (skin-to-skin contact with parents). For medical professionals, technical expertise is essential, but using that expertise in the context of therapeutic and nurturing relationships forms the cornerstone of quality healthcare in the NICU.

For Babies

The NICU is a stressful place for newborns. Due to their still-developing nervous systems, infants experience hyper- and hypo-arousal stress responses when exposed to bright lights and unfamiliar sounds, unnatural positioning, sudden handling by medical staff, and painful medical procedures.[1] Separation from the mother adds to the baby's distress due to mammalian protest-despair biology, which is the instinctive biopsychological reaction of newborn mammals when they are removed from their natural habitat of life-sustaining maternal warmth, nutrition, and safety.[2] None of these aspects of intensive care are conducive to stabilization, growth, brain development, or immune function for any infant, much less vulnerable newborns. Research has confirmed that, by compromising the infant's early nervous system development, the harsh environment of the NICU results in long-term physical and mental health problems and developmental disabilities.[1]

As a medical professional, your relationship expertise contributes to the quality of babies' lives in the NICU and improves long-term outcomes. Relationship expertise involves being attuned and responsive to each baby's unique needs, not just for medical intervention but also for soothing, comfort, and support. As you provide intensive medical care, reflect on how you carry out medical procedures. Do you find that you tune out the baby's distress, or do you strive to prevent, reduce, or eliminate it? When you only focus on carrying out the technical aspects of medical procedures as quickly and effectively as possible, this can compound the baby's stress. "Stressful but quick" may seem efficient and necessary to you, but for the baby, it may set off a chain reaction of hormonal and metabolic sequelae that is difficult to recover from and is not conducive to medical stabilization, recovery, or healing. Even simple or routine caregiving tasks, such as diaper changes, heel sticks, or tubing adjustments, can cause unnecessary stress when done in invasive, painful, or intrusive ways. In contrast, you can approach the baby with a nurturing mindset by attending and responding to subtle signs of stress, even during a medical crisis. You can be efficient and effective without being hurried or insensitive to the baby's overwhelm and suffering. Depending on the infant's unique sensitivities and thresholds, you can soothe or circumvent, or, even better, *prevent* distress with/by

- gentle touch,

- a soft, soothing voice,

- measured pacing,

- appropriate timing,

- shielding the eyes from bright lights,

- covering the ears to block out sharp or loud sounds,

- warmth and containment or swaddling,

- supportive positioning, and

- adequate pain medication.

Your therapeutic relationship with each baby enables you to attune to signs of discomfort, overwhelm, and distress and respond according to their unique cues, tolerance levels, needs, and preferences. Besides improving neonatal outcomes, your focus on relationships can also enhance the culture of the NICU, all of which boosts your resilience and job satisfaction.[3]

There is one more vital strategy for providing relationship-based care to babies, and it is the most neuroprotective and neuroessential: involving parents in their baby's care.[4] In particular, kangaroo mother care (KMC), a type of newborn care involving skin-to-skin contact with the mother or another caregiver, optimizes infant physiologic stabilization and neurodevelopment by enlisting the parent-infant relationship, bonding, breastfeeding, and attachment.[5,6] Several decades of research have provided clinical evidence that the parents' touch and soothing presence can promote breastfeeding and the baby's weight gain, temperature maintenance, and oxygen saturation levels. KMC can also reduce infection, shorten hospital stays, and improve growth, healing, and long-term outcomes for NICU infants, including preventing the significantly disabling consequences of stress on the infant's immature nervous system.[1-4,6-9]

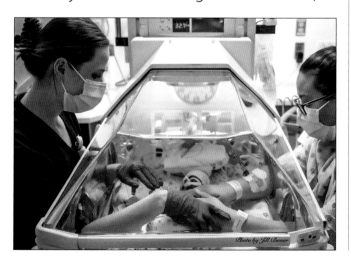

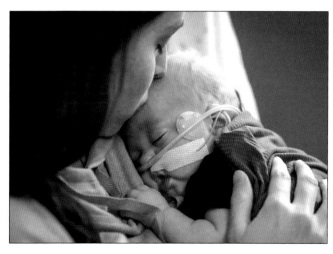

As more worldwide research focuses on *kangaroo mother care immediately after birth*, the results resoundingly reinforce earlier conclusions that newborns should not be separated from their mothers.[2] In the absence of imminently life-threatening conditions, babies who receive immediate KMC stabilize faster than babies admitted to the NICU and are more likely to survive *and thrive*—to need less cardio-respiratory support, to be successful breastfeeders, to grow faster, to require fewer antibiotics, and to leave the hospital earlier.[6,10]

For Parents

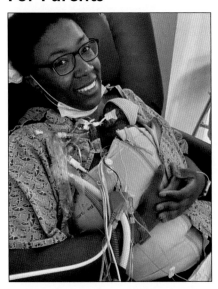

Just as intensive care can be stressful for babies, it is stressful for parents. Parents long to feel close to their babies, but hospitalization and critical medical conditions are barriers that can feel insurmountable.[11] It is normal and natural for parents to feel distressed, overwhelmed, disoriented, fearful, and uncertain about how to approach their baby. These emotions are not due to a lack of bonding but rather an indication of parents' struggling with developing parental identity and learning to become a different kind of parent to a different kind of baby. Indeed, a parent's caution is often a sign of a their caring and emotional investment in their baby's well-being and best interests.

Relationship-based care, particularly family-integrated care, addresses parents' caution by actively and implicitly encouraging their engagement, including learning how to read and respond to their baby, shared decision-making, and positive parent-infant caregiving experiences.[12] Parental involvement fosters parental identity, confidence, competence, emotional coping, and bonding.[13] As mentioned earlier, a key component is kangaroo care, which helps parents understand and *feel* how intimately necessary they are to their baby's care, growth, and development. The research on family-integrated care and kangaroo care shows significant benefits for parents, including increased parental self-efficacy, exclusive breastfeeding upon discharge, improved parent-infant relationships, improved infant developmental outcomes, and reduced parental stress and anxiety—all of which benefit parents *and* their babies.[11-14]

Just as your relationship with each baby enables you to attend to and respond in ways that support healing, growth, and development, your relationship with each parent enables you to support them as they grow and develop into their role as mother or father to this child. In fact, your encouraging attitude toward parents and their involvement is key to their success in the NICU *and beyond*. As you strive to build relationships with parents, here are some tips to remember:

- Assume that even though parents may be emotionally numb or overwhelmed at times, they are competent people and devoted to their baby. With your support, they can adjust to the situation, cope with their grief, and learn the caregiving skills that match their baby's individual needs.

- Reach out in a spirit of collaboration, as this welcomes and includes parents as central members of their baby's caregiving team.

- Think of parents as "parenting," not "visiting," and integrate them as their baby's primary caregivers.

- As you establish a warm rapport with parents, support them as they struggle and learn. Your compassion, patience, and confidence in them build their trust in you—and themselves—and enhance your ability to teach and model caregiving skills.

- Your responsive, soothing care of their baby is reassuring to parents because your sensitivity reinforces their nurturing instincts and helps them trust leaving their baby in your care.

- As you and the parents become attuned to their baby, you can mutually share observations and ideas, showing parents that you value their insights.

- Making room for parents to be parents facilitates their growth into effective soothers, competent decision-makers, and confident caregivers for their babies.

Your goal is not simply to discharge a healthy baby but to discharge a healthy baby to parents who feel devoted and ready to assume total care of their infant. When you facilitate the parents' relationship with their baby, you are fortifying their parental identity, competence, attunement, and confidence, which provides the foundation for successful parenting and developmental outcomes.

Deborah L. Davis, Ph.D., is a developmental psychologist, researcher, and writer, whose books include *Empty Cradle, Broken Heart* (Fulcrum, 4th ed., 2024) and *A Gift of Time* (Johns Hopkins University Press, 2nd ed., 2023). She also blogs for Psychology Today. Mara Tesler Stein, Psy.D., is a clinical psychologist, consultant, trainer, and founder of the Touchstone Institute. Both Davis and Stein specialize in the emotional aspects of grief, trauma, and adjustment around pregnancy, infancy, and parenting. They've co-authored two books: *Parenting Your Premature Baby and Child: The Emotional Journey* (Fulcrum, 2004) and *Intensive Parenting: Surviving the Emotional Journey through the NICU* (Fulcrum, 2012).

References

1. Als H, McAnulty GB. The newborn individualized developmental care and assessment program (NIDCAP) with kangaroo mother care (KMC): Comprehensive care for preterm infants. *Curr Womens Health Rev*. 2011;7(3):288-301.

2. Bergman NJ, Linley LL, Fawcus SR. Randomized controlled trial of skin-to-skin contact from birth versus conventional incubator for physiological stabilization in 1200- to 2199-gram newborns. *Acta Paediatr*. 2004;93(6):779-785.

3. Grunberg VA, Vranceanu AM, Lerou PH. Caring for our caretakers: Building resiliency in NICU parents and staff. *Eur J Pediatr*. 2022;181(9):3545-3548.

4. Bergman NJ, Ludwig RJ, Westrup B, Welch MG. Nurturescience versus neuroscience: A case for rethinking perinatal mother-infant behaviors and relationship. *Birth Defects Res*. 2019;111(15):1110-1127.

5. Altimier L, Phillips R. Neuroprotective care of extremely preterm Infants in the first 72 hours after birth. *Crit Care Nurs Clin North Am*. 2018;30(4):563-583.

6. WHO Immediate KMC Study Group. Immediate "kangaroo mother care" and survival of infants with low birth weight. *N Engl J Med*. 2021;384(21):2028-2038.

7. Conde-Agudelo A, Díaz-Rossello JL. Kangaroo mother care to reduce morbidity and mortality in low birthweight infants. *Cochrane Database Syst Rev*. 2016;2016(8):CD002771.

8. Samsudin S, Chui PL, Ahmad Kamar A, Abdullah KL, Yu CW, Mohamed Z. The impact of structured kangaroo care education on premature infants' weight gain, breastfeeding and length of hospitalization in Malaysia. *J Multidiscip Healthc*. 2023;(16):1023-1035.

9. Forde D, Deming DD, Tan JC, et al. Oxidative stress biomarker decreased in preterm neonates treated with kangaroo mother care. *Biol Res Nurs*. 2020;22(2):188-196.

10. Chi Luong K, Long Nguyen T, Huynh Thi DH, Carrara HPO, Bergman NJ. Newly born low birthweight infants stabilise better in skin-to-skin contact than when separated from their mothers: A randomised controlled trial. *Acta Paediatr*. 2016;105(4):381-390.

11. Fernández Medina IM, Granero-Molina J, Fernández-Sola C, Hernández-Padilla JM, Camacho Ávila M, López Rodríguez MDM. Bonding in neonatal intensive care units: Experiences of extremely preterm infants' mothers. *Women Birth*. 2018;31(4):325-330.

12. Franck LS, Waddington C, O'Brien K. Family integrated care for preterm infants. *Crit Care Nurs Clin North Am*. 2020;32(2):149-165.

13. Thomson G, Flacking R, George K, et al. Parents' experiences of emotional closeness to their infants in the neonatal unit: A meta-ethnography. *Early Hum Dev*. 2020;(149):105155.

14. O'Brien K, Robson K, Bracht M, et al. Effectiveness of family integrated care in neonatal intensive care units on infant and parent outcomes: A multicentre, multinational, cluster-randomised controlled trial. *Lancet Child Adolesc Health*. 2018;2(4):245-254.

Appendix 6.2 **Recognizing and Supporting Parents Through Traumatic Stress and Grief**

Contributed by Celeste Poe, Ph.D., PMH-C, NICU Psychologist

The need for intensive care of critically ill newborns is often considered a crisis or trauma for parents and families. No parent is completely prepared for this crisis, and in addition to the traumatic stress that ensues, many parents feel grief and loss throughout their infant's medical journey. By definition, trauma can include witnessing the near death of a loved one,[1] and grief can follow any significant loss, including non-death-related losses.[2] The extent to which traumatic stress and grief impact someone will vary across different parents and families. Some parents and families come into our care with past experiences of trauma or loss, often exacerbating their traumatic stress and grief. It is crucial for providers to have tools to recognize traumatic stress and grief and feel comfortable in providing sensitive and attuned care.

Traumatic Stress

Traumatic stress can happen to any parent, with almost half of the parents of critically ill infants experiencing it to some degree.[3] Many factors can contribute to a parent's experience of traumatic stress, including having experienced a traumatic birth, the severity of their infant's medical condition, and characteristics of the NICU environment.[4] Traumatic stress can impact an individual's functioning in several areas, including their thinking, emotional processing, bodily functioning, and behaviors.[1] Symptoms of traumatic stress can be demonstrated on a

spectrum of mild to severe and can be organized into four major categories.

1. Re-Experiencing

The first major category of symptoms describes how a crisis or traumatic event can "re-visit" or stay with an individual even after the event or parts of the event have occurred. Traumatic events can include a traumatic birth experience, witnessing a code event, learning of a potentially life-limiting diagnosis, etc. Re-experiencing can occur through disturbing nightmares or flashbacks about the event or through intrusive thoughts that feel difficult to block out and cause distress. Re-experiencing can also occur as the result of reminders or triggers in the environment that can cause emotional or physical distress, such as anxiety, sadness, a pounding heart, shortness of breath, and sweating.

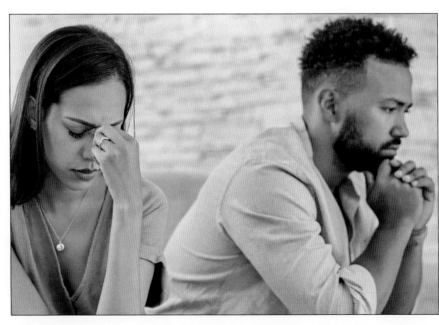

2. Negative Thoughts and Feelings

The second major category of symptoms details how a traumatic event can impact an individual's feelings and perspectives of themselves, others, and the world. This situation can occur through negative feelings, such as anger or guilt, a lack of interest in doing things they used to enjoy, or difficulty experiencing positive emotions like joy. Parents experiencing these feelings may demonstrate fatigue despite getting sleep or appear to have a flat affect, such as having no or very limited facial expressions.

3. Arousal and Reactivity

The third major category of symptoms describes how traumatic stress impacts the nervous system and an individual's ability to regulate their emotions. During and following traumatic events, individuals commonly report a sense of restlessness and an inability for their bodies to settle down. Symptoms of arousal and reactivity include an increased startle response and hypervigilance, irritability, reckless behaviors, and difficulty concentrating and sleeping. Parents in this state may be pacing, have difficulty sitting still, or seem constantly on edge.

4. Avoidance

The fourth major category of symptoms is avoidance, or the tendency to want to push away distressing thoughts, emotions, or memories. Dissociation can also be a form of escape from extreme emotional distress, where a parent may disconnect from their thoughts or feelings or describe feeling "out of their body" or as if what is happening "isn't real." Feelings of avoidance may at times contradict what a parent's true desires are, such as desperately wanting to visit their infant in the NICU but finding it extremely challenging to do so, given significant feelings of anxiety or stress when coming into the hospital or being at the bedside for long periods. For this reason, it's essential that when a parent's engagement seems limited, we consider whether avoidance and traumatic stress could be playing a role.

Grief and Loss

While grief is commonly experienced in the context of bereavement following the death of a loved one, grief can also be the result of other significant losses. Even when a baby survives, parents of critically ill infants often experience several forms of loss throughout their infant's medical care.[5]

For nearly all parents, navigating issues related to prematurity, critical illness, and prolonged hospitalization come with several ambiguous losses, or losses unrelated to death that can represent an end to one's hopes or possibilities and may be hard to describe.[6] Examples of these ambiguous forms of loss include feeling "robbed" of the pregnancy or birth experience one planned for, the absence of highly anticipated moments like holding a newborn for the first time immediately following birth, or the imagined child that may now have an unexpected developmental trajectory.

Changes to a previously held or imagined parental role are inevitable when a newborn or infant is in critical care. Parents often report needing to "ask permission" to do things with their infant, questioning who is "in charge," or feeling hesitant to ask questions or advocate for themselves.[7] While most limitations to the parental role during critical care cannot be avoided, understanding and empathizing with the impact of this loss on parents can help providers find opportunities to highlight the parental role and the value parents hold within their infant's care.

When a newborn or infant is not expected to live, processing the transition into comfort care can understandably be challenging for parents and will likely take time. It is important to note that access to palliative care is not always available for parents. In these cases, it can be helpful to support parents' understanding of what they can expect throughout their infant's end-of-life journey while providing reassurance of the lack of suffering and assuaging guilt when appropriate. In addition, many parents report the complexity of experiencing anticipatory grief while also trying to hold out hope for their infant's recovery.

While a natural and adaptive response to loss, grief—like traumatic stress—can impact parents on cognitive, emotional, physical, and behavioral levels. Parents may report symptoms of re-experiencing, such as intrusive thoughts or grief triggers, negative thoughts and feelings like depression or guilt, arousal and reactivity like irritability and difficulty sleeping, and avoidance in thinking or talking about the loss.

How Can You Support Parents Through Traumatic Stress and Grief?

Traumatic stress and grief can be all-encompassing experiences, impacting parents on multiple levels and often making ideal engagement and participation in their infant's care challenging. Difficulties with concentration, remembering details, and getting quality sleep, as well as constantly feeling on edge can certainly impact parents' ability to think and communicate clearly with staff.[8] It is important that perinatal caregivers consider how traumatic stress and grief may be playing a role for a parent or family and remain curious about what supports would be helpful for parents during this crisis.

Tips

- Remember that coping with grief and trauma are both universal and individual experiences. This definition means that while trauma and grief are both a part of the human experience following a crisis, each parent and family will experience and cope with their traumatic stress and grief in ways unique to them.

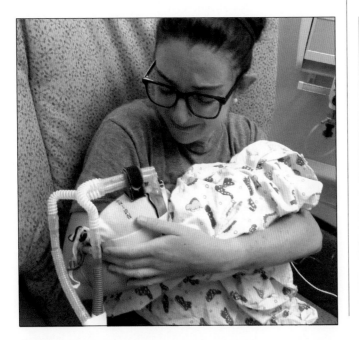

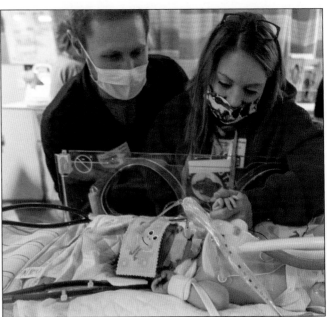

- Often, in a crisis, parents do not feel like themselves and may have difficulty understanding their own emotions and behaviors. Empathic listening and supporting parents in feeling seen and heard can bring them a great deal of relief and help them process their emotions.

- It is common for experiences of grief and traumatic stress to impact daily functioning, including basic self-care such as hygiene, prioritizing sleep and rest, and ensuring proper nutrition and hydration. Significantly, impairments in basic care can also exacerbate difficulties in managing traumatic stress and grief. Gentle guidance around how to balance care for both the infant and self is very helpful for parents.

- Given potential difficulties with remembering and processing information, communication from providers should be as clear, consistent, and transparent as possible. During lengthy or complex discussions, pausing for breaks or asking parents to repeat back their understanding can ensure comprehension and retention of information. Finding ways to provide reassurance as appropriate can be extremely relieving for parents.

- It can be helpful to consider what environmental factors may be contributing to emotional or physical trauma or grief triggers, including the sights and sounds within the hospital. For example, parents may be triggered by their infant's appearance, the sights and sounds of medical equipment, discussions of past medical events, or barriers to comforting or soothing their infant. You can help by anticipating and minimizing triggers when possible. Learn from and collaborate with parents to identify triggers and strategies for grounding and calming during distress, such as engaging in deep breathing, taking breaks, or leaning on their social support system.

- Experiences of grief and loss will change over time. Still, grief has no definitive timeline, and sometimes suggesting to a parent that "it will get better with time" after a baby dies can feel dismissive, given the significance and acuity of the pain immediately following the death of their baby.

Celeste H. Poe, Ph.D., PMH-C, is a licensed clinical psychologist certified in perinatal mental health. She is the Director of the NICU Psychology Program at Lucile Packard Children's Hospital within the Stanford School of Medicine. Dr. Poe specializes in infant and early childhood mental health as well as grief and trauma throughout the perinatal period. Her work is centered on providing psychological support to parents of medically fragile infants before, during, and after a NICU admission.

References

1. American Psychiatric Association. *Diagnostic and Statistical Manual of Mental Disorders*. 5th ed. American Psychiatric Association Publishing; 2013. Accessed March 25, 2024.

2. Ratcliffe MJ, Richardson LF. Grief over non-death losses: A phenomenological perspective. *Passion: Journal of the European Philosophical Society for the Study of Emotions*. 2023;1(1):50–67.

3. Malouf R, Harrison S, Burton HA, et al. Prevalence of anxiety and post-traumatic stress (PTS) among the parents of babies admitted to neonatal units: A systematic review and meta-analysis. *EClinical Medicine*. 2022;(43):101233.

4. Sharp M, Huber N, Ward LG, Dolbier C. NICU-specific stress following traumatic childbirth and its relationship with posttraumatic stress. *J Perinat Neonatal Nurs*. 2021;35(1):57-67.

5. Golish TD, Powell KA. Ambiguous loss': Managing the dialectics of grief associated with premature birth. *J Soc Pers Relat*. 2003;20(3):309-334.

6. Wilson C, Cook C. Ambiguous loss and post-traumatic growth: Experiences of mothers whose school-aged children were born extremely prematurely. *J Clin Nurs*. 2018;27(7-8), e1627-e1639.

7. Al Maghaireh DAF, Abdullah KL, Chan CM, Piaw CY, & Al Kawafha MM. Systematic review of qualitative studies exploring parental experiences in the Neonatal Intensive Care Unit. *J Clin Nurs*. 2016;25(19-20):2745-2756.

8. Friedman J, Friedman SH, Collin M, Martin RJ. Staff perceptions of challenging parent–staff interactions and beneficial strategies in the Neonatal Intensive Care Unit. *Acta Paediatrica*. 2018;107(1):33-39.

Appendix 6.3 Emotional Support for Newborns and Their Parents

Contributed by Dr. Raylene Phillips, MD, MA, FAAP, FABM, IBCLC

Support for Stable Newborns, Their Mothers, and Their Families[1]

The first hour after birth is a once-in-a-lifetime experience that should be honored and protected.

- Even an uncomplicated birth is a huge transition for all newborns. To best support this transition from intrauterine to extrauterine life, immediately place the stable newborn on the mother's chest (or another parent's chest if the mother is not available or is not stable) while being dried and assessed. If the infant remains stable (and the mother is also stable), they should be kept in uninterrupted skin-to-skin contact (SSC) until after their first feeding.

- Routine care (weight, foot/hand printing, Vitamin K, and eye ointment treatments) should be done only after the baby's first feeding (or the first hour after birth) is completed. Bathing can be delayed to support an optimal transition from intrauterine to extrauterine life.

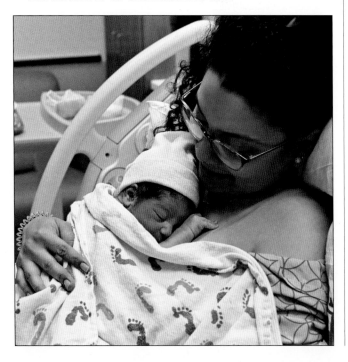

- Uninterrupted SSC of the newborn with their mother (or other parent) supports improved physiologic stability (temperature, respiration, heart rate, blood pressure, glucose level), increases maternal/parental bonding and attachment behaviors, protects the newborn from the stress of separation from the mother/parent, supports optimal infant brain development, and increases breastfeeding initiation and duration.

- If the baby or mother requires medical care and SSC must be interrupted, the baby should be returned to SSC with the mother (or significant other if the mother is unavailable) as soon as possible.

Support for Preterm or Sick Newborns and Their Parents

- Remember that every newborn has just exited the warm, quiet, and supportive environment of the womb where they were in constant physical, hormonal, and psychological contact with their mother. Any baby needing resuscitation and transport or admission to intensive care will find themselves in a very different environment than developmentally expected, which is unavoidably stressful. However, you can moderate and reduce this stress by protecting babies from direct bright lights and loud sounds (including loud voices) and providing soft boundaries, gentle handling, and contact with parents (perhaps most important).

- Separation of newborns from their mothers always leads to an increased stress response for the babies (and their mothers). Whenever possible, placing the newborn (of any gestational age) in SSC with the mother after birth will help stabilize the baby, even if there is mild respiratory distress. If the baby needs more aggressive resuscitation or intubation, facilitating SSC as soon as possible will support physiological stability for both the baby and the parent and will also support their developing bonds of attachment.

- When the mother is not available for SSC, the father or significant other can be encouraged to hold the baby in SSC even if the baby is on CPAP or intubated. This step can also help support the baby's physiologic stability and promote the father-infant bonds of attachment.

- If the baby must be admitted to the NICU and the mother had planned to breastfeed their baby, support them in early hand expression or pumping and send any drops of colostrum to the NICU for oral care or early feeding. Mother's breast milk is like "medicine" to preterm and sick babies.

- If the baby needs transport to another NICU and the mother had planned to breastfeed their baby (and their medical condition permits), encourage them to hand express or pump before the neonatal transport team departs with the baby. Sending their milk with the baby allows the opportunity to provide something very personal, and even a few drops of colostrum should be welcomed by the receiving NICU nurse for oral care or trophic feeds.

- Talking directly to babies in a soft, gentle, and comforting voice can help reduce their stress. A 33-week gestation fetus (and possibly younger) is known to be responsive to their mother's voice and prefers it over other female voices or sounds.[2] At 32 weeks gestation, the fetus shows more stability (with higher heart variability) when their

mother communicates *directly to* them than if the mother communicates with another adult nearby *about* the baby.[3] Preterm infants in the NICU at 32 weeks corrected gestational age are known to make vocalizations, and they make even more vocalizations when their parents are talking directly to them at the bedside than when no one is talking directly to them.[4]

- When the mother is not available, the partner/significant other can be encouraged to talk to their newborn even during resuscitation or stabilization, and often, their familiar voice can help to stabilize the baby.

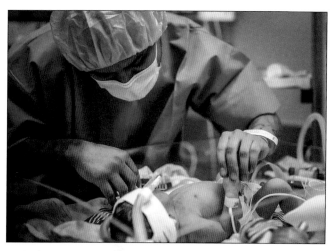

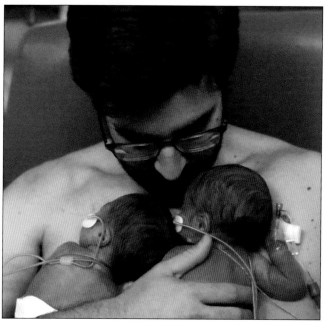

Emotional Support

E

- Recognize that SSC is not just a "nice" thing to do for babies and parents. There is well-documented evidence that SSC contributes to a NICU infant's physiological stability, improves infant sleep (and thus brain development and growth), helps to heal the emotional wounds from mother-infant separation, and helps mothers recover from the loss of an expected "healthy-outcome" pregnancy. Physical connection with kangaroo care, hand hugging, and other forms of positive touch is critically important for continuing the emotional connections that began when the baby was in the womb. These early emotional connections form the basis for bonding and attachment, which are crucial for lifelong emotional health and well-being.

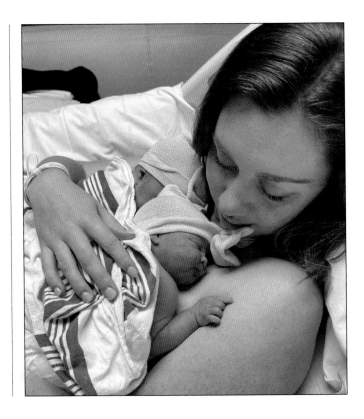

Dr. Raylene Phillips, MD, MA, FAAP, FABM, IBCLC, is the Medical Director of Neonatal Services and Pediatric Department Chair at Loma Linda University Medical Center – Murrieta. She is also an Associate Professor of Pediatrics/Neonatology at Loma Linda University School of Medicine and Director of Breastfeeding/Lactation at Loma Linda University Children's Hospital in Loma Linda, California. During her career as a neonatologist, she has developed a passion for supporting early parent-infant connections and helping others understand the impact of the birth experience on the long-term emotional health and well-being of the child.

References

1. Phillips R. The sacred hour: Uninterrupted skin-to-skin contact immediately after birth. *Newborn Infant Nurs Rev.* 2013;13(2):67-72.

2. Webb AR, Heiler HT, Benson CB, Lahav A. Mother's voice and heartbeat sounds elicit auditory plasticity in the human brain before full gestation. *Proc Natl Acad Sci U S A.* 2015;112(10):3152-7.

3. Busnel M-C, Volff T, Ribeiro A, et al. Communication between mother and infant (fetus or newborn). *Infant Ment Health J.* 2006;27(3A):738.

4. Caskey M, Stephens B, Tucker R, Vohr B. Adult talk in the NICU with preterm infants and developmental outcomes. *Pediatrics.* 2014;133(3):e578-84.

Quality Improvement Module

Sugar

Temperature

Airway

Blood Pressure

Lab Work

Emotional Support

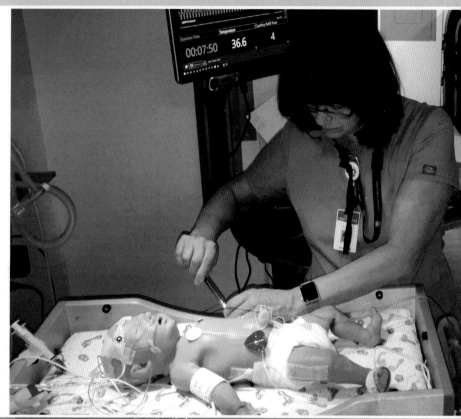

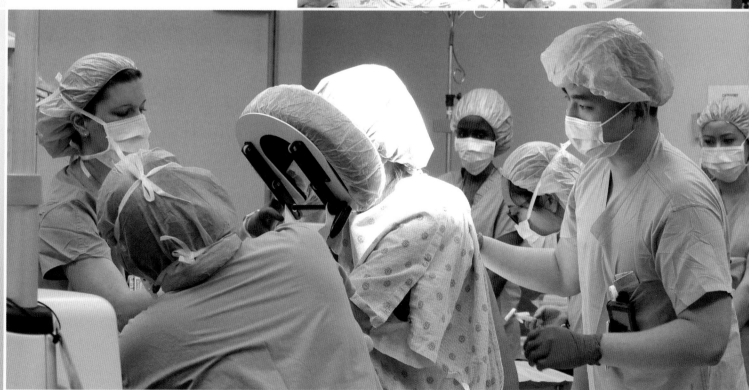

Quality Improvement—Module Objectives

Upon completion of this module, participants will gain an increased understanding of:

1. Methods to enhance patient safety and reduce medical errors and preventable adverse events in the vulnerable neonatal population.

2. The importance of effective communication and teamwork to prevent harm and improve patient safety.

3. Simulation-based education as a strategy to improve patient safety.

4. Self-assessment and post-event debriefing to evaluate care provided to patients.

Introduction

Improving patient outcomes and reducing errors and adverse events is the goal of everyone involved with healthcare delivery. A uniform, standardized process of care and a comprehensive team approach can improve patient safety, processes for delivering quality care, and, ultimately, infant outcomes.[1,2] The six S.T.A.B.L.E. modules you have just completed focused on the importance of assessing patient history, signs, laboratory and test data, and developing a team plan of care. It is essential to remember that sick infants require continual reassessment because their status may change rapidly. The goal of S.T.A.B.L.E. education is to provide important, evidence-based information to improve the delivery of safe, quality care to sick, vulnerable infants.

In the United States, as many as 400,000 patients die every year as a result of preventable causes, and many survivors of errors suffer life-long disability.[3] This number of deaths is much higher than was originally reported by the Institute of Medicine in their landmark publication *To Err is Human*.[4] Mechanisms known to reduce errors include standardizing processes of care, avoiding reliance on memory, and communicating in clear, direct ways.[1,4-7]

The Situation, Background, Assessment, Recommendation (SBAR) form of structured communication is used to reduce potential errors associated with miscommunication or a lack of information.[8,9] The SBAR technique also achieves an important goal of standardizing communication regarding an infant's condition.[10] SBAR has its roots in the military and was designed to facilitate quick communication of critical information to the leader. Table 7.1 contains a summary of the components of SBAR communication.

colspan table

Start each interaction with the medical care provider by INTRODUCING yourself and the patient you are calling about.

Example:
"Hi Dr. Smith, this is <u>your name</u>, and I'm the nurse taking care of baby girl Jones in Bed 16. She's the 39-week gestation baby that was admitted for TEF last night. I'm calling because I'm concerned about her increased respiratory distress. At the beginning of my shift, she was on 40% oxygen and saturating in the mid-90s, but ever since we started her IV an hour ago, her oxygen requirement has gone up to 60%, and she is retracting now. I'd like for you to come to the bedside to assess her."

	INFORMATION TO PROVIDE	
SITUATION Concise statement of the problem—What is happening with the patient?	Admitting diagnosis or reason for admission	
	Age	
	Weight	
	Gender	
	Signs/symptoms of concern (the reason you are calling)	
BACKGROUND Information pertinent to your concern—What is the clinical background?	Brief summary of significant medical history	
	Vital signs and status	
	Labs—normal & critical findings	
	Medications or treatments given	
	Previous orders received	
	Tests—ordered and results known or pending	
	IV status and fluids	
	Maternal history (if applicable)	
	Other information pertinent to the present illness	
ASSESSMENT Synthesis of relevant information you have analyzed—What you think the problem is or what you have found	Respiratory	Neurological
	Cardiovascular	GI / GU
	Endocrine / Labs	Infection
	Family psychosocial / social (as applicable)	Lines/tubes
	Other systems pertinent to the present illness	
RECOMMENDATION Action requested or recommended to address the problem	Overall impressions and/or concerns—be specific	
	Make recommendations for change(s) in the plan of care or request new orders	
	Identify the plan of care	
	Wrap Up: When does the physician//HCP want to be notified again?	
	For what changes does the physician/HCP want to be notified?	
	If you want the physician/HCP to come to the bedside, state that request and ask when you can expect them to arrive.	

READ BACK all verbal orders or repeat back your understanding of the expectations.

Table 7.1. Components of SBARR communication. Adapted from TeamSTEPPS at www.ahrq.gov/teamsteppstools.

The Importance of Optimal Communication and Team Training[11-15]

Given the complex and dynamic nature of hospitals, combined with the unpredictability of patient outcomes, errors do occur. While healthcare systems, procedures, and guidelines are intended to provide optimal patient care, there are often unexpected shortcomings. Healthcare professionals face unforeseen challenges that threaten patient safety on a daily basis. Some suggestions to reduce errors include knowing how to invoke the "chain of command;" consistently using clear, unambiguous communication; using standardized processes of care; being prepared with knowledge, equipment, and skills for situations that will arise; and participating in post-assessment evaluation of care that was delivered, focusing on what went well and what could have been done differently.

Communication

Written and verbal communication must be clear, unambiguous, and timely. When a verbal order is given, it should be repeated back to the person giving the order to ensure it was heard correctly (i.e., closed-loop communication). As seen in Table 7.1, the SBAR conversation should end with a readback of all verbal orders or repeating back understanding of expectations. The S.T.A.B.L.E. Program added an additional "R" to represent repeat back orders received or the plan of care agreed upon with the medical care provider. A handwritten order or prescription should be legible and not include medical abbreviations that may be easily mistaken for other words.

In the United States, the hospital accreditation agency The Joint Commission published a Sentinel Event report of 93 cases of infant death and 16 cases of permanent disability.[16] Communication issues topped the list of identified root causes (72%), with 55% of the facilities citing organizational culture as a barrier to effective communication and teamwork (i.e., intimidation and hierarchy, failure to function as a team, and failure to follow the chain of communication). Numerous risk reduction strategies were identified by The Joint Commission, including conducting team training in perinatal areas to teach staff to work together and communicate more effectively.

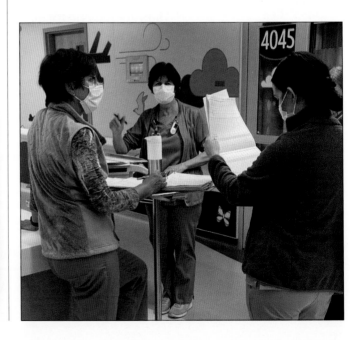

Know How to Activate and Use the Chain of Command

Every healthcare facility has a "chain of command" or a "chain of communication" in place to help employees resolve disputes and advocate for patients. This chain is designed to identify personnel with progressively higher authority within a department or facility who can be approached to help resolve disputes. For example, a nurse concerned about a physician's order would first discuss their concern with the physician. If they were not satisfied with the response and felt carrying out the order would not be in the patient's best interest, they could then discuss their concern with the charge nurse. The charge nurse can help the nurse discuss the problem with the physician. If both are not satisfied that the problem is being addressed, the charge nurse can then notify the nursing supervisor, who can then go to the medical director of the unit and so on up the chain until the dispute is satisfactorily resolved. Knowing how to access the chain of command includes knowing when to invoke it, the line of authority, and the steps to move up. Most hospitals have safety initiatives in place, such as safety rounds, safety committees, anonymous reporting phone lines or anonymous electronic reporting (of concerns), and quality department personnel available for private consultation should you have concerns to discuss.

Simulation-Based Training: Being Prepared for Situations That Arise[17-31]

Neonatology and newborn care is a dynamic and ever-changing field. One of the most exciting changes in the past decade has been the integration of simulation-based education into neonatal training. Simulation that mimics the situations encountered clinically allows for the practice of cognitive (knowledge and decision-making), technical (skills carried out to stabilize or resuscitate the patient), and behavioral (communication and teamwork) skills by interprofessional participants—nurses, physicians, respiratory therapists, licensed practical nurses, nurse aides, and other allied health professionals. A major benefit of simulation training is the ability to learn on a manikin and with workplace teammates without any consequence of patient harm.

Simulation-based education offers a valuable opportunity to improve patient safety. By practicing patient care via realistic clinical scenarios, participants will be challenged with dynamic decision-making under stress, experience firsthand the impact of communication and interactions between team members on patient care and outcomes, and understand the challenges of selecting and correctly using resources and information during time-pressured emergencies.

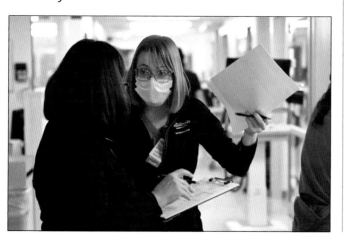

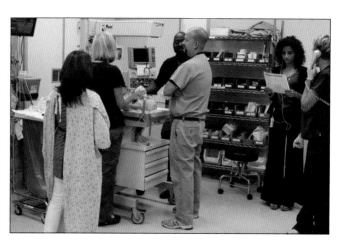

Debriefing

Simply performing a simulation will not fix the problem. Fundamental in achieving experiential learning is the opportunity for participants to debrief at the end of each clinical scenario. During debriefing, participants analyze, discuss, and make sense of what just happened.[32,33] It is important for the debriefer (the person facilitating the debriefing) to seek training in simulation methodology and debriefing since the effect of a poorly run simulation experience or poorly conducted debriefing will dilute the intended effect of the simulation experience and may even be harmful to the participants.

A core principle of simulation-based education is ensuring *psychological safety* is maintained so that participants feel 'safe' to make mistakes or openly discuss, without embarrassment or rejection, the thought processes that went into their decisions and actions. A core goal of simulation is to apply what is learned theoretically and demonstrate the ability to synthesize clinical data within a time-pressured emergency in a safe environment. Developing scenarios based on real-life situations facilitates the further development of teamwork, problem-solving, and communication skills. Learning and practicing through simulation can translate to more effective handling of challenging clinical situations and emergencies when encountered.

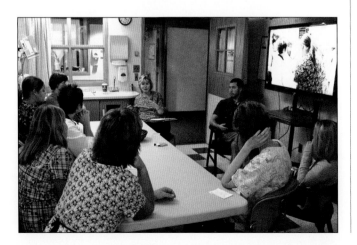

Human Factors[26,34-46]

Human factors were first identified in the aviation industry in the 1970s and have since permeated through other high-risk industries, including healthcare. They are known to play a part in the occurrence of adverse critical clinical events and include areas such as the following:

- Lack of effective leadership

- Lack of effective teamwork as evidenced by individuals working independently of each other, without coordination

- Use of hierarchical methods of communication that inhibit contributions from less experienced or less confident staff

Consider the potential effect of poor leadership and teamwork where, in a crisis, individuals work independently of each other and without direction or coordination. Confusing, unclear, or hierarchical communication (fear of speaking up because of one's perceived lower position in healthcare or being intimidated by the leader) is a recipe for errors and poor patient outcomes. These human factors must be considered if educational strategies such as simulation are to be successful. Effective stabilization of the infant requires all those involved to work **respectfully** and **collaboratively**. There is increasing evidence that an understanding of human behavior under stressful conditions may also give insight into how further improvements can be made.

Standardized Processes of Care: The S.T.A.B.L.E. Program

Training maternal-child and neonatal healthcare providers in The S.T.A.B.L.E. Program will help achieve several goals. First, it will help promote teamwork by bringing everyone together on the same page so the team can work effectively and in concert with each other. Second, it will allow for the evaluation of care and enable the identification of deviations from program guidelines. At times, it is necessary to change or modify the care provided to infants; however, inappropriate deviations are easier to identify when everyone uses the same approach.

Post-Assessment Evaluation of Care and Debriefing[5,13,23,34,39,47-53]

Evaluation of care provided to an infant is essential to improving patient safety. Look for potential causes of poor or inadequate care and the types of errors that were committed (e.g., preventative, diagnostic, and treatment). Try to include the healthcare team members involved in the case in a debriefing and/or a formal morbidity and mortality conference. Consult experts in neonatology, cardiology, surgery, and/or pathology when needed. Case review can be considered for the following events, acknowledging that other situations may also arise that merit review:

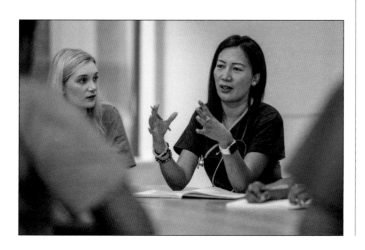

- An infant is expected to be well but is unexpectedly sick and requires transport. Review the adequacy of the stabilization care provided. See page 270 for the Pre-transport Stabilization Self-Assessment Tool to guide the review.

- An error occurs during the delivery of care.

  o An error is defined as using a wrong plan to achieve an aim (an error of planning) or failure to complete a planned action as intended (an error of execution).[4]

  o A *preventable adverse event* or *near-miss* is identified. A preventable adverse event is defined as an injury caused by medical intervention or management rather than the underlying disease or condition of the patient.[14] A near-miss event is an error detected and corrected before it reaches the patient and causes harm.[54]

- Patient care should be reviewed when an infant becomes sicker than was expected or when other unanticipated issues arise, including complications that lengthen hospitalization or lead to death.

The following is a suggestion for closing an actual patient debrief: *"Thank you all for attending. I know this was a stressful situation (and may not have been the outcome we wanted). I appreciate that everyone pulled together to try to obtain the best outcome. I appreciate that we identified areas where we can improve, and we will work toward accomplishing those goals. Again, I value the opportunity to work with each of you. If anyone wants to discuss anything further, my door remains open."*

Questions to Ask When Evaluating Stabilization Care

- Start the debrief or discussion by asking the team, "What did we do well?"

- Did we encounter problems that affected our ability to stabilize the infant?

    o Did we have the equipment we needed, and did we know how to use it?

    o Did we have the personnel with the proper experience and/or skills to carry out the necessary stabilization?

    o Did personnel respond promptly to a call for help?

    o Are there education deficits that need to be addressed?

    o Are there protocols or procedures that need to be developed to guide future care?

- How did we perform as a team?

- What could we do to improve our performance?

- Was the patient well-stabilized?

- Are there any care processes that must be improved if there is another patient with similar circumstances?

- Was patient care delivered in a safe and error-free manner?

- Can we identify any preventable errors or adverse events?

- What was the patient outcome?

Asking yourself and your team whether anything could have been done differently or better will promote discussion about how to improve care the next time an infant is sick

and needs to be stabilized and/or transported to a neonatal intensive care unit. In addition, this important review process is beneficial for identifying simulation education activities that may help prepare for similar future events.

The Pre-Transport Stabilization Self-Assessment Tool (PSSAT)

When an infant requires transport, it is helpful to comprehensively assess the stabilization care provided prior to transport. Again, it is most effective and beneficial if the infant's caregivers are involved with the assessment. The PSSAT data collection tool found on page 271 may be used during the debriefing of perinatal caregivers involved with a neonatal transport to assess the timeliness and completeness of stabilization care. The time "A" and "B" recordings should be completed by the birth hospital providers (referring), and the time "C" recordings should be completed by the transport team and the referring facility together if time allows. The PSSAT may also be used for developing future simulations, case reviews within the unit or joint case reviews with the transport team, and interdepartmental discussions of logistical issues during stabilization (e.g., getting medications from the pharmacy in a timely manner, performing diagnostic tests or communicating with specialists about test results). Directions for using the PSSAT are found on page 270. The PSSAT form may also be downloaded from the S.T.A.B.L.E. website at http://www.stableprogram.org under the Student menu.

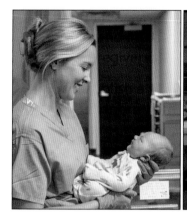
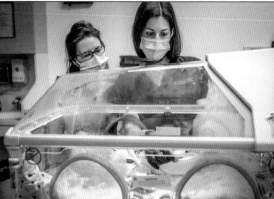
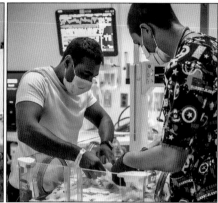

A message from the Program Author and Founder, Dr. Kris Karlsen

The care you provide has the power to improve the lives of babies and their families. The knowledge you share has the power to teach others for generations to come. The questions you answer from more novice staff will carry forward long after you retire. Please view every question you receive and answer you give as directly relating to patient safety. We have an opportunity to make a difference for children and their families, and I recognize it sometimes feels overwhelming to make it through our incredibly busy, complicated, and stressful days. After a 45-year career in the NICU as a nurse practitioner and educator of S.T.A.B.L.E. and other curricula, I can look back and know those extra moments I gave to teach a nurse, therapist, resident, or family were worth it. Go forward and do the best you can each and every day. With admiration for all you do, thank you for *Improving Neonatal Outcomes – With Education.*

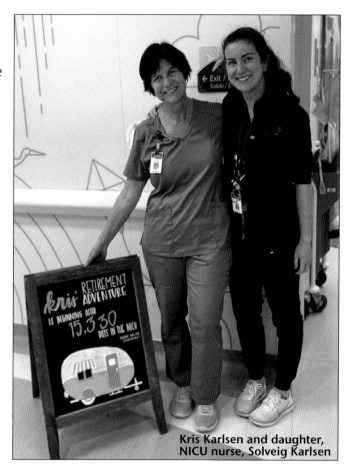

Kris Karlsen and daughter, NICU nurse, Solveig Karlsen

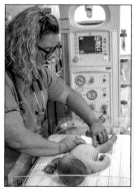
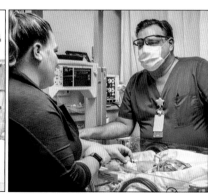
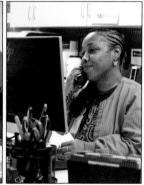
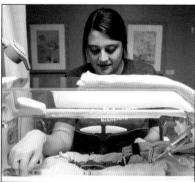

Directions for Using the Pre-transport Stabilization Self-Assessment Tool

1. Either during pre-transport stabilization care or immediately after the infant is transported, complete the demographic information in the Patient Information section of the form.

2. Under Indications for Referral, select all suspected or confirmed diagnoses that apply at the time of referral.

3. Times A, B, and C are used repetitively on the first and second pages of the form. Record the vital signs, physical exam, and stabilization procedures that were performed:

   - At the time the transport team was called (transport was requested) = Time A

   - Upon the arrival of the transport team to your nursery = Time B

   - Upon the departure of the transport team = Time C

     o The transport team should help complete the Time C items unless the infant is unstable and time does not allow. In that case, if at all possible, ask the team to leave a copy of their stabilization record so you can complete the Time C items.

4. Completion of this form will allow evaluation of stabilization care by looking at three specific time intervals:

   - What stabilization actions were taken at the time it was determined the infant was sick?

   - What stabilization actions were taken while awaiting the team's arrival?

   - What stabilization actions were completed by the team?

   - The following scenarios are possible:

     o When the team arrives, stabilization is complete, so they only need to assess the baby, attach the transport equipment, and move the baby into the incubator.

     o The team arrives quickly and completes the stabilization procedures you did not have time to complete.

     o The team arrives and determines that additional care is needed, and therefore, further actions are taken (such as intubating the patient, inserting lines, changing an ET tube, administering certain medications, etc.).

   - By recording these actions, it is hoped that the nursing and medical leadership team will be able to assess the adequacy of pre-transport (or transfer) stabilization care.

   - In addition, this important review process may be beneficial for identifying simulation education activities that may help prepare for similar future events.

If you have trouble filling out the form or need additional expertise to answer the questions on the third page of the form, consult your neonatal transport team or the transport team coordinator or medical director for assistance. An optimally performed stabilization is the goal of community caregivers and transport teams alike!

Pre-transport Stabilization Self-Assessment Tool (PSSAT)

PARENT INFORMATION

Birth weight: ☐☐☐☐ grams **Birth order:** _____ of _____

Growth: AGA SGA LGA **Gender:** Male Female Ambiguous

Estimated Gest. Age: ☐☐ - ☐ / ☐ weeks/days (ex: 34-3/7)

Baby admitted from: ☐ Labor & Delivery ☐ Mother-baby unit ☐ Nursery ☐ Emergency room

Resuscitation at birth: Suction Blow-by oxygen CPAP CPAP & PPV Intubation & PPV Chest compressions

Resuscitation meds (list): _____

Other meds (list): _____

Apgar at 1 minute: ☐☐ 5 min: ☐☐ 10 min: ☐☐ 15 min: ☐☐ 20 min: ☐☐

Indications for referral (circle all that apply)

Prematurity Respiratory distress Sepsis Cardiac Metabolic Genetic Neurologic Hematologic Surgical Birth depression

Other (explain): _____

TIME

Age of baby in Days and Hours after birth – **at time transport team called** _____ Days _____ Hours

A **Transport team called** _____ AM PM

B **Transport team arrived at nursery** _____ AM PM

C **Transport team departed nursery** _____ AM PM

Note: these times will be used throughout this form. When answering questions, evaluate the parameter closest to time A, B, and C.

Time patient died; transport aborted _____ AM PM (complete remainder of form even if patient died)

VITAL SIGNS

	Temperature °C °F	Axillary or Rectal	Heart Rate	Respiratory Rate	Blood Pressure Systolic/Diastolic	Mean	Method (RA, LA, RL, LL) or Arterial
Time A	_____	_____	☐	☐	☐ / ☐	☐	_____
Time B	_____	_____	☐	☐	☐ / ☐	☐	_____
Time C	_____	_____	☐	☐	☐ / ☐	☐	_____

PHYSICAL EXAM

Perfusion/Pulses

	Capillary Refill Time (sec.) over chest	over knee		Pulses	Pulses equal upper & lower	(If no, explain)
Time A	_____	_____ sec.		Normal Decreased Increased	YES NO	_____
Time B	_____	_____ sec.		Normal Decreased Increased	YES NO	_____
Time C	_____	_____ sec.		Normal Decreased Increased	YES NO	_____

Retractions

	Severity (circle all that apply)	Location (circle all that apply)	O2 Saturation	FiO2
Time A	Mild Moderate Severe Gasping	Substernal Intercostal Subcostal	☐ %	☐ %
Time B	Mild Moderate Severe Gasping	Substernal Intercostal Subcostal	☐ %	☐ %
Time C	Mild Moderate Severe Gasping	Substernal Intercostal Subcostal	☐ %	☐ %

Level of consciousness

	Response to noxious stimuli (circle all that apply)	Other (explain)
Time A	Withdraws/good tone, cries Lethargic, no cry Seizure(s) No response, comatose	_____
Time B	Withdraws/good tone, cries Lethargic, no cry Seizure(s) No response, comatose	_____
Time C	Withdraws/good tone, cries Lethargic, no cry Seizure(s) No response, comatose	_____

Paralytic used (i.e. pavulon)? Yes No Reason given: _____

Time/dose of all Opioids given past 24 hrs (list type) _____

Time/dose of all Sedatives given past 24 hrs (list type) _____

Pre-transport Stabilization Self-Assessment Tool (PSSAT)

Use Time **A B C** from page 1	**Time A** _____	**Time B** _____	**Time C** _____
IV in place?	Y N Location _____	Y N Location _____	Y N Location _____
IV fluid infusing?	Y N Type _____ Rate ml/kg/day _____	Y N Type _____ Rate ml/kg/day _____	Y N Type _____ Rate ml/kg/day _____
UVC in place?	Y N Tip location _____	Y N Tip location _____	Y N Tip location _____
UAC in place?	Y N Tip location _____	Y N Tip location _____	Y N Tip location _____
Glucose – closest to 15 – 30 minutes of this time	Y N Value mg/dL _____	Y N Value mg/dL _____	Y N Value mg/dL _____
Glucose bolus given?	Y N Fluid _____ Amount _____	Y N Fluid _____ Amount _____	Y N Fluid _____ Amount _____
Oxygen in use?	Y N % _____	Y N % _____	Y N % _____
Pulse oximetry on?	Y N O$_2$ sat _____	Y N O$_2$ sat _____	Y N O$_2$ sat _____
CPAP in use?	Y N Type _____ Pressure _____	Y N Type _____ Pressure _____	Y N Type _____ Pressure _____
PPV provided?	Y N Pressures _____ Rate _____	Y N Pressures _____ Rate _____	Y N Pressures _____ Rate _____
Tracheal intubation?	Y N Cm at lip _____	Y N Cm at lip _____	Y N Cm at lip _____
ET tube properly secured?	Y N	Y N	Y N
Chest tube in place?	Y N	Y N	Y N
Chest needle or cath placed?	Y N	Y N	Y N
Volume bolus?	Y N Type _____ Amount _____	Y N Type _____ Amount _____	Y N Type _____ Amount _____
On dopamine?	Y N Dose mcg/kg/min _____	Y N Dose mcg/kg/min _____	Y N Dose mcg/kg/min _____
CBC with differential done?	Y N	Y N	Y N
Blood culture drawn?	Y N	Y N	Y N
Antibiotics given?	Y N	Y N	Y N Additional antibiotic or dose given?
On radiant warmer on ISC?	Y N	Y N	Y N
In incubator on ISC?	Y N	Y N	Y N
In incubator on air temp?	Y N	Y N	Y N

(Left margin label: STABILIZATION PROCEDURES)

BLOOD GASSES

Time	Indicate CBG, ABG, Venous						Ventilation settings PIP/PEEP	Rate	FiO$_2$	Method B/M? Prongs? Hood Intubated
_____ AM PM	☐	pH ____	pCO$_2$ ____	pO$_2$ ____	HCO$_3$ ____	BE ____	____ / ____	____	____ %	_____
_____ AM PM	☐	pH ____	pCO$_2$ ____	pO$_2$ ____	HCO$_3$ ____	BE ____	____ / ____	____	____ %	_____
_____ AM PM	☐	pH ____	pCO$_2$ ____	pO$_2$ ____	HCO$_3$ ____	BE ____	____ / ____	____	____ %	_____

Pre-transport Stabilization Self-Assessment Tool (PSSAT)

SPECIFIC INTERVENTIONS

Airway

ET tube location (cm marking **at the lip**) when Team arrived: _____ cm

Was ET tube location readjusted **prior** to the transport team arrival?   Y   N   Explain: _____

Was ET tube location readjusted **after** transport team arrival?   Y   N   Explain: _____

Was patient **re-intubated** by the transport team?   Y   N   Explain: _____

Other: _____

Antibiotics

Time _____ AM PM   Order for antibiotics given   **Order was** (Circle one)   Written   Verbally given

Time _____ AM PM   Blood culture obtained

Time _____ AM PM   Antibiotic 1 begun (name/dose) _____

Time _____ AM PM   Antibiotic 2 begun (name/dose) _____

Other stabilization efforts not yet described: _____

_____

SELF-EVALUATION QUESTIONS

Healthcare providers involved with this stabilization (to be completed by initial healthcare facility providers). Healthcare provider who requested the transport: ☐ Family practice   ☐ Pediatrician   ☐ Neonatologist   ☐ Midwife   ☐ Nurse Practitioner   ☐ Physician Assistant

Was physician or primary healthcare provider PRESENT at patient's bedside or in nursery at the time of transport team arrival?

☐ Yes   ☐ No (If no, explain): _____

TIME consultations made: _____ AM PM Family practice called   _____ AM PM Pediatrician called   _____ AM PM Neonatologist called

Provide name or initials of other healthcare providers involved with this stabilization:

Nurse (RN) _____

RT _____   LPN _____   Nurse Assistant _____   Other: _____

1. We feel our strengths with this stabilization effort were: _____

_____

The following people should be commended: _____

_____

2. We feel our weaknesses with this stabilization effort were: _____

_____

3. We encountered the following barriers that altered our ability to work as a team: _____

_____

4. We wish we had the opportunity to learn more about (list all educational needs): _____

_____

5. We encountered the following problems that affected our ability to perform the stabilization we would like to perform (include equipment malfunction or equipment not available, slow response times from other healthcare departments, uncertainty about the diagnosis, communication issues, etc). _____

_____

_____

6. The next time we have to stabilize a sick neonate, we would change the following: _____

_____

NAME OF PERSON completing this form & date: _____

1. Srinivasan C, Sachdeva R, Morrow WR, et al. Standardized management improves outcomes after the Norwood procedure. *Congenit Heart Dis*. 2009;4(5):329-37.

2. Spector JM, Villanueva HS, Brito ME, Sosa PG. Improving outcomes of transported newborns in Panama: Impact of a nationwide neonatal provider education program. *J Perinatol*. 2009;29(7):512-6.

3. Verónica R, Gallo L, Medina D, et al. Safe neonatal transport in the state of Jalisco: Impact of the S.T.A.B.L.E. program on morbidity and mortality. *Bol Med Hosp Infant Mex*. 2011;68(1):31-35.

4. Insoft R, Schwartz HP, Romito J, Alexander SN. Outreach education. *Guidelines for Air and Ground Transport of Neonatal and Pediatric Patients*. American Academy of Pediatrics; 2016: 257-266.

5. Bellezza F. Mnemonic devices: Classification, characteristics, and criteria. *Review of Educational Research*. 1981;51(2):247-275.

6. Taylor RM, Price-Douglas W. The S.T.A.B.L.E. Program: Postresuscitation/pretransport stabilization care of sick infants. *J Perinat Neonatal Nurs*. 2008;22(2):159-65.

7. Kendall AB, Scott PA, Karlsen KA. The S.T.A.B.L.E.(R) Program: The evidence behind the 2012 update. *J Perinat Neonatal Nurs*. 2012;26(2):147-57.

8. Ljungblad LW, Skovdahl K, McCormack B, Dahl B. "Keep it simple"—Co-creation of a tailored newborn resuscitation course for midwifery students. *Adv Med Educ Pract*. 2022;13:81-93.

9. Aziz K, Lee HC, Escobedo MB, et al. Part 5: Neonatal resuscitation: 2020 American Heart Association guidelines for cardiopulmonary resuscitation and emergency cardiovascular care. *Circulation*. 2020;142(16_suppl_2):S524-S550.

10. Weiner G, Zaichkin J. *Textbook of Neonatal Resuscitation*. 8th ed. American Academy of Pediatrics; 2021.

11. Karlsen KA, Trautman M, Price-Douglas W, Smith S. National survey of neonatal transport teams in the United States. *Pediatrics*. 2011;128(4):685-91.

12. Spillane NT, Chivily C, Andrews T. Short-term outcomes in term and late preterm neonates admitted to the well-baby nursery after resuscitation in the delivery room. *J Perinatol*. 2019;39(7):983-989.

13. Redpath S, Shah PS, Moore GP, et al. Do transport factors increase the risk of severe brain injury in outborn infants <33 weeks gestational age? *J Perinatol*. 2020;40(3):385-393.

14. Sawyer T, Lee HC, Aziz K. Anticipation and preparation for every delivery room resuscitation. *Semin Fetal Neonatal Med*. 2018;23(5):312-320.

15. Gould J, Medoff-Cooper B, Donovan E, Startk A. Applying quality improvement principles in caring for the high-risk infant. In: Berns SD, Kott A, eds. *Toward Improving the Outcome of Pregnancy III: Enhancing Perinatal Health Through Quality, Safety and Performance Initiatives*. March of Dimes Foundation; 2011: 76-86.

16. Yousef N, Moreau R, Soghier L. Simulation in neonatal care: Towards a change in traditional training? *Eur J Pediatr*. 2022;181(4):1429-1436.

17. American Academy of Pediatrics. Maternal and neonatal interhospital transfer. *Guidelines for Perinatal Care*. 8th ed. AAP; 2017: 113-130.

18. Chien LY, Whyte R, Aziz K, Thiessen P, Matthew D, Lee SK, Canadian Neonatal Network. Improved outcome of preterm infants when delivered in tertiary care centers. *Obstet Gynecol*. 2001;98(2):247-52.

19. Cifuentes J, Bronstein J, Phibbs CS, Phibbs RH, Schmitt SK, Carlo WA. Mortality in low birth weight infants according to level of neonatal care at hospital of birth. *Pediatrics*. 2002;109(5):745-51.

20. Rojas M, Flaherty A, Furlong Brown H, Rush T. Perinatal transport and levels of care. In: Gardner S, Carter B, Enzman-Hines M, Niermeyer S, eds. *Merenstein & Gardner's Handbook of Neonatal Intensive Care: An Interprofessional Approach*. 9th ed. Elsevier; 2021: 45-66.

21. Meguerdichian D. Complications in late pregnancy. *Emerg Med Clin North Am*. 2012;30(4):919-36.

22. Ledger WJ. Identification of the high risk mother and fetus—Does it work? *Clin Perinatol*. 1980;7(1):125-34.

23. Aboudi D, Shah SI, La Gamma EF, Brumberg HL. Impact of neonatologist availability on preterm survival without morbidities. *J Perinatol*. 2018;38(8):1009-1016.

24. Zayegh A, Stewart M, Delzoppo C, Sheridan B. Improving transport time for babies with antenatally diagnosed transposition of the great arteries reduces the need for ECMO. *J Perinatol*. 2020;40(10):1570-1575.

25. Sawyer T, Loren D, Halamek LP. Post-event debriefings during neonatal care: Why are we not doing them, and how can we start? *J Perinatol*. 2016;36(6):415-9.

26. Gougoulis A, Trawber R, Hird K, Sweetman G. 'Take 10 to talk about it': Use of a scripted, post-event debriefing tool in a neonatal intensive care unit. *J Paediatr Child Health*. 2020;56(7):1134-1139.

27. Koenig JS, Davies AM, Thach BT. Coordination of breathing, sucking, and swallowing during bottle feedings in human infants. *J Appl Physiol*. 1990;69(5):1623-9.

28. Pickler RH. A model of feeding readiness for preterm infants. *Neonatal Intensive Care*. 2004;17(4):31-36.

29. dos Santos Mezzacappa MA, Collares EF. Gastric emptying in premature newborns with acute respiratory distress. *J Pediatr Gastroenterol Nutr*. 2005;40(3):339-44.

30. Billimoria ZC, Woodward GA. Neonatal transport. In: Gleason CA, Sawyer T, eds. *Avery's Diseases of the Newborn*. 11th ed. Elsevier; 2024: 217-229.

31. Valentine GC, Wallen LD. Neonatal bacterial sepsis and meningitis. In: Gleason CA, Sawyer T, eds. *Avery's Diseases of the Newborn*. 11th ed. Elsevier; 2024: 439-449.

32. Munshi UK, Clark DA. Development of the gastrointestinal circulation in the fetus and newborn. In: Polin RA, Abman SH, Rowitch DH, Benitz WE, eds. *Fetal and Neonatal Physiology*. 6th ed. Elsevier; 2022: 517-520.

33. Philipps AF. Oxygen consumption and general carbohydrate metabolism of the fetus. In: Polin RA, Abman SH, Rowitch DH, Benitz WE, eds. *Fetal and Neonatal Physiology*. 6th ed. Elsevier; 2022: 368-382.

34. Paulusova E, Matasova K, Zibolenova J, Lucanova L, Kocvarova L, Zibolen M. Very early postnatal changes in splanchnic circulation in term infants. *Pediatr Radiol*. 2014;44(3):274-8.

35. Wild KT, Rintoul NE, Puder M, Hansen AR. Surgical conditions in the newborn. In: Eichenwald EC, Hansen AR, Martin CR, Stark AR, eds. *Cloherty and Stark's Manual of Neonatal Care*. 9th ed. Wolters Kluwer; 2023: 982-1012.

36. Karpen H, Poindexter B. Enteral nutrition. In: Gleason CA, Sawyer T, eds. *Avery's Diseases of the Newborn*. 11th ed. Elsevier; 2024: 871-887.

37. Poindexter BB, Martin CR. Nutritional support for the preterm infant. In: Martin RJ, Fanaroff AA, Walsh MC, eds. *Fanaroff and Martin's Neonatal-Perinatal Medicine: Diseases of the Fetus and Infant*. 12th ed. Elsevier; 2025: 720-737.

38. Srinath A, Rudolph JA. Nutrition and gastroenterology. In: Zitelli BJ, McIntire SC, Nowalk AJ, Garrison J, eds. *Zitelli and Davis' Atlas of Pediatric Physical Diagnosis*. 8th ed. Elsevier; 2023: 399-423.

39. Flynn-O'Brien KT, Rice-Townsend SE. Structural anomalies of the gastrointestinal tract. In: Gleason CA, Sawyer T, eds. *Avery's Diseases of the Newborn*. 11th ed. Elsevier; 2024: 897-911.

40. Dingeldein M. Selected gastrointestinal anomalies in the neonate. In: Martin RJ, Fanaroff AA, Walsh MC, eds. *Fanaroff and Martin's Neonatal-Perinatal Medicine: Diseases of the Fetus and Infant*. 12th ed. Elsevier; 2025: 1626-1652.

41. Mahe MM, Helmrath MA, Shroyer NF. Organogenesis of the gastrointestinal tract. In: Polin RA, Abman SH, Rowitch DH, Benitz WE, eds. *Fetal and Neonatal Physiology*. 6th ed. Elsevier; 2022: 845-854.

42. Taylor JA, Neu J. Disorders of the gastrointestinal tract. In: Boardman JP, Groves AM, Ramasethu J, eds. *Avery & MacDonald's Neonatology: Pathophysiology and Management of the Newborn*. 10th ed. Wolters Kluwer; 2021: 546-563.

43. Hall JE, Hall ME. Cerebral blood flow, cerebrospinal fluid, and brain metabolism. *Guyton and Hall Textbook of Medical Physiology E-book*. 14th ed. Elsevier; 2021: 777-784.

44. Rozance PJ, McGowan JE, Price-Douglas W, Hay WW. Glucose homeostasis. In: Gardner S, Carter, BS, Enzman-Hines, M., Niermeyer, S., eds. *Merenstein & Gardner's Handbook of Neonatal Intensive Care*. 9th ed. Elsevier; 2021: 431-458.

45. Hawkes CP, Stanescu DE, Stanley CA. Pathophysiology of neonatal hypoglycemia. In: Polin RA, Abman SH, Rowitch DH, Benitz WE, eds. *Fetal and Neonatal Physiology*. 6th ed. Elsevier; 2022: 1624-1632.

46. Menni F, de Lonlay P, Sevin C, et al. Neurologic outcomes of 90 neonates and infants with persistent hyperinsulinemic hypoglycemia. *Pediatrics*. 2001;107(3):476-9.

47. Burns CM, Rutherford MA, Boardman JP, Cowan FM. Patterns of cerebral injury and neurodevelopmental outcomes after symptomatic neonatal hypoglycemia. *Pediatrics*. 2008;122(1):65-74.

48. Harding JE, Harris DL, Hegarty JE, Alsweiler JM, McKinlay CJ. An emerging evidence base for the management of neonatal hypoglycaemia. *Early Hum Dev*. 2017;104:51-56.

49. Sharma A, Davis A, Shekhawat PS. Hypoglycemia in the preterm neonate: Etiopathogenesis, diagnosis, management and long-term outcomes. *Transl Pediatr*. 2017;6(4):335-348.

50. Choi H-y. Peripheral intravenous line placement. In: Ramasethu J, Seo S, eds. *MacDonald's Atlas of Procedures in Neonatology*. 6th ed. Wolters Kluwer; 2020: 188-193.

51. Sax H, Allegranzi B, Uckay I, Larson E, Boyce J, Pittet D. 'My five moments for hand hygiene': A user-centered design approach to understand, train, monitor and report hand hygiene. *J Hosp Infect*. 2007;67(1):9-21.

52. McKinney A, Steanson K, Lebar K. A standardized training program in ultrasound-guided intravenous line placement: Improving nurses' confidence and success. *Adv Neonatal Care*. 2023;23(1):17-22.

53. Vaughn A, Choi H-Y. Management of extravasation injuries. In: Ramasethu J, Seo S, eds. *MacDonald's Atlas of Procedures in Neonatology*. 6th ed. Wolters Kluwer; 2020: 194-198.

54. Corbett M, Marshall D, Harden M, Oddie S, Phillips R, McGuire W. Treating extravasation injuries in infants and young children: A scoping review and survey of UK NHS practice. *BMC Pediatr*. 2019;19(1):6.

55. Chan KM, Chau JPC, Choi KC, et al. Clinical practice guideline on the prevention and management of neonatal extravasation injury: A before-and-after study design. *BMC Pediatr*. 2020;20(1):445.

56. Restieaux M, Maw A, Broadbent R, Jackson P, Barker D, Wheeler B. Neonatal extravasation injury: Prevention and management in Australia and New Zealand—A survey of current practice. *BMC Pediatr*. 2013;13:34.

57. Marchetti JM, Blaine T, Shelly CE, et al. Effective use of extended dwell peripheral intravenous catheters in neonatal intensive care patients. *Adv Neonatal Care*. 2023;23(1):93-101.

58. Chenoweth KB, Guo JW, Chan B. The extended dwell peripheral intravenous catheter is an alternative method of NICU intravenous access. *Adv Neonatal Care*. 2018;18(4):295-301.

59. Choi H-Y, Rivera A, Chahine AA. Central venous catheterization. In: Ramasethu J, Seo S, eds. *MacDonald's Atlas of Procedures in Neonatology*. 6th ed. Wolters Kluwer; 2020: 233-252.

60. Srinivasan HB, Tjin ATA, Galang R, Hecht A, Srinivasan G. Migration patterns of peripherally inserted central venous catheters at 24 hours postinsertion in neonates. *Am J Perinatol*. 2013;30(10):871-4.

61. Sharpe EL. Neonatal peripherally inserted central catheter practices and their association with demographics, training, and radiographic monitoring: Results from a national survey. *Adv Neonatal Care*. 2014;14(5):329-35.

62. Coit AK, Kamitsuka MD, Pediatrix Medical G. Peripherally inserted central catheter using the saphenous vein: Importance of two-view radiographs to determine the tip location. *J Perinatol*. 2005;25(10):674-6.

63. Gorski LA, Hadaway L, Hagle ME, et al. Infusion therapy standards of practice, 8th ed. *J Infus Nurs*. 2021;44(1S Suppl 1):S1-S224.

64. Sharpe EL, Curry S, Wyckoff MM. *Peripherally Inserted Central Catheters: Guideline for Practice*. 4th ed., National Association of Neonatal Nurses; 2022.

65. Goldwasser B, Baia C, Kim M, Taragin BH, Angert RM. Non-central peripherally inserted central catheters in neonatal intensive care: Complication rates and longevity of catheters relative to tip position. *Pediatr Radiol*. 2017;47(12):1676-1681.

66. Wrightson DD. Peripherally inserted central catheter complications in neonates with upper versus lower extremity insertion sites. *Adv Neonatal Care*. 2013;13(3):198-204.

67. Blackburn S. Carbohydrate, fat, and protein metabolism. In: Blackburn ST, ed. *Maternal, Fetal, Neonatal Physiology: A Clinical Perspective*. 5th ed. Elsevier; 2018: 543-570.

68. Wernimont SA, Norris AW. Glucose metabolism in the fetus and newborn, and methods for its investigation. In: Polin RA, Abman SH, Rowitch DH, Benitz WE, eds. *Fetal and Neonatal Physiology*. 6th ed. Elsevier; 2022: 358-368.

69. Sweet CB, Grayson S, Polak M. Management strategies for neonatal hypoglycemia. *J Pediatr Pharmacol Ther*. 2013;18(3):199-208.

70. Nyp M, Brunkhorst JL, Reavey D, Pallotto EK. Fluid and electrolyte management. In: Gardner SL, Carter BS, Enzman-Hines M, Niermeyer S, eds. *Merenstein & Gardner's Handbook of Neonatal Intensive Care*. 9th ed. Elsevier; 2021: 407-430.

71. Carter N, Chalk BS. Neonatology. In: Kleinman K, Mcdaniel L, Molloy M, eds. *The Harriet Lane Handbook*. 22nd ed. Elsevier; 2021: 447-471.

72. Whitesel E. Fluid and electrolyte management. In: Eichenwald EC, Hansen AR, Martin CR, Stark AR, eds. *Cloherty and Stark's Manual of Neonatal Care*. 9th ed. Wolters Kluwer; 2023: 301-317.

73. Barrero-Castillero A, Simmons R. Hypoglycemia and hyperglycemia. In: Eichenwald EC, Hansen AR, Martin CR, Stark AR, eds. *Cloherty and Stark's Manual of Neonatal Care*. 9th ed. Wolters Kluwer; 2023: 318-332.

74. Garg M, Devaskar SU. Disorders of carbohydrate metabolism in the neonate. In: Martin RJ, Fanaroff AA, Walsh MC, eds. *Fanaroff and Martin's Neonatal-Perinatal Medicine: Diseases of the Fetus and Infant*. 12th ed. Elsevier; 2025: 1672-1696.

75. Buchanan TA, Kitzmiller JL. Metabolic interactions of diabetes and pregnancy. *Annu Rev Med*. 1994;45:245-60.

76. Cheung NW. The management of gestational diabetes. *Vasc Health Risk Manag*. 2009;5(1):153-64.

77. Elliott BD, Schenker S, Langer O, Johnson R, Prihoda T. Comparative placental transport of oral hypoglycemic agents in humans: A model of human placental drug transfer. Comparative study. *Am J Obstet Gynecol*. 1994;171(3):653-60.

78. Langer O, Conway DL, Berkus MD, Xenakis EM, Gonzales O. A comparison of glyburide and insulin in women with gestational diabetes mellitus. *NEJM*. 2000;343(16):1134-8.

79. Philipps AF, Dubin JW, Raye JR. Response of the fetal and newborn lamb to glucose and tolbutamide infusions. *Pediatr Res*. 1979;13(12):1375-8.

80. ACOG practice bulletin no. 190: Gestational diabetes mellitus. *Obstet Gynecol*. 2018;131(2):e49-e64.

81. ElSayed NA, Aleppo G, Aroda VR, et al. 15. Management of diabetes in pregnancy: Standards of care in diabetes—2023. *Diabetes Care*. 2023;46(Supplement_1):S254-S266.

82. Wexler DJ. Sulfonylureas and meglitinides in the treatment of type 2 diabetes mellitus. In: Nathan DM, Rubinow K, eds. *UpToDate-Lexidrug*. Wolters Kluwer; Updated October 31, 2022. Accessed March 19, 2024. https://online-lexi-com (requires facility or individual subscription).

83. Glipizide (Lexi-Drugs). *UpToDate-Lexidrug*. Wolters Kluwer; Updated March 15, 2024. Accessed March 19, 2024. https://online-lexi-com (requires facility or individual subscription).

84. Glyburide (glibenclamide): Drug information. *UpToDate-Lexidrug*. Wolters Kluwer; Updated 2024. Accessed March 19, 2024. https://online-lexi-com (requires facility or individual subscription).

85. Bergman B, Bokstrom H, Borga O, Enk L, Hedner T, Wangberg B. Transfer of terbutaline across the human placenta in late pregnancy. *Eur J Respir Dis Suppl*. 1984;134:81-6.

86. Main EK, Main DM, Gabbe SG. Chronic oral terbutaline tocolytic therapy is associated with maternal glucose intolerance. *Am J Obstet Gynecol*. 1987;157(3):644-7.

87. Angel JL, O'Brien WF, Knuppel RA, Morales WJ, Sims CJ. Carbohydrate intolerance in patients receiving oral tocolytics. *Am J Obstet Gynecol*. 1988;159(3):762-6.

88. Warburton D, Parton L, Buckley S, Cosico L, Saluna T. Effects of beta-2 agonist on hepatic glycogen metabolism in the fetal lamb. *Pediatr Res*. 1988;24(3):330-2.

89. de Bruin R, van Dalen SL, Franx SJ, et al. The risk for neonatal hypoglycemia and bradycardia after beta-blocker use during pregnancy or lactation: A systematic review and meta-analysis. *Int J Environ Res Public Health*. 2022;19(15):9616.

90. Kubota K, Inai K, Shimada E, Shinohara T. alpha/beta- and beta-Blocker exposure in pregnancy and the risk of neonatal hypoglycemia and small for gestational age. *Circ J*. 2023;87(4):569-577.

91. Collins R, Yusuf S, Peto R. Overview of randomised trials of diuretics in pregnancy. *Br Med J (Clin Res Ed)*. 1985;290(6461):17-23.

92. Kallen B. Neonate characteristics after maternal use of antidepressants in late pregnancy. *Arch Pediatr Adolesc Med*. 2004;158(4):312-6.

93. Andersohn F, Schade R, Suissa S, Garbe E. Long-term use of antidepressants for depressive disorders and the risk of diabetes mellitus. *Am J Psychiatry*. 2009;166(5):591-8.

94. Costantine MM, Saad A, Saade G. Obstetric management of prematurity. In: Martin RJ, Fanaroff AA, Walsh MC, eds. *Fanaroff and Martin's Neonatal-Perinatal Medicine: Diseases of the Fetus and Infant*. 12th ed. Elsevier; 2025: 318-351.

95. Sifianou P, Thanou V, Karga H. Metabolic and hormonal effects of antenatal betamethasone after 35 weeks of gestation. *J Pediatr Pharmacol Ther*. 2015;20(2):138-43.

96. Pettit KE, Tran SH, Lee E, Caughey AB. The association of antenatal corticosteroids with neonatal hypoglycemia and hyperbilirubinemia. *J Matern Fetal Neonatal Med*. 2014;27(7):683-6.

97. Dude AM, Yee LM, Henricks A, Eucalitto P, Badreldin N. Neonatal hypoglycemia after antenatal late preterm steroids in individuals with diabetes. *J Perinatol*. 2021;41(12):2749-2753.

98. McElwee ER, Wilkinson K, Crowe R, et al. Latency of late preterm steroid administration to delivery and risk of neonatal hypoglycemia. *Am J Obstet Gynecol MFM*. 2022;4(5):100687.

99. Shrivastava VK, Garite TJ, Jenkins SM, et al. A randomized, double-blinded, controlled trial comparing parenteral normal saline with and without dextrose on the course of labor in nulliparas. *Am J Obstet Gynecol*. 2009;200(4):379.e1-6.

100. Luna B, Feinglos MN. Drug-induced hyperglycemia. *JAMA*. 2001;286(16):1945-8.

101. Chlorthalidone. In: American Pharmacists Association, ed. *Lexicomp Pediatric & Neonatal Dosage Handbook*. 24th ed. Wolters Kluwer; 2017: 421-422.

102. Insulin, glucagon, and diabetes mellitus. In: Hall JE, Hall ME, eds. *Guyton and Hall Textbook of Medical Physiology E-book*. 14th ed. Elsevier; 2021: 973-989.

103. Hubbard EM, Hay WW, Jr. The term newborn: Hypoglycemia. *Clin Perinatol*. 2021;48(3):665-679.

104. Kaiser JR, Bai S, Rozance PJ. Newborn plasma glucose concentration nadirs by gestational-age group. *Neonatology*. 2018;113(4):353-359.

105. Guemes M, Rahman SA, Hussain K. What is a normal blood glucose? *Arch Dis Child*. 2016;101(6):569-574.

106. Herrera E, Ortega-Senavilla H. Lipids as an energy source for the premature and term neonate. In: Polin RA, Abman SH, Rowitch DH, Benitz WE, eds. *Fetal and Neonatal Physiology*. 6th ed. Elsevier; 2022: 332-339.

107. Puchalski ML, Russell TL, Karlsen KA. Neonatal hypoglycemia: Is there a sweet spot? *Crit Care Nurs Clin North Am*. 2018;30(4):467-480.

108. Arnold HE, Parsons KV, Jain L. The late preterm infant. In: Martin RJ, Fanaroff AA, Walsh MC, eds. *Fanaroff and Martin's Neonatal-Perinatal Medicine: Diseases of the Fetus and Infant*. 12th ed. Elsevier; 2025: 704-719.

109. Karnati S, Kollikonda S, Abu-Shaweesh J. Late preterm infants—Changing trends and continuing challenges. *Int J Pediatr Adolesc Med*. 2020;7(1):36-44.

110. Lubow JM, How HY, Habli M, Maxwell R, Sibai BM. Indications for delivery and short-term neonatal outcomes in late preterm as compared with term births. *Am J Obstet Gynecol*. 2009;200(5):e30-3.

111. American College of Obstetricians and Gynecologists' Committee on Obstetric Practice, Gyamfi-Bannerman C, Gantt AB, Miller RS, Society for Maternal-Fetal Medicine. Committee opinion no. 831: Medically indicated late-preterm and early-term deliveries. *Obstet Gynecol*. 2021;138(1):e35-e39.

112. Burgess JL, Unal ER, Nietert PJ, Newman RB. Risk of late-preterm stillbirth and neonatal morbidity for monochorionic and dichorionic twins. *Am J Obstet Gynecol*. 2014;210(6):578 e1-9.

113. Martin JA, Hamilton BE, Michelle JK, Osterman MHS. Births in the United States, 2022. NCHS data brief, no 477. National Center for Health Statistics. August 2023. Accessed January 11, 2024.

114. Richards JL, Kramer MS, Deb-Rinker P, et al. Temporal trends in late preterm and early term birth rates in 6 high-income countries in North America and Europe and association with clinician-initiated obstetric interventions. *JAMA*. 2016;316(4):410-9.

115. Ely DM, Driscoll AK. Infant mortality in the United States, 2020: Data from the Period Linked Birth/Infant Death file. *Natl Vital Stat Rep*. 2022;71(5):1-17.

116. Vohr B. Long-term outcomes of moderately preterm, late preterm, and early term infants. *Clin Perinatol*. 2013;40(4):739-51.

117. McGowan JE, Alderdice FA, Holmes VA, Johnston L. Early childhood development of late-preterm infants: A systematic review. *Pediatrics*. 2011;127(6):1111-24.

118. Lubow JM, How HY, Habli M, Maxwell R, Sibai BM. Indications for delivery and short-term neonatal outcomes in late preterm as compared with term births. Comparative study. *Am J Obstet Gynecol*. 2009;200(5):e30-3.

119. Mitha A, Chen R, Altman M, Johansson S, Stephansson O, Bolk J. Neonatal morbidities in infants born late preterm at 35-36 weeks of gestation: A Swedish nationwide population-based study. *J Pediatr*. 2021;233:43-50 e5.

120. Simmons R. Abnormalities of fetal growth. In: Gleason CA, Sawyer T, eds. *Avery's Diseases of the Newborn*. 11th ed. Elsevier; 2024: 33-41.

121. Kuhn-Riordon K, Lee YK, Styne DM. Endocrine factors affecting neonatal growth. In: Polin RA, Abman SH, Rowitch DH, Benitz WE, eds. *Fetal and Neonatal Physiology*. 6th ed. Elsevier; 2022: 224-241.

122. Devaskar SU, Janzen C, Calkins KL. Fetal growth restriction: A complex interplay between the intrauterine and maternal environment. In: Martin RJ, Fanaroff AA, Walsh MC, eds. *Fanaroff and Martin's Neonatal-Perinatal Medicine: Diseases of the Fetus and Infant*. 12th ed. Elsevier; 2025: 259-273.

123. Mejri A, Dorval VG, Nuyt AM, Carceller A. Hypoglycemia in term newborns with a birth weight below the 10th percentile. *Paediatr Child Health*. 2010;15(5):271-5.

124. Bhat MA, Kumar P, Bhansali A, Majumdar S, Narang A. Hypoglycemia in small for gestational age babies. Comparative study. *Indian J Pediatr*. 2000;67(6):423-7.

125. Wallenstein MB, Harper LM, Odibo AO, et al. Fetal congenital heart disease and intrauterine growth restriction: A retrospective cohort study. *J Matern Fetal Neonatal Med*. 2012;25(6):662-5.

126. Kesavan K, Devaskar SU. Intrauterine growth restriction: Postnatal monitoring and outcomes. *Pediatr Clin North Am*. 2019;66(2):403-423.

127. Chang J, Mestan K. Placental function in intrauterine growth restriction. In: Polin RA, Abman SH, Rowitch DH, Benitz WE, eds. *Fetal and Neonatal Physiology*. 6th ed. Elsevier; 2022: 137-149.

128. Olsen IE, Groveman SA, Lawson ML, Clark RH, Zemel BS. New intrauterine growth curves based on United States data. *Pediatrics*. 2010;125(2):e214-24.

129. Timpson W, Barrero-Castillero A. The high-risk newborn: Antcipation, evaluation, management, and outcome. In: Eichenwald EC, Hansen AR, Martin CR, Stark AR, eds. *Cloherty and Stark's Manual of Neonatal Care*. 9th ed. Wolters Kluwer; 2023: 78-93.

130. Cartwright RD, Anderson NH, Sadler IC, Harding JE, McCowan LME, McKinlay CJD. Neonatal morbidity and small and large size for gestation: A comparison of birthweight centiles. *J Perinatol*. 2020;40(5):732-742.

131. Brady JM, Barnes-Davis ME, Poindexter BB. The high-risk infant. In: Kliegman RM, St. Geme III JW, Blum NJ, Shah SS, Tasker RC, Wilson KM, Behrman RE, eds. *Nelson Textbook of Pediatrics E-Book*. 21st ed. Elsevier; 2020: 897-909.

132. Harris DL, Weston PJ, Harding JE. Incidence of neonatal hypoglycemia in babies identified as at risk. *J Pediatr*. 2012;161(5):787-91.

133. Das UG, Sysyn GD. Abnormal fetal growth: Intrauterine growth retardation, small for gestational age, large for gestational age. *Pediatr Clin North Am*. 2004;51(3):639-54, viii.

134. Fay E, Simmons L, Brown C. Maternal diabetes. In: Gleason CA, Sawyer T, eds. *Avery's Diseases of the Newborn*. 11th ed. Elsevier; 2024: 67-81.

135. O'Brien K. Neonatal effects of maternal diabetes. In: Eichenwald EC, Hansen AR, Martin CR, Stark AR, eds. *Cloherty and Stark's Manual of Neonatal Care*. 9th ed. Wolters Kluwer; 2023: 949-961.

136. Rozance PJ, Hay WW, Jr. New approaches to management of neonatal hypoglycemia. *Matern Health Neonatol Perinatol*. 2016;(2):3.

137. Katz LL, Stanley CA. Disorders of glucose and other sugars. In: Spitzer AR, ed. *Intensive Care of the Fetus & Neonate*. 2nd ed. Elsevier Mosby; 2005: 1167-1178.

138. Weiner MR, Gurevich P, Shinwell ES, Yogev Y. Pregnancy complicated by diabetes mellitus. In: Martin RJ, Fanaroff AA, Walsh MC, eds. *Fanaroff and Martin's Neonatal-Perinatal Medicine: Diseases of the Fetus and Infant*. 12th ed. Elsevier; 2025: 307-317.

139. Metzger BE, Lowe LP, Dyer AR, et al. Hyperglycemia and adverse pregnancy outcome (HAPO) study: Associations with neonatal anthropometrics. *Diabetes*. 2009;58(2):453-9.

140. Vora N, Bianchi DW. Genetic considerations in the prenatal diagnosis of overgrowth syndromes. *Prenat Diagn*. 2009;29(10):923-9.

141. Dolin CD. Maternal diabetes mellitus. In: Eichenwald EC, Hansen AR, Martin CR, Stark AR, eds. *Cloherty and Stark's Manual of Neonatal Care*. 9th ed. Wolters Kluwer; 2023: 15-21.

142. Macrosomia: ACOG practice bulletin, number 216. *Obstet Gynecol*. 2020;135(1):e18-e35.

143. Balest AL, Riley MM, O'Donnell B, Zarit JS. Neonatology. In: Zitelli BJ, McIntire SC, Nowalk AJ, Garrison J, eds. *Zitelli and Davis' Atlas of Pediatric Physical Diagnosis*. 8th ed. Elsevier; 2023: 43-70.

144. Abramowicz JS, Ahn JT. Fetal macrosomia. In: Levine D, Barss VA, eds. *UpToDate*. Wolters Kluwer; Updated July 12, 2022. Accessed December 28, 2022. https://www.uptodate.com/contents/fetal-macrosomia

145. Gabbe SG, Landon MB, Warren-Boulton E, Fradkin J. Promoting health after gestational diabetes: A National Diabetes Education Program call to action. *Obstet Gynecol*. 2012;119(1):171-6.

146. American Diabetes Association. Diagnosis and classification of diabetes mellitus. *Diabetes Care*. 2010;33 Suppl 1:S62-9.

147. American Diabetes Association. 14. Management of diabetes in pregnancy: Standards of medical care in diabetes—2019. *Diabetes Care*. 2019;42(Suppl 1):S165-S172.

148. Heideman WH, Middelkoop BJ, Nierkens V, et al. Changing the odds. What do we learn from prevention studies targeted at people with a positive family history of type 2 diabetes? *Prim Care Diabetes*. 2011;5(4):215-21.

149. Aune D, Saugstad OD, Henriksen T, Tonstad S. Maternal body mass index and the risk of fetal death, stillbirth, and infant death: A systematic review and meta-analysis. *JAMA*. 2014;311(15):1536-46.

150. Monaco-Brown M, Lawrence DA. Obesity and maternal-placental-fetal immunology and health. *Front Pediatr*. 2022;10:859885.

151. Azher S, Pinheiro JMB, Philbin B, Gifford J, Khalak R. The Impact of Maternal Obesity on NICU and Newborn Nursery Costs. *Front Pediatr*. 2022;10:863165.

152. Kureshi A, Khalak R, Gifford J, Munshi U. Maternal obesity-associated neonatal morbidities in early newborn period. *Front Pediatr*. 2022;10:867171.

153. Kokhanov A. Congenital bbnormalities in the infant of a diabetic mother. *Neoreviews*. 2022;23(5):e319-e327.

154. Herrick CJ, Puri R, Rahaman R, Hardi A, Stewart K, Colditz GA. Maternal race/ethnicity and postpartum diabetes screening: A systematic review and meta-analysis. *J Womens Health (Larchmt)*. 2020;29(5):609-621.

155. Kahn R, Fonseca V. Translating the A1C assay. Comment editorial. *Diabetes Care*. 2008;31(8):1704-7.

156. Eyth E, Naik R. Hemoglobin A1C. StatPearls [Internet]. March 15, 2022. Accessed December 25, 2022. https://www.ncbi.nlm.nih.gov/books/NBK549816/

157. ElSayed NA, Aleppo G, Aroda VR, et al. 2. Classification and diagnosis of diabetes: Standards of care in diabetes—2023. *Diabetes Care*. 2023;46(Supplement_1):S19-S40.

158. Arimitsu T, Kasuga Y, Ikenoue S, et al. Risk factors of neonatal hypoglycemia in neonates born to mothers with gestational diabetes. *Endocr J*. 2023;70(5):511-517.

159. Finneran MM, Kiefer MK, Ware CA, et al. The use of longitudinal hemoglobin A1c values to predict adverse obstetric and neonatal outcomes in pregnancies complicated by pregestational diabetes. *Am J Obstet Gynecol MFM*. 2020;2(1):100069.

160. Maresh MJ, Holmes VA, Patterson CC, et al. Glycemic targets in the second and third trimester of pregnancy for women with type 1 diabetes. *Diabetes Care*. 2015;38(1):34-42.

161. Rios DR, El-Khuffash AF, McNamara PJ. Oxygen transport and delivery. In: Polin RA, Abman SH, Rowitch DH, Benitz WE, eds. *Fetal and Neonatal Physiology*. 6th ed. Elsevier; 2022: 684-696.

162. Hall JE, Hall ME. Metabolism of carbohydrates and formation of adenosine triphosphate. In: Hall JE, Hall ME, eds. *Guyton and Hall Textbook of Medical Physiology E-book*. 14th ed. Elsevier; 2021: 843-852.

163. Keszler M, Abubakar K. Physiologic principles. In: Keszler M, Gautham KS, eds. *Goldsmith's Assisted Ventilation of the Neonate*. 7th ed. Elsevier; 2022: 11-32.

164. Turner DA, Cheifetz IM. Shock. In: Kliegman RM, St. Geme III JW, Blum NJ, Shah SS, Tasker RC, Wilson KM, Behrman RE, eds. *Nelson Textbook of Pediatrics E-Book*. 21st ed. Elsevier; 2020: 572-583.

165. Basu SK, Kaiser JR, Guffey D, Minard CG, Guillet R, Gunn AJ, CoolCap Study G. Hypoglycaemia and hyperglycaemia are associated with unfavourable outcome in infants with hypoxic ischaemic encephalopathy: A post hoc analysis of the CoolCap Study. *Arch Dis Child Fetal Neonatal Ed*. 2016;101(2):F149-55.

166. Tam EW, Haeusslein LA, Bonifacio SL, et al. Hypoglycemia is associated with increased risk for brain injury and adverse neurodevelopmental outcome in neonates at risk for encephalopathy. *J Pediatr*. 2012;161(12):88-93.

167. Groenendaal F, De Vries LS. Hypoxic-ischemic encephalopathy. In: Martin RJ, Fanaroff AA, Walsh MC, eds. *Fanaroff and Martin's Neonatal-Perinatal Medicine: Diseases of the Fetus and Infant*. 12th ed. Elsevier; 2025: 1059-2166.

168. Tan JKG, Minutillo C, McMichael J, Rao S. Impact of hypoglycaemia on neurodevelopmental outcomes in hypoxic ischaemic encephalopathy: A retrospective cohort study. *BMJ Paediatr Open*. 2017;1(1):e000175.

169. Basu SK, Ottolini K, Govindan V, et al. Early glycemic profile is associated with brain injury patterns on magnetic resonance imaging in hypoxic ischemic encephalopathy. *J Pediatr*. 2018;203:137-143.

170. Glasgow MJ, Harding JE, Edlin R. Cost analysis of cot-side screening methods for neonatal hypoglycaemia. *Neonatology*. 2018;114(2):155-162.

171. Woo HC, Tolosa L, El-Metwally D, Viscardi RM. Glucose monitoring in neonates: Need for accurate and non-invasive methods. *Arch Dis Child Fetal Neonatal Ed*. 2014;99(2):F153-7.

172. Thornton PS, Stanley CA, De Leon DD, et al. Recommendations from the Pediatric Endocrine Society for Evaluation and Management of Persistent Hypoglycemia in Neonates, Infants, and Children. *J Pediatr*. 2015;167(2):238-45.

173. Wada Y, Nakamura T, Kaneshige M, et al. Evaluation of two glucose meters and interference corrections for screening neonatal hypoglycemia. *Pediatr Int*. 2015;57(4):603-7.

174. Harris DL, Weston PJ, Gamble GD, Harding JE. Glucose profiles in healthy term infants in the first 5 days: The glucose in well babies (GLOW) study. *J Pediatr*. 2020;223:34-41 e4.

175. Narvey MR, Marks SD. The screening and management of newborns at risk for low blood glucose. *Paediatr Child Health*. 2019;24(8):536-554.

176. Harris DL, Weston PJ, Signal M, Chase JG, Harding JE. Dextrose gel for neonatal hypoglycaemia (the Sugar Babies Study): A randomised, double-blind, placebo-controlled trial. *Lancet*. 2013;382(9910):2077-83.

177. Gomella TL, Eyal FG, Bany-Mohammed F. Hypoglycemia. In: Gomella TL, Eyal FG, Bany-Mohammed F, eds. *Gomella's Neonatology: Management, Procedures, On-Call Problems, Diseases, and Drugs*. 8th ed. McGraw Hill; 2020: 587-602.

178. Werny D, Huang A, Tenney J, Pihoker C. Neonatal hypoglycemia and hyperglycemia. In: Gleason CA, Sawyer T, eds. *Avery's Diseases of the Newborn*. 11th ed. Elsevier; 2024: 1254-1268.

179. Rozance PJ. Pathogenesis, screening, and diagnosis of neonatal hypoglycemia. In: Garcia-Prats JA, Wolfsdorf JI, Tehrani N, eds. *UpToDate*. Wolters Kluwer; Updated April 17, 2023. Accessed December 26, 2023. https://www.uptodate.com/contents/pathogenesis-screening-and-diagnosis-of-neonatal-hypoglycemia

180. Arhan E, Ozturk Z, Serdaroglu A, Aydin K, Hirfanoglu T, Akbas Y. Neonatal hypoglycemia: A wide range of electroclinical manifestations and seizure outcomes. *Eur J Paediatr Neurol*. 2017;21(5):738-744.

181. Fong CY, Harvey AS. Variable outcome for epilepsy after neonatal hypoglycaemia. *Dev Med Child Neurol*. 2014;56(11):1093-9.

182. Caraballo RH, Sakr D, Mozzi M, et al. Symptomatic occipital lobe epilepsy following neonatal hypoglycemia. *Pediatr Neurol*. 2004;31(1):24-9.

183. Lucas A, Morley R, Cole TJ. Randomised trial of early diet in preterm babies and later intelligence quotient. *BMJ*. 1998;317(7171):1481-7.

184. Filan PM, Inder TE, Cameron FJ, Kean MJ, Hunt RW. Neonatal hypoglycemia and occipital cerebral injury. *J Pediatr*. 2006;148(4):552-555.

185. Alkalay AL, Flores-Sarnat L, Sarnat HB, Moser FG, Simmons CF. Brain imaging findings in neonatal hypoglycemia: Case report and review of 23 cases. *Clin Pediatr (Phila)*. 2005;44(9):783-90.

186. Gataullina S, DE Lonlay P, Dellatolas G, et al. Topography of brain damage in metabolic hypoglycaemia is determined by age at which hypoglycaemia occurred. *Dev Med Child Neurol*. 2013;55(2):162-6.

187. Gataullina S, DE lonlay P, Lemaire E, et al. Seizures and epilepsy in hypoglycaemia caused by inborn errors of metabolism. *Dev Med Child Neurol*. 2015;57(2):194-9.

188. Barkovich AJ, Ali FA, Rowley HA, Bass N. Imaging patterns of neonatal hypoglycemia. *AJNR Am J Neuroradiol*. 1998;19(3):523-8.

189. Wickstrom R, Skiold B, Petersson G, Stephansson O, Altman M. Moderate neonatal hypoglycemia and adverse neurological development at 2-6 years of age. *Eur J Epidemiol*. 2018;33(10):1011-1020.

190. Yalcin EU, Genc HM, Bayhan A, Anik Y, Kara B. Neurodevelopmental outcome in patients with typical imaging features of injury as a result of neonatal hypoglycemia. *Noro Psikiyatr Ars*. 2022;59(4):296-302.

191. McKinlay CJ, Alsweiler JM, Anstice NS, et al. Association of neonatal glycemia with neurodevelopmental outcomes at 4.5 years. *JAMA Pediatr*. 2017;171(10):972-983.

192. Kaiser JR, Bai S, Gibson N, et al. Association between transient newborn hypoglycemia and fourth-grade achievement test proficiency: A population-based study. *JAMA Pediatr*. 2015;169(10):913-21.

193. Dai DWT, Franke N, McKinlay CJD, et al. Executive function and behaviour problems in school-age children born at risk of neonatal hypoglycaemia. *Dev Med Child Neurol*. 2023;65(9):1226-1237.

194. Rozance PJ, Wolfsdorf JI. Hypoglycemia in the Newborn. *Pediatr Clin North Am*. 2019;66(2):333-342.

195. Tas E, Garibaldi L, Muzumdar R. Glucose homeostasis in newborns: An endocrinology perspective. *Neoreviews*. 2020;21(1):e14-e29.

196. Srinivasan G, Pildes RS, Cattamanchi G, Voora S, Lilien LD. Plasma glucose values in normal neonates: A new look. *J Pediatr*. 1986;109(1):114-7.

197. Hoseth E, Joergensen A, Ebbesen F, Moeller M. Blood glucose levels in a population of healthy, breast fed, term infants of appropriate size for gestational age. *Arch Dis Child Fetal Neonatal Ed*. 2000;83(2):F117-9.

198. Cornblath M, Hawdon JM, Williams AF, et al. Controversies regarding definition of neonatal hypoglycemia: Suggested operational thresholds. *Pediatrics*. 2000;105(5):1141-5.

199. Rozance PJ. Management and outcome of neonatal hypoglycemia. In: Garcia-Prats JA, Wolfsdorf JI, Tehrani N, eds. *UpToDate*. Wolters Kluwer; Updated February 28, 2023. Accessed December 26, 2023. https://www.uptodate.com/contents/management-and-outcome-of-neonatal-hypoglycemia

200. Stanley CA, Rozance PJ, Thornton PS, et al. Re-evaluating "transitional neonatal hypoglycemia": Mechanism and implications for management. *J Pediatr*. 2015;166(6):1520-5 e1.

201. Kishnani PS, Chen Y-T. Defects in metabolism of carbohydrates. In: Kliegman RM, St. Geme III JW, Blum NJ, Shah SS, Tasker RC, Wilson KM, Behrman RE, eds. *Nelson Textbook of Pediatrics*. 21st ed. Elsevier; 2020: 777-806.

202. De Cosio AP, Thornton P. Current and emerging agents for the treatment of hypoglycemia in patients with congenital hyperinsulinism. *Paediatr Drugs*. 2019;21(3):123-136.

203. Miralles RE, Lodha A, Perlman M, Moore AM. Experience with intravenous glucagon infusions as a treatment for resistant neonatal hypoglycemia. *Arch Pediatr Adolesc Med*. 2002;156(10):999-1004.

204. Kasirer Y, Dotan O, Mimouni FB, Wasserteil N, Hammerman C, Bin-Nun A. The use of intramuscular glucagon to prevent IV glucose infusion in early neonatal hypoglycemia. *J Perinatol*. 2021;41(5):1158-1165.

205. Marasch J, McClary JD. Appendix A.2 drug dosing table. In: Fanaroff AA, Fanaroff JM, eds. *Klaus and Fanaroff's Care of the High-Risk Neonate*. 7th ed. Elsevier; 2020: 456-473.

206. Gomella TL, Eyal FG, Bany-Mohammed F. Medications used in the neonatal intensive care unit. In: Gomella TL, Eyal FG, Bany-Mohammed F, eds. *Gomella's Neonatology: Management, Procedures, On-Call Problems, Diseases, and Drugs*. 8th ed. McGraw Hill; 2020: 1225-1316.

207. Edwards T, Liu G, Battin M, et al. Oral dextrose gel for the treatment of hypoglycaemia in newborn infants. *Cochrane Database Syst Rev*. 2022;3(3):CD011027.

208. Gregory K, Turner D, Benjamin CN, et al. Incorporating dextrose gel and feeding in the treatment of neonatal hypoglycaemia. *Arch Dis Child Fetal Neonatal Ed.* 2020;105(1):45-49.

209. Rawat M, Chandrasekharan P, Turkovich S, et al. Oral dextrose gel reduces the need for intravenous dextrose therapy in neonatal hypoglycemia. *Biomed Hub.* 2016;1(3):1-9.

210. Revenis ME, Soghier L. Intraosseous infusions. In: Ramasethu J, Seo S, eds. *MacDonald's Atlas of Procedures in Neonatology.* 6th ed. Wolters Kluwer; 2020: 453-458.

211. Weiner GM, Jeanette Z. Lesson 7: Medications. In: GM W, J Z, eds. *Textbook of Neonatal Resuscitation.* 8th ed. American Academy of Pediatrics; 2021: 179-212.

212. Part 9: Management of shock. In: Samson RA, Schexnayder SM, Hazinski MF, et al., eds. *Pediatric Advanced Life Support Provider Manual.* American Heart Association; 2016: 197-238.

213. Percy A. Procedures. In: Kleinman K, Mcdaniel L, Molloy M, eds. *The Harriet Lane Handbook.* 22nd ed. Elsevier; 2021:61-97.

214. Harcke HT, Curtin RN, Harty MP, et al. Tibial intraosseous insertion in pediatric emergency care: A review based upon postmortem computed tomography. *Prehosp Emerg Care.* 2020;24(5):665-671.

215. Nagler J, Krauss B. Videos in clinical medicine. Intraosseous catheter placement in children. *N Engl J Med.* 2011;364(8):e14.

216. Venous access: Intraosseous infusion. In: Gomella TL, Eyal FG, Bany-Mohammed F, eds. *Gomella's Neonatology: Management, Procedures, On-Call Problems, Diseases, and Drugs.* 8th ed. McGraw Hill; 2020: 403-407.

217. Maxien D, Wirth S, Peschel O, et al. Intraosseous needles in pediatric cadavers: Rate of malposition. *Resuscitation.* 2019;145:1-7.

218. Voigt J, Waltzman M, Lottenberg L. Intraosseous vascular access for in-hospital emergency use: A systematic clinical review of the literature and analysis. *Pediatr Emerg Care.* 2012;28(2):185-99.

219. Scrivens A, Reynolds PR, Emery FE, et al. Use of intraosseous needles in neonates: A systematic review. *Neonatology.* 2019;116(4):305-314.

220. Veldhoen ES, de Vooght KM, Slieker MG, Versluys AB, Turner NM. Analysis of bloodgas, electrolytes and glucose from intraosseous samples using an i-STAT((R)) point-of-care analyser. *Resuscitation.* 2014;85(3):359-63.

221. Peguet O, Beissel A, Chassery C, Gueugniaud PY, Bouchut JC. Intraosseous devices in small children: The need for a clearly defined strategy. *Resuscitation.* 2020;146:281-282.

222. Fuchs Z, Scaal M, Haverkamp H, Koerber F, Persigehl T, Eifinger F. Anatomical investigations on intraosseous access in stillborns—Comparison of different devices and techniques. *Resuscitation.* 2018;127:79-82.

223. Paxton JH, Knuth TE, Klausner HA. Proximal humerus intraosseous infusion: A preferred emergency venous access. *J Trauma.* 2009;67(3):606-11.

224. Philbeck TE, Miller LJ, Montez D, Puga T. Hurts so good. Easing IO pain and pressure. *JEMS.* 2010;35(9):58-62, 65-6, 68.

225. Lidocaine (systemic) and (dosing: pediatric). *UpToDate-Lexidrug.* Wolters Kluwer; Updated 2024. Accessed March 19, 2024. https://online-lexi-com (requires facility or individual subscription).

226. Olsen SL, Oschman A, Tracy K. Total parenteral nutrition. In: Gardner S, Carter BS, Enzman-Hines M., Niermeyer S., eds. *Merenstein & Gardner's Handbook of Neonatal Intensive Care.* 9th ed. Elsevier; 2021: 459-479.

227. Ramel SE, Georgieff MK. Nutrition. In: Boardman JP, Groves AM, Ramasethu J, eds. *Avery & MacDonald's Neonatology: Pathophysiolgy and Management of the Newborn.* 8th ed. Wolters Kluwer; 2021: 258-277.

228. Seo S. Umbilical vein catheterization. In: Ramasethu J, Seo S, eds. *McDonald's Atlas of Procedures in Neonatology.* 6th ed. Wolters Kluwer; 2020: 217-223.

229. Young A, Harrison K, Sellwood MW. How to use... Imaging for umbilical venous catheter placement. *Arch Dis Child Educ Pract Ed.* 2019;104(2):88-96.

230. Ades A, Leeman KT. Neonatal procedures: Basic principles and considerations. In: Eichenwald EC, Hansen AR, Martin CR, Stark AR, eds. *Cloherty and Stark's Manual of Neonatal Care.* 9th ed. Wolters Kluwer; 2023: 1050-1075.

231. Karber BC, Nielsen JC, Balsam D, Messina C, Davidson D. Optimal radiologic position of an umbilical venous catheter tip as determined by echocardiography in very low birth weight newborns. *J Neonatal Perinatal Med.* 2017;10(1):55-61.

232. Hoellering AB, Koorts PJ, Cartwright DW, Davies MW. Determination of umbilical venous catheter tip position with radiograph. *Pediatr Crit Care Med.* 2014;15(1):56-61.

233. Butler GC, Al-Assaf N, Tarrant A, Ryan S, El-Khuffash A. Using lateral radiographs to determine umbilical venous catheter tip position in neonates. *Ir Med J.* 2014;107(8):256-8.

234. Sharma D, Farahbakhsh N, Tabatabaii SA. Role of ultrasound for central catheter tip localization in neonates: A review of the current evidence. *J Matern Fetal Neonatal Med.* 2019;32(14):2429-2437.

235. Hoellering A, Tshamala D, Davies MW. Study of movement of umbilical venous catheters over time. *J Paediatr Child Health.* 2018;54(12):1329-1335.

236. Venous access: Umbilical vein catheterization. In: Gomella TL, Eyal FG, Bany-Mohammed F, eds. *Gomella's Neonatology: Management, Procedures, On-Call Problems, Diseases, and Drugs.* 8th ed. McGraw Hill; 2020: 417-423.

237. Coe K, Bradshaw WT, Tanaka DT. Physiologic monitoring. In: Gardner S, Carter, BS, Enzman-Hines, M., Niermeyer, S., eds. *Merenstein & Gardner's Handbook of Neonatal Intensive Care.* 9th ed. Elsevier; 2021: 165-185.

238. Nash P. Umbilical catheters, placement, and complication management. *J Infus Nurs.* 2006;29(6):346-52.

239. Bradshaw WT, Furdon SA. A nurse's guide to early detection of umbilical venous catheter complications in infants. *Adv Neonatal Care.* 2006;6(3):127-38; quiz 139-41.

240. Sims ME. Legal briefs: Venous catheter tips need to stay out of the heart. *Neoreviews.* 2019;20(9):e543-e547.

241. Levit OL, Shabanova V, Bizzarro MJ. Umbilical catheter-associated complications in a level IV neonatal intensive care unit. *J Perinatol.* 2020;40(4):573-580.

242. Coley BD, Seguin J, Cordero L, Hogan MJ, Rosenberg E, Reber K. Neonatal total parenteral nutrition ascites from liver erosion by umbilical vein catheters. *Pediatr Radiol.* 1998;28(12):923-7.

243. El Ters N, Claassen C, Lancaster T, et al. Central versus low-lying umbilical venous catheters: A multicenter study of practices and complications. *Am J Perinatol.* 2019;36(11):1198-1204.

244. Grizelj R, Vukovic J, Bojanic K, et al. Severe liver injury while using umbilical venous catheter: Case series and literature review. *Am J Perinatol.* 2014;31(11):965-74.

Ⓢ Introduction and Sugar Module

245. Smith L, Dills R. Survey of medication administration through umbilical arterial and venous catheters. *Am J Health Syst Pharm*. 2003;60(15):1569-72.

246. Seo S. Umbilical artery catheterization. In: Ramasethu J, Seo S, eds. *MacDonald's Atlas of Procedures in Neonatology*. 6th ed. Wolters Kluwer; 2020: 199-216.

247. Arterial access: Umbilical artery catheterization. In: Gomella TL, Eyal FG, Bany-Mohammed F, eds. *Gomella's Neonatology: Management, Procedures, On-Call Problems, Diseases, and Drugs*. 8th ed. McGraw Hill; 2020: 312-322.

248. Shukla H, Ferrara A. Rapid estimation of insertional length of umbilical catheters in newborns. *Am J Dis Child*. 1986;140(8): 786-8.

249. Wright IM, Owers M, Wagner M. The umbilical arterial catheter: A formula for improved positioning in the very low birth weight infant. Randomized controlled trial. *Pediatr Crit Care Med*. 2008;9(5):498-501.

250. Travers C, Ambalavanan N. Blood gases: Technical aspects and interpretation. In: Keszler M, Gautham KS, eds. *Goldsmith's Assisted Ventilation of the Neonate*. 7th ed. Elsevier; 2022: 93-110.

251. Kulali F, Calkavur S, Oruc Y, Demiray N, Devrim I. Impact of central line bundle for prevention of umbilical catheter-related bloodstream infections in a neonatal intensive care unit: A pre-post intervention study. *Am J Infect Control*. 2019;47(4):387-390.

252. Bierlaire S, Danhaive O, Carkeek K, Piersigilli F. How to minimize central line-associated bloodstream infections in a neonatal intensive care unit: A quality improvement intervention based on a retrospective analysis and the adoption of an evidence-based bundle. *Eur J Pediatr*. 2021;180(2):449-460.

253. Plooij-Lusthusz AM, van Vreeswijk N, van Stuijvenberg M, Bos AF, Kooi EMW. Migration of umbilical venous catheters. *Am J Perinatol*. 2019;36(13):1377-1381.

254. Dubbink-Verheij GH, Visser R, Tan R, Roest AAW, Lopriore E, Te Pas AB. Inadvertent migration of umbilical venous catheters often leads to malposition. *Neonatology*. 2019;115(3):205-210.

255. Kaushal S, Ramasethu J. Peripheral arterial catheterization. In: Ramasethu J, Seo S, eds. *MacDonald's Atlas of Procedures in Neonatology*. 6th ed. Wolters Kluwer; 2020: 224-232.

256. Barrington KJ. Umbilical artery catheters in the newborn: Effects of heparin. *Cochrane Database Syst Rev*. 2000;1999(2):CD000507.

257. Gialamas S, Stoltz Sjostrom E, Diderholm B, Domellof M, Ahlsson F. Amino acid infusions in umbilical artery catheters enhance protein administration in infants born at extremely low gestational age. *Acta Paediatr*. 2022;111(3):536-545.

258. Jackson JK, Biondo DJ, Jones JM, et al. Can an alternative umbilical arterial catheter solution and flush regimen decrease iatrogenic hemolysis while enhancing nutrition? A double-blind, randomized, clinical trial comparing an isotonic amino acid with a hypotonic salt infusion. *Pediatrics*. 2004;114(2):377-83.

259. Zenk KE, Noerr B, Ward R. Severe sequelae from umbilical arterial catheter administration of dopamine. *Neonatal Network*. 1994;13(5):89-91.

260. Brown MS, Phibbs RH. Spinal cord injury in newborns from use of umbilical artery catheters: Report of two cases and a review of the literature. *J Perinatol*. 1988;8(2):105-10.

261. Furdon SA, Horgan MJ, Bradshaw WT, Clark DA. Nurses' guide to early detection of umbilical arterial catheter complications in infants. *Adv in Neonatal Care*. 2006;(6):242-256.

262. Saxonhouse MA. Thrombosis in the neonatal intensive care unit. *Clin Perinatol*. 2015;42(3):651-73.

263. Saxonhouse MA, Hinson A. Management of vascular spasm and thrombosis. In: Ramasethu J, Seo S, eds. *McDonald's Atlas of Procedures in Neonatology*. 6th ed. Wolters Kluwer; 2020: 274.

264. Schulz G, Keller E, Haensse D, Arlettaz R, Bucher HU, Fauchere JC. Slow blood sampling from an umbilical artery catheter prevents a decrease in cerebral oxygenation in the preterm newborn. *Pediatrics*. 2003;111(1):e73-6.

265. Roll C, Huning B, Kaunicke M, Krug J, Horsch S. Umbilical artery catheter blood sampling volume and velocity: Impact on cerebral blood volume and oxygenation in very-low-birthweight infants. *Acta Paediatr*. 2006;95(1):68-73.

266. Mintzer JP, Parvez B, La Gamma EF. Umbilical arterial blood sampling alters cerebral tissue oxygenation in very low birth weight neonates. *J Pediatr*. 2015;167(5):1013-7.

267. Mintzer JP, Messina C. Cerebral oxygenation during umbilical arterial blood sampling in very low birth weight neonates. *J Perinatol*. 2018;38(4):368-373.

268. Butt WW, Gow R, Whyte H, Smallhorn J, Koren G. Complications resulting from use of arterial catheters: Retrograde flow and rapid elevation in blood pressure. *Pediatrics*. 1985;76(2):250-4.

269. Davies MW, Mehr S, Morley CJ. The effect of draw-up volume on the accuracy of electrolyte measurements from neonatal arterial lines. In vitro. *Journal of Paediatrics and Child Health*. 2000;36(2):122-4.

270. Wohlmuth C. The pathophysiology of twin-twin transfusion syndrome, twin-anemia polycythemia sequence, and twin-reversed arterial perfusion. In: Polin RA, Abman SH, Rowitch DH, Benitz WE, eds. *Fetal and Neonatal Physiology*. 6th ed. Elsevier; 2022:b1582-1588.

271. Lazebnik N, Ozean T, Lazebnik RS. Perinatal ultrasound. In: Martin RJ, Fanaroff AA, Walsh MC, eds. *Fanaroff and Martin's Neonatal-Perinatal Medicine: Diseases of the Fetus and Infant*. 12th ed. Elsevier; 2025: 171-211.

Ⓣ Temperature Module

1. Ting JY, Synnes AR, Lee SK, Shah PS, Canadian Neonatal Network, Canadian Neonatal Follow-Up Network. Association of admission temperature and death or adverse neurodevelopmental outcomes in extremely low-gestational age neonates. *J Perinatol*. 2018;38(7):844-849.

2. Kato S, Iwata O, Iwata S, et al. Admission temperature of very low birth weight infants and outcomes at three years old. *Sci Rep*. 2022;12(1):11912.

3. Lyu Y, Shah PS, Ye XY, et al. Association between admission temperature and mortality and major morbidity in preterm infants born at fewer than 33 weeks' gestation. *JAMA Pediatr*. 2015;169(4):e150277.

4. Ramaswamy VV, de Almeida MF, Dawson JA, et al. Maintaining normal temperature immediately after birth in late preterm and term infants: A systematic review and meta-analysis. *Resuscitation*. 2022;(180):81-98.

5. American Academy of Pediatrics and American Heart Association. Lesson 3: Initial steps of newborn care. In: Weiner GM, Zaichkin J, eds. *Textbook of Neonatal Resuscitation*. 8th ed. American Academy of Pediatrics; 2021: 33-63.

6. Conde-Agudelo A, Díaz-Rossello JL. Kangaroo mother care to reduce morbidity and mortality in low birthweight infants. *Cochrane Database Syst Rev*. 2016;2016(8):CD002771.

7. Ukke GG, Diriba K. Prevalence and factors associated with neonatal hypothermia on admission to neonatal intensive care units in Southwest Ethiopia—A cross-sectional study. *PLoS One*. 2019;14(6):e0218020.

8. Chiu WT, Lu YH, Chen YT, et al. Reducing intraventricular hemorrhage following the implementation of a prevention bundle for neonatal hypothermia. *PLoS One*. 2022;17(9):e0273946.

9. Laptook AR, Salhab W, Bhaskar B, Neonatal Research Network. Admission temperature of low birth weight infants: Predictors and associated morbidities. *Pediatrics*. 2007;119(3):e643-9.

10. Blackburn S. Thermoregulation. In: Blackburn ST, ed. *Maternal, Fetal, Neonatal Physiology: A Clinical Perspective*. 5th ed. Elsevier; 2018: 639-660.

11. Trevisanuto D, Testoni D, de Almeida MFB. Maintaining normothermia: Why and how? *Semin Fetal Neonatal Med*. 2018;23(5):333-339.

12. Heiderich AE, Leone TA. Resuscitation and initial stabilization. In: Fanaroff AA, Fanaroff JM, eds. *Klaus and Fanaroff's Care of the High-Risk Neonate*. 7th ed. Elsevier; 2020: 44-57.

13. Lakshminrusimha S, Keszler M. Diagnosis and management of persistent pulmonary hypertension of the newborn. In: Keszler M, Gautham KS, eds. *Goldsmith's Assisted Ventilation of the Neonate*. Elsevier; 2022: 427-444.

14. Agren J. Thermal environment of the intensive care nursery. In: Martin RJ, Fanaroff AA, Walsh MC, eds. *Fanaroff and Martin's Neonatal-Perinatal Medicine: Diseases of the Fetus and Infant*. 12th ed. Elsevier; 2025: 594-603.

15. World Health Organization, Maternal and Newborn Health/Safe Motherhood, eds. *Thermal Protection of the Newborn: A Practical Guide*. World Health Organization; 1997.

16. Aziz K, Lee HC, Escobedo MB, et al. Part 5: Neonatal resuscitation 2020 American Heart Association guidelines for cardiopulmonary resuscitation and emergency cardiovascular care. *Pediatrics*. 2021;147(Suppl 1):e2020038505E.

17. Sahni R. Temperature control in newborn infants. In: Polin RA, Abman SH, Rowitch DH, Benitz WE, eds. *Fetal and Neonatal Physiology*. 6th ed. Elsevier; 2022: 423-445.

18. Wilson E, Maier RF, Norman M, et al. Admission hypothermia in very preterm infants and neonatal mortality and morbidity. *J Pediatr*. 2016;(175):61-67.e4.

19. Mathur NB, Krishnamurthy S, Mishra TK. Evaluation of WHO classification of hypothermia in sick extramural neonates as predictor of fatality. Evaluation Studies. *J Trop Pediatr*. 2005;51(6):341-5.

20. Fanaroff AA, Lissauer T, Fanaroff JM. Physical examination of the newborn infant and the physical environment. In: Fanaroff AA, Fanaroff JM, eds. *Klaus and Fanaroff's Care of the High-Risk Neonate*. 7th ed. Elsevier; 2020: 58-79.

21. Ramasethu J. The preterm infant. In: Boardman J, Groves A, Ramasethu J, eds. *Avery & MacDonald's Neonatology: Pathophysiology and Management of the Newborn*. 8th ed. Wolters Kluwer; 2021: 325-341.

22. Chatson K. Temperature control. In: Eichenwald EC, Hansen AR, Martin CR, Stark AR, eds. *Cloherty and Stark's Manual of Neonatal Care*. 9th ed. Wolters Kluwer; 2023: 188-196.

23. Knobel RB, Holditch-Davis D, Schwartz TA, Wimmer JE Jr., Extremely low birth weight preterm infants lack vasomotor response in relationship to cold body temperatures at birth. *J Perinatol*. 2009;29(12):814-21.

24. Lyon AJ, Pikaar ME, Badger P, McIntosh N. Temperature control in very low birthweight infants during first five days of life. *Arch Dis Child Fetal Neonatal Ed*. 1997;76(1):F47-50.

25. Skiold B, Stewart M, Theda C. Predictors of unfavorable thermal outcome during newborn emergency retrievals. *Air Med J*. 2015;34(2):86-91.

26. Billimoria ZC, Woodward GA. Neonatal transport. In: Gleason CA, Sawyer T, eds. *Avery's Diseases of the Newborn*. 11th ed. Elsevier; 2024: 217-229.

27. Chabra S, Anderson JE, Javid PJ. Abdominal wall defects. In: Gleason CA, Sawyer T, eds. *Avery's Diseases of the Newborn*. 11th ed. Elsevier; 2024: 913-924.

28. Dean B, Doherty D. Congenital malformations of the central nervous system. In: Gleason CA, Sawyer T, eds. *Avery's Diseases of the Newborn*. 11th ed. Elsevier; 2024: 787-807.

29. Wild KT, Rintoul NE, Puder M, Hansen AR. Surgical conditions in the newborn. In: Eichenwald EC, Hansen AR, Martin CR, Stark AR, eds. *Cloherty and Stark's Manual of Neonatal Care*. 9th ed. Wolters Kluwer; 2023: 982-1012.

30. Ohliger S. Anesthesia in the neonate. In: Martin RJ, Fanaroff AA, Walsh MC, eds. *Fanaroff and Martin's Neonatal-Perinatal Medicine: Diseases of the Fetus and Infant*. 12th ed. Elsevier; 2025: 665-686.

31. Lenhardt R. The effect of anesthesia on body temperature control. *Front Biosci (Schol Ed)*. 2010;2(3):1145-54.

32. Sessler DI. Perioperative thermoregulation and heat balance. *Lancet*. 2016;387(10038):2655-2664.

33. Kamholz KL, McGovern JM. Care of the normal newborn. In: Boardman J, Groves A, Ramasethu J, eds. *Avery & MacDonald's Neonatology: Pathophysiology and Management of the Newborn*. 8th ed. Wolters Kluwer; 2021: 237-249.

34. Gardner SL, Cammack BH. Heat balance. In: Gardner S, Carter BS, Enzman-Hines M, Niermeyer S, eds. *Merenstein & Gardner's Handbook of Neonatal Intensive Care*. 9th ed. Elsevier; 2021: 137-164.

35. Law JB, Hodson A. Temperature regulation. In: Gleason CA, Sawyer T, eds. *Avery's Diseases of the Newborn*. 11th ed. Elsevier; 2024: 192-198.

36. Baumgart S. Iatrogenic hyperthermia and hypothermia in the neonate. *Clin Perinatol*. 2008;35(1):183-97, ix-x.

37. Hall JE, Hall ME. Body temperature regulation and fever. In: Hall JE, Hall ME, eds. *Guyton and Hall Textbook of Medical Physiology*. 14th ed. Elsevier; 2021: 901-912.

38. Merklin RJ. Growth and distribution of human fetal brown fat. *Anat Rec*. 1974;178(3):637-45.

39. Nedergaard J, Cannon B. Brown adipose tissue. In: Polin RA, Abman SH, Rowitch DH, Benitz WE, eds. *Fetal and Neonatal Physiology*. 6th ed. Elsevier; 2022: 323-332.

40. McCall EM, Alderdice F, Halliday HL, Vohra S, Johnston L. Interventions to prevent hypothermia at birth in preterm and/or low birth weight infants. *Cochrane Database Syst Rev*. 2018;2(2):CD004210.

Temperature Module

41. National Association of Neonatal Nurses. *Thermoregulation in the Care of Infants: Guideline for Practice.* National Association of Neonatal Nurses; 2021.

42. McCarthy LK, Molloy EJ, Twomey AR, Murphy JF, O'Donnell CP. A randomized trial of exothermic mattresses for preterm newborns in polyethylene bags. *Pediatrics.* 2013;132(1):e135-41.

43. WHO Immediate KMC Study Group, Arya S, Naburi H, et al. Immediate "kangaroo mother care" and survival of infants with low birth weight. *N Engl J Med.* 2021;384(21):2028-2038.

44. Jani P, Mishra U, Buchmayer J, et al. Thermoregulation and golden hour practices in extremely preterm infants: An international survey. *Pediatr Res.* 2023;93(6):1701-1709.

45. Bhavsar SR, Kabra NS, Avasthi BS, et al. Efficacy and safety of polythene wrap in preventing hypothermia in preterm and low birth weight neonates during transport: A randomized controlled trial. *Perinatology.* 2015;16(1):23-30.

46. Vohra S, Roberts RS, Zhang B, Janes M, Schmidt B. Heat loss prevention (HeLP) in the delivery room: A randomized controlled trial of polyethylene occlusive skin wrapping in very preterm infants. *J Pediatr.* 2004;145(6):750-3.

47. Knobel R, Holditch-Davis D. Thermoregulation and heat loss prevention after birth and during neonatal intensive-care unit stabilization of extremely low-birthweight infants. *J Obstet Gynecol Neonatal Nurs.* 2007;36(3):280-7.

48. McCall EM, Alderdice F, Halliday HL, Vohra S, Johnston L. Interventions to prevent hypothermia at birth in preterm and/or low birth weight infants. *Cochrane Database Syst Rev.* 2018;2(2):CD004210.

49. Meyer MP, Hou D, Ishrar NN, Dito I, te Pas AB. Initial respiratory support with cold, dry gas versus heated humidified gas and admission temperature of preterm infants. *J Pediatr.* 2015;166(2):245-50.e1.

50. Laptook AR, Watkinson M. Temperature management in the delivery room. *Semin Fetal Neonatal Med.* 2008;13(6):383-91.

51. Meyer MP, Owen LS, te Pas AB. Use of heated humidified gases for early stabilization of preterm infants: A meta-analysis. *Front Pediatr.* 2018;(6):319.

52. Jia Y-S, Lin Z-L, Lv H, Li Y-M, Green R, Lin J. Effect of delivery room temperature on the admission temperature of premature infants: A randomized controlled trial. *J Perinatol.* 2013;33(4):264-7.

53. American Academy of Pediatrics and American Heart Association. Anticipating and preparing for resuscitation. In: Weiner GM, Zaichkin J, eds. *Textbook of Neonatal Resuscitation.* 8th ed. American Academy of Pediatrics; 2021: 13-32.

54. Duryea EL, Nelson DB, Wyckoff MH, et al. The impact of ambient operating room temperature on neonatal and maternal hypothermia and associated morbidities: A randomized controlled trial. *Am J Obstet Gynecol.* 2016;214(4):505.e1-505.e7.

55. Caka SY, Gozen D. Effects of swaddled and traditional tub bathing methods on crying and physiological responses of newborns. *J Spec Pediatr Nurs.* 2018;23(1).

56. Association of Women's Health Obstetric and Neonatal Nurses (AWHONN) and National Associaton of Neonatal Nurses (NANN). *Neonatal Skin Care: Evidence-Based Clinical Practice Guideline.* 4th ed. AWHONN; 2018.

57. Edraki M, Paran M, Montaseri S, Razavi Nejad M, Montaseri Z. Comparing the effects of swaddled and conventional bathing methods on body temperature and crying duration in premature infants: A randomized clinical trial. *J Caring Sci.* 2014;3(2):83-91.

58. Brogan J, Rapkin G. Implementing evidence-based neonatal skin care with parent-performed, delayed immersion baths. *Nurs Womens Health.* 2017;21(6):442-450.

59. American Academy of Pediatrics and The American College of Obstetricians and Gynecologists. Care of the newborn. In: Kilpatrick SJ, Papile L-A, Macones GA, eds. *Guidelines for Perinatal Care.* American Academy of Pediatrics; 2017: 347-408.

60. Nolt D, O'Leary ST, Aucott SW. Risks of infectious diseases in newborns exposed to alternative perinatal practices. *Pediatrics.* 2022;149(2):e2021055554.

61. Nelson NP, Jamieson DJ, Murphy TV. Prevention of perinatal hepatitis B virus transmission. *J Pediatric Infect Dis Soc.* 2014;3 Suppl 1(Suppl 1):S7-S12.

62. Narendran V. The skin of the neonate. In: Martin RJ, Fanaroff AA, Walsh MC, eds. *Fanaroff and Martin's Neonatal-Perinatal Medicine: Diseases of the Fetus and Infant.* 12th ed. Elsevier; 2025: 1992-2026.

63. Garg M, Devaskar SU. Disorders of carbohydrate metabolism in the neonate. In: Martin RJ, Fanaroff AA, Walsh MC, eds. *Fanaroff and Martin's Neonatal-Perinatal Medicine: Diseases of the Fetus and Infant.* 12th ed. Elsevier; 2025: 1672-1696.

64. Mandell E, Steinhorn RH, Abman SH. Persistent pulmonary hypertension. In: Gleason CA, Sawyer T, eds. *Avery's Diseases of the Newborn.* 11th ed. Elsevier; 2024: 703-715.

65. Keszler M, Abubakar K. Physiologic principles. In: Keszler M, Gautham KS, eds. *Goldsmith's Assisted Ventilation of the Neonate.* 7th ed. Elsevier; 2022: 10-32.

66. Konopova P, Janota J, Termerova J, Burianova I, Paulova M, Zach J. Successful treatment of profound hypothermia of the newborn. *Acta Paediatr.* 2009;98(1):190-2.

67. Rech Morassutti F, Cavallin F, Zaramella P, Bortolus R, Parotto M, Trevisanuto D. Association of rewarming rate on neonatal outcomes in extremely low birth weight infants with hypothermia. *J Pediatr.* 2015;167(3):557-61.e1-2.

68. Jain P, Dalal JS, Gathwala G. Rapid vs. slow rewarming for management of moderate to severe hypothermia in low-birth-weight pre-term neonates—An open label randomized controlled trial. *J Trop Pediatr.* 2021;67(1):fmaa098.

69. Thoresen M, Whitelaw A. Cardiovascular changes during mild therapeutic hypothermia and rewarming in infants with hypoxic-ischemic encephalopathy. *Pediatrics.* 2000;106(1 Pt 1):92-9.

70. McCarthy LK, O'Donnell CPF. Comparison of rectal and axillary temperature measurements in preterm newborns. *Arch Dis Child Fetal Neonatal Ed.* 2021;106(5):509-513.

71. te Pas AB, Lopriore E, Dito I, Morley CJ, Walther FJ. Humidified and heated air during stabilization at birth improves temperature in preterm infants. *Pediatrics.* 2010;125(6):e1427-32.

72. Whitelaw A, Thoresen M. Brain injury at term. In: Boardman JP, Groves AM, Ramasethu J, eds. *Avery & MacDonald's Neonatology: Pathophysiolgy and Management of the Newborn.* 10th ed. Wolters Kluwer; 2021: 792-803.

73. Mietzsch U, Juul SE. Neonatal encephalopathy. In: Gleason CA, Sawyer T, eds. *Avery's Diseases of the Newborn*. 11th ed. Elsevier; 2024: 827-842.

74. Berlin S. Diagnostic imaging of the neonate. In: Martin RJ, Fanaroff AA, Walsh MC, eds. *Fanaroff and Martin's Neonatal-Perinatal Medicine: Diseases of the Fetus and Infant*. 11th ed. Elsevier; 2020: 608-633.

75. Bonifacio SL, Hutson S. The term newborn: Evaluation for hypoxic-ischemic encephalopathy. *Clin Perinatol*. 2021;48(3):681-695.

76. Hansen AR, Soul JS. Perinatal asphyxia and hypoxic-ischemic encephalopathy. In: Eichenwald EC, Hansen AR, Martin CR, Stark AR, eds. *Cloherty and Stark's Manual of Neonatal Care*. 9th ed. Wolters Kluwer; 2023: 825-846.

77. Groenendaal F, De Vries LS. Hypoxic-ischemic encephalopathy. In: Martin RJ, Fanaroff AA, Walsh MC, eds. *Fanaroff and Martin's Neonatal-Perinatal Medicine: Diseases of the Fetus and Infant*. 12th ed. Elsevier; 2025: 1059-1084.

78. Inder TE, Matthews LG. Neonatal brain disorders. In: Fanaroff AA, Fanaroff JM, eds. *Klaus and Fanaroff's Care of the High-Risk Neonate*. 7th ed. Elsevier; 2020: 386-408.

79. Hall AS, Reavey DA. Neurologic disorders. In: Gardner SL, Carter BS, Enzman-Hines M, Niermeyer S, eds. *Merenstein & Gardner's Handbook of Neonatal Intensive Care*. 9th ed. Elsevier; 2021: 929-968.

80. Laventhal NT, Barks JDE. Beyond the clinical trials: Off-protocol therapeutic hypothermia. *Clin Perinatol*. 2022;49(1):137-147.

81. Natarajan G, Laptook A, Shankaran S. Therapeutic hypothermia: How can we optimize this therapy to further improve outcomes? *Clin Perinatol*. 2018;45(2):241-255.

82. Chalak L. New horizons in mild hypoxic-ischemic encephalopathy: A standardized algorithm to move past conundrum of care. *Clin Perinatol*. 2022;49(1):279-294.

83. Laptook AR, Shankaran S, Tyson JE, et al. Effect of therapeutic hypothermia initiated after 6 hours of age on death or disability among newborns with hypoxic-ischemic encephalopathy: A randomized clinical trial. *Jama*. 2017;318(16):1550-1560.

84. McAdams R, Traudt C. Brain injury in the term infant. In: Gleason CA, Juul SE, eds. *Avery's Diseases of the Newborn*. 10th ed. Elsevier; 2018: 897-909.

85. Wyatt JS, Gluckman PD, Liu PY, et al. Determinants of outcomes after head cooling for neonatal encephalopathy. *Pediatrics*. 2007;119(5):912-21.

86. Laptook A, Tyson J, Shankaran S, et al. Elevated temperature after hypoxic-ischemic encephalopathy: Risk factor for adverse outcomes. *Pediatrics*. 2008;122(3):491-9.

87. Laptook AR, McDonald SA, Shankaran S, et al. Elevated temperature and 6- to 7-year outcome of neonatal encephalopathy. *Ann Neurol*. 2013;73(4):520-8.

88. Owji ZP, Gilbert G, Saint-Martin C, Wintermark P. Brain temperature is increased during the first days of life in asphyxiated newborns: Developing brain injury despite hypothermia treatment. *AJNR Am J Neuroradiol*. 2017;38(11):2180-2186.

89. Basu SK, Kaiser JR, Guffey D, Minard CG, Guillet R, Gunn AJ, CoolCap Study Group. Hypoglycaemia and hyperglycaemia are associated with unfavourable outcome in infants with hypoxic-ischaemic encephalopathy: A post hoc analysis of the CoolCap Study. *Arch Dis Child Fetal Neonatal Ed*. 2016;101(2):F149-55.

90. Chouthai NS, Sobczak H, Khan R, Subramanian D, Raman S, Rao R. Hyperglycemia is associated with poor outcome in newborn infants undergoing therapeutic hypothermia for hypoxic-ischemic encephalopathy. *J Neonatal Perinatal Med*. 2015;8(2):125-31.

91. Tam EW, Haeusslein LA, Bonifacio SL, et al. Hypoglycemia is associated with increased risk for brain injury and adverse neurodevelopmental outcome in neonates at risk for encephalopathy. *J Pediatr*. 2012;161(1):88-93.

92. Guellec I, Ancel PY, Beck J, et al. Glycemia and neonatal encephalopathy: Outcomes in the LyTONEPAL (Long-Term Outcome of Neonatal Hypoxic EncePhALopathy in the Era of Neuroprotective Treatment With Hypothermia) cohort. *J Pediatr*. 2023;(257):113350.

93. Pinchefsky EF, Hahn CD, Kamino D, et al. Hyperglycemia and glucose variability are associated with worse brain function and seizures in neonatal encephalopathy: A prospective cohort study. *J Pediatr*. 2019;(209):23-32.

94. Guemes M, Rahman SA, Hussain K. What is a normal blood glucose? *Arch Dis Child*. 2016;101(6):569-574.

95. American Pediatric Society. Common treatment for brain injury not effective for some newborns. Medical Press. April 28, 2023. Accessed September 29, 2023. https://medicalxpress.com/news/2023-04-common-treatment-brain-injury-effective.html

96. Finder M, Boylan GB, Twomey D, Ahearne C, Murray DM, Hallberg B. Two-year neurodevelopmental outcomes after mild hypoxic-ischemic encephalopathy in the era of therapeutic hypothermia. *JAMA Pediatr*. 2020;174(1):48-55.

97. Chalak LF, Nguyen KA, Prempunpong C, et al. Prospective research in infants with mild encephalopathy identified in the first six hours of life: Neurodevelopmental outcomes at 18-22 months. *Pediatr Res*. 2018;84(6):861-868.

A Airway Module

1. Lakshminrusimha S, Keszler M. Diagnosis and management of persistent pulmonary hypertension of the newborn. In: Keszler M, Gautham KS, eds. *Goldsmith's Assisted Ventilation of the Neonate*. Elsevier; 2022: 427-444.

2. Di Fiore JM, Travers CP, Carlo WA. Assessment of neonatal pulmonary function. In: Martin RJ, Fanaroff AA, Walsh MC, eds. *Fanaroff and Martin's Neonatal-Perinatal Medicine: Diseases of the Fetus and Infant*. 12th ed. Elsevier; 2025: 1210-1225.

3. Dyess N, Kinsella J, Parker T. Acute neonatal respiratory disorders. In: Gleason CA, Sawyer T, eds. *Avery's Diseases of the Newborn*. 11th ed. Elsevier; 2024: 594-612.

4. Dyet L, Crowley R. Physical assessment and classification. In: Boardman J, Groves A, Ramasethu J, eds. *Avery & MacDonald's Neonatology: Pathophysiology and Management of the Newborn*. 8th ed. Wolters Kluwer; 2021: 214-237.

5. Johnson L. Assessment of the newborn history and physical examination of the newborn. In: Eichenwald EC, Hansen AR, Martin CR, Stark AR, eds. *Cloherty and Stark's Manual of Neonatal Care*. 9th ed. Wolters Kluwer; 2023: 94-105.

6. Bhandari V. Nasal intermittent positive pressure ventilation in the newborn: Review of literature and evidence-based guidelines. *J Perinatol*. 2010;30(8):505-12.

7. Mahmoud RA, Roehr CC, Schmalisch G. Current methods of non-invasive ventilatory support for neonates. *Paediatr Respir Rev*. 2011;12(3):196-205.

A Airway Module

8. Manley BJ, Davis PG, Yoder BA, Owen LS. Noninvasive respiratory support. In: Keszler M, Gautham KS, eds. *Goldsmith's Assisted Ventilation of the Neonate*. 7th ed. Elsevier; 2022: 200-220.

9. Durand D, Courtney S. Neonatal respiratory therapy. In: Gleason CA, Sawyer T, eds. *Avery's Diseases of the Newborn*. 11th ed. Elsevier; 2024: 559-579.

10. Gardner S, Enzman-Hines M, Nyp M. Respiratory diseases. In: Gardner S, Carter, BS, Enzman-Hines, M., Niermeyer, S., eds. *Merenstein & Gardner's Handbook of Neonatal Intensive Care*. 9th ed. Elsevier; 2021: 729-835.

11. Mathew B, Lakshminrusimha S. Noninvasive monitoring of gas exchange. In: Keszler M, Gautham KS, eds. *Goldsmith's Assisted Ventilation of the Neonate*. 7th ed. Elsevier; 2022: 110-123.

12. Levin J, Rhein L. Blood gas and pulmonary function monitoring. In: Eichenwald EC, Hansen AR, Martin CR, Stark AR, eds. *Cloherty and Stark's Manual of Neonatal Care*. 9th ed. Wolters Kluwer; 2023: 439-447.

13. Di Fiore J, Raffay T. Neonatal cardiorespiratory monitoring. In: Martin RJ, Fanaroff AA, Walsh MC, eds. *Fanaroff and Martin's Neonatal-Perinatal Medicine: Diseases of the Fetus and Infant*. 12th ed. Elsevier; 2025: 622-633.

14. Shepherd E, Nelin L. Physical examination. In: Keszler M, Gautham KS, eds. *Goldsmith's Assisted Ventilation of the Neonate*. 7th ed. Elsevier; 2022: 69-75.

15. Apnea and bradycardia (A's and B's): On call. In: Gomella TL, Eyal FG, Bany-Mohammed F, eds. *Gomella's Neonatology: Management, Procedures, On-Call Problems, Diseases, and Drugs*. 8th ed. McGraw Hill Medical; 2020: 442-459.

16. Travers C, Ambalavanan N. Blood gases: Technical aspects and interpretation. In: Keszler M, Gautham KS, eds. *Goldsmith's Assisted Ventilation of the Neonate*. 7th ed. Elsevier; 2022: 93-110.

17. Keszler M, Abubakar K. Physiologic principles. In: Keszler M, Gautham KS, eds. *Goldsmith's Assisted Ventilation of the Neonate*. 7th ed. Elsevier; 2022: 10-32.

18. Azhibekov T, Friedlich PS, Seri I. Regulation of acid-base balance in the fetus and newborn. In: Polin RA, Abman SH, Rowitch DH, Benitz WE, eds. *Fetal and Neonatal Physiology*. 6th ed. Elsevier; 2022: 1076-1080.

19. Yoder BA, Grubb PH. Mechanical ventilation: Disease-specific strategies. In: Keszler M, Gautham KS, eds. *Goldsmith's Assisted Ventilation of the Neonate*. 7th ed. Elsevier; 2022: 287-302.

20. American Heart Association. Part 9: Recognizing shock. In: Kadlec KD, McBride ME, Meeks R, et al., eds. *Pediatric Advanced Life Support Provider Manual eBook*. American Heart Association; 2020: e12-e17.

21. Hynes KM, Mottram CD. Pulmonary function testing and bedside pulmonary mechanics. In: Walsh BK, ed. *Neonatal and Pediatric Respiratory Care*. Elsevier; 2019: 65-88.

22. Guttentag S. Respiratory distress syndrome. In: Eichenwald EC, Hansen AR, Martin CR, Stark AR, eds. *Cloherty and Stark's Manual of Neonatal Care*. 9th ed. Wolters Kluwer; 2023: 458-468.

23. Maresh A, Harrington A, Midulla P, Modi V. Surgical management of the airway and lungs. In: Boardman J, Groves A, Ramasethu J, eds. *Avery & MacDonald's Neonatology: Pathophysiology and Management of the Newborn*. Wolters Kluwer; 2021: 399-417.

24. Yost GC, Young PC, Buchi KF. Significance of grunting respirations in infants admitted to a well-baby nursery. *Arch Pediatr Adolesc Med*. 2001;155(3):372-5.

25. Gardner S, Cammack B. Heat balance. In: Gardner S, Carter BS, Enzman-Hines M, Niermeyer S, eds. *Merenstein & Gardner's Handbook of Neonatal Intensive Care*. 9th ed. Elsevier; 2021:137-164.

26. Saxonhouse M, Hinson A. Polycythemia. In: Eichenwald EC, Hansen AR, Martin CR, Stark AR, eds. *Cloherty and Stark's Manual of Neonatal Care*. 9th ed. Wolters Kluwer; 2023: 640-647.

27. Walsh BK. Oxygen administration. In: Walsh BK, ed. *Neonatal and Pediatric Respiratory Care*. Elsevier; 2019: 149-163.

28. Vento M. Oxygen therapy. In: Keszler M, Gautham KS, eds. *Goldsmith's Assisted Ventilation of the Neonate*. 7th ed. Elsevier; 2022: 184-195.

29. Oatts J, De Alba Campomanes A, Binenbaum G. Eye and vision disorders. In: Martin RJ, Fanaroff AA, Walsh MC, eds. *Fanaroff and Martin's Neonatal-Perinatal Medicine: Diseases of the Fetus and Infant*. 12th ed. Elsevier; 2025: 1391-1413.

30. Mandell E, Steinhorn RH, Abman SH. Persistent pulmonary hypertension. In: Gleason CA, Sawyer T, eds. *Avery's Diseases of the Newborn*. 11th ed. Elsevier; 2024: 703-715.

31. Cyanotic congenital heart defects. In: Park MK, Salamat M, eds. *Park's Pediatric Cardiology for Practitioners*. 7th ed. Elsevier; 2021: 160-223.

32. Polin RA, Hooven TA, Randis TM. Perinatal infections and chorioamnionitis. In: Martin RJ, Fanaroff AA, Walsh MC, eds. *Fanaroff and Martin's Neonatal-Perinatal Medicine: Diseases of the Fetus and Infant*. Elsevier; 2025: 414-424.

33. Karlsen KA, Cowley CG. *S.T.A.B.L.E. Cardiac Module: Recognition and Stabilization of Neonates with Severe CHD*. 2nd ed. S.T.A.B.L.E., Inc.; 2021.

34. Respiratory insufficiency-pathophysiology, diagnosis, oxygen therapy. In: Hall JE, Hall ME, eds. *Guyton and Hall Textbook of Medical Physiology E-Book*. 14th ed. Elsevier; 2021: 541-549.

35. Hall JE, Hall ME. Metabolism of carbohydrates and formation of adenosine triphosphate. In: Hall JE, Hall ME, eds. *Guyton and Hall Textbook of Medical Physiology E-book*. 14th ed. Elsevier; 2021: 843-852.

36. Smallwood C. Noninvasive monitoring in neonatal and pediatric care. In: Walsh BK, ed. *Neonatal and Pediatric Respiratory Care*. Elsevier; 2019: 135-148.

37. Levesque BM, Pollack P, Griffin BE, Nielsen HC. Pulse oximetry: What's normal in the newborn nursery? *Pediatr Pulmonol*. 2000;30(5):406-12.

38. Harigopal S, Satish HP, Taktak AF, Southern KW, Shaw NJ. Oxygen saturation profile in healthy preterm infants. *Arch Dis Child Fetal Neonatal Ed*. 2011;96(5):F339-42.

39. Ravert P, Detwiler TL, Dickinson JK. Mean oxygen saturation in well neonates at altitudes between 4498 and 8150 feet. *Adv Neonatal Care*. 2011;11(6):412-7.

40. Bakr AF, Habib HS. Normal values of pulse oximetry in newborns at high altitude. *J Trop Pediatr*. 2005;51(3):170-3.

41. Patel R, Josephson C. Anemia. In: Eichenwald EC, Hansen AR, Martin CR, Stark AR, eds. *Cloherty and Stark's Manual of Neonatal Care*. 9th ed. Wolters Kluwer; 2023: 629-639.

42. Karlsen KA, Cowley CG. *S.T.A.B.L.E. - Cardiac Module: Recognition and Stabilization of Neonates with Severe CHD*. 2nd ed. S.T.A.B.L.E., Inc.; 2021.

43. Abubakar MK. Continuous blood gas monitoring. In: Ramasethu J, Seo S, eds. *MacDonald's Atlas of Procedures in Neonatology*. 6th ed. Wolters Kluwer; 2020: 91-100.

44. Rios DR, El-Khuffash AF, McNamara PJ. Oxygen transport and delivery. In: Polin RA, Abman SH, Rowitch DH, Benitz WE, eds. *Fetal and Neonatal Physiology*. 6th ed. Elsevier; 2022: 684-696.

45. Tung S. Pulmonology and sleep medicine. In: Kleinman K, Mcdaniel L, Molloy M, eds. *The Harriet Lane Handbook*. 22nd ed. Elsevier; 2021: 586-605.

46. Wright CJ, Posencheg MA, Seri I. Fluid, electrolyte, and acid-base balance. In: Gleason CA, Sawyer T, eds. *Avery's Diseases of the Newborn*. 11th ed. Elsevier; 2024: 231-252.

47. Andersen OS. Blood acid-base alignment nomogram. Scales for pH, pCO2 base excess of whole blood of different hemoglobin concentrations, plasma bicarbonate, and plasma total-CO2. *Scand J Clin Lab Invest*. 1963;(15):211-7.

48. Walsh BK. Monitoring of gas exchange in the NICU. In: Walsh BK, ed. *Neonatal and Pediatric Respiratory Care*. Elsevier; 2019: 699-721.

49. Arterial blood gases. In: Pagana K, Pagana T, Pagana T, eds. *Mosby's Manual of Diagnostic and Laboratory Tests*. 7th ed. Elsevier; 2022: 103-111.

50. Harsten A, Berg B, Inerot S, Muth L. Importance of correct handling of samples for the results of blood gas analysis. *Acta Anaesthesiol Scand*. 1988;32(5):365-8.

51. Sood P, Paul G, Puri S. Interpretation of arterial blood gas. *Indian J Crit Care Med*. 2010;14(2):57-64.

52. Crowley MA. Spectrum of neonatal respiratory disorders. In: Martin RJ, Fanaroff AA, Walsh MC, eds. *Fanaroff and Martin's Neonatal-Perinatal Medicine: Diseases of the Fetus and Infant*. Elsevier; 2025: 1271-2166.

53. Gillion V, Jadoul M, Devuyst O, Pochet JM. The patient with metabolic alkalosis. *Acta Clin Belg*. 2019;74(1):34-40.

54. Noori S, Friedlich PS, Seri I. Pathophysiology of shock in the fetus and neonate. In: Polin RA, Abman SH, Rowitch DH, Benitz WE, Fox WW, eds. *Fetal and Neonatal Physiology*. 6th ed. Elsevier; 2022: 1662-1671.

55. Noori S, Seri I. Cardiovascular compromise in the newborn infant. In: Gleason CA, Sawyer T, eds. *Avery's Diseases of the Newborn*. 11th ed. Elsevier; 2024: 675-701.

56. Nicks BA. Acute lactic acidosis. Medscape. Updated September 26, 2022. Accessed January 11, 2024. https://emedicine.medscape.com/article/768159-overview

57. Zaidi AN, Daniels CJ. Myocardial ischemia in the pediatric population. In: Allen HD, Shaddy RE, Penny DJ, Feltes TF, Cetta F, eds. *Moss and Adams' Heart Disease in Infants, Children, and Adolescents*. 9th ed. Wolters Kluwer; 2016: 1455-1463.

58. American Heart Association. Part 10: Managing shock. In: Kadlec KD, McBride ME, Meeks R, et al., eds. *Pediatric Advanced Life Support Provider Manual eBook*. American Heart Association; 2020: e13-e17.

59. Konczal L. Inborn errors of metabolism. In: Martin RJ, Fanaroff AA, Walsh MC, eds. *Fanaroff and Martin's Neonatal-Perinatal Medicine: Diseases of the Fetus and Infant*. 12th ed. Elsevier; 2025: 1790-1872.

60. Davis AL, Carcillo JA, Aneja RK, et al. American College of Critical Care Medicine clinical practice parameters for hemodynamic support of pediatric and neonatal septic shock. *Crit Care Med*. 2017;45(6):1061-1093.

61. Soul JS. Intracranial hemorrhage and white matter injury/periventricular leukomalacia. In: Eichenwald EC, Hansen AR, Martin CR, Stark AR, eds. *Cloherty and Stark's Manual of Neonatal Care*. 9th ed. Wolters Kluwer; 2023: 796-824.

62. Crowley MA, Martin RJ. Respiratory problems. In: Fanaroff AA, Fanaroff JM, eds. *Klaus and Fanaroff's Care of the High-Risk Neonate*. 7th ed. Elsevier; 2020: 190-210.

63. Carlo WA, Ambalavanan N. Assisted ventilation. In: Fanaroff AA, Fanaroff JM, eds. *Klaus and Fanaroff's Care of the High-Risk Neonate*. 7th ed. Elsevier; 2020: 211-226.

64. American Academy of Pediatrics and American Heart Association. Lesson 4: Positive-pressure ventilation. In: Weiner GM, Zaichkin J, eds. *Textbook of Neonatal Resuscitation*. 8th ed. AAP; 2021: 65-116.

65. Abnormal blood gas. In: Gomella TL, Eyal FG, Bany-Mohammed F, eds. *Gomella's Neonatology: Management, Procedures, On-Call Problems, Diseases, and Drugs*. 8th ed. McGraw Hill; 2020: 431-442.

66. Donn S, Stepanovich G, Attar M. Assisted ventilation and its complications. In: Martin RJ, Fanaroff AA, Walsh MC, eds. *Fanaroff and Martin's Neonatal-Perinatal Medicine: Diseases of the Fetus and Infant*. 12th ed. Elsevier; 2025: 1240-1270.

67. Owen L, Davis P. Role of positive-pressure ventilation in neonatal resuscitation. In: Martin RJ, Fanaroff AA, Walsh MC, eds. *Fanaroff and Martin's Neonatal-Perinatal Medicine: Diseases of the Fetus and Infant*. Elsevier; 2025: 545-558.

68. Eichenwald EC, Hatch LD. Mechanical ventilation. In: Eichenwald EC, Hansen AR, Martin CR, Stark AR, eds. *Cloherty and Stark's Manual of Neonatal Care*. 9th ed. Wolters Kluwer; 2023: 418-438.

69. American Heart Association. Part 8: Managing respiratory distress and failure. In: Kadlec KD, McBride ME, Meeks R, et al., eds. *Pediatric Advanced Life Support Provider Manual eBook*. American Heart Association; 2020: e11.

70. Katakam L. Complications of respiratory support. In: Keszler M, Gautham KS, eds. *Goldsmith's Assisted Ventilation of the Neonate*. 7th ed. Elsevier; 2022: 499-503.

71. Gupta AO, Dirnberger DR. Thoracostomy. In: Ramasethu J, Seo S, eds. *MacDonald's Atlas of Procedures in Neonatology*. 6th ed. Wolters Kluwer; 2020: 307-320.

72. Benheim A, North J. Pericardiocentesis. In: Ramasethu J, Seo S, eds. *MacDonald's Atlas of Procedures in Neonatology*. 6th ed. Wolters Kluwer; 2020: 321-326.

73. Ades A, Johnston L. Endotracheal intubation. In: Ramasethu J, Seo S, eds. *MacDonald's Atlas of Procedures in Neonatology*. 6th ed. Wolters Kluwer; 2020: 281-293.

74. Keszler M. Overview of assisted ventilation. In: Keszler M, Gautham KS, eds. *Goldsmith's Assisted Ventilation of the Neonate*. 7th ed. Elsevier; 2022: 220-231.

75. American Heart Association. Part 7: Recognizing respiratory distress and failure. In: Kadlec KD, McBride ME, Meeks R, et al., eds. *Pediatric Advanced Life Support Provider Manual eBook*. American Heart Association; 2020: e10-e17.

76. Singh N, Sawyer T, Johnston LC, et al. Impact of multiple intubation attempts on adverse tracheal intubation associated events in neonates: A report from the NEAR4NEOS. *J Perinatol*. 2022;42(9):1221-1227.

77. Miller KE, Singh N. Association of multiple tracheal intubation attempts with clinical outcomes in extremely preterm infants: A retrospective single-center cohort study. *J Perinatol*. 2022;42(9):1216-1220.

References

(A) Airway Module

78. American Academy of Pediatrics and American Heart Association. Lesson 3: Initial steps of newborn care. In: Weiner GM, Zaichkin J, eds. *Textbook of Neonatal Resuscitation*. 8th ed. AAP; 2021: 33-63.

79. American Academy of Pediatrics and American Heart Association. Lesson 6: Chest compressions. In: Weiner GM, Zaichkin J, eds. *Textbook of Neonatal Resuscitation*. 8th ed. AAP; 2021: 159-178.

80. American Academy of Pediatrics and American Heart Association. Lesson 5: Endotracheal intubation. In: Weiner GM, Zaichkin J, eds. *Textbook of Neonatal Resuscitation*. 8th ed. AAP; 2021: 117-157.

81. Owen LS, Weiner G, Davis PG. Delivery room stabilization and respiratory support. In: Keszler M, Gautham KS, eds. *Goldsmith's Assisted Ventilation of the Neonate*. 7th ed. Elsevier; 2022: 151-171.

82. Pinheiro JMB, Munshi UK, Chowdhry R. Strategies to improve neonatal intubation safety by preventing endobronchial placement of the tracheal tube—Literature review and experience at a tertiary center. *Children (Basel)*. 2023;10(2): 361.

83. Tochen ML. Orotracheal intubation in the newborn infant: A method for determining depth of tube insertion. *J Pediatr*. 1979;95(6):1050-1.

84. Kempley ST, Moreiras JW, Petrone FL. Endotracheal tube length for neonatal intubation. *Resuscitation*. 2008;77(3):369-73.

85. Berlin SC, Carr CB. Diagnostic imaging of the neonate. In: Martin RJ, Fanaroff AA, Walsh MC, eds. *Fanaroff and Martin's Neonatal-Perinatal Medicine: Diseases of the Fetus and Infant*. 12th ed. Elsevier; 2025: 634-664.

86. Park MK, Salamat M. History taking. In: Park MK, Salamat M, eds. *Park's Pediatric Cardiology for Practitioners*. 7th ed. Elsevier; 2021:2-5.

87. Andropoulos DB, Dunbar BS, Shekerdemian LS, Checchia PA, Chang AC. Cardiovascular intensive care. In: Shaddy RE, Penny DJ, Feltes TF, Cetta F, Mital S, eds. *Moss and Adams' Heart Disease in Infants, Children, and Adolescents*. 10th ed. Wolters Kluwer; 2022: 627-677.

88. Singh Y, Chee Y-H, Gahlaut R. Evaluation of suspected congenital heart disease. *Paediatrics and Child Health*. 2015;25(1):7-12.

89. Park MK, Salamat M. Physical examination. In: Park MK, Salamat M, eds. *Park's Pediatric Cardiology for Practitioners*. 7th ed. Elsevier; 2021: 6-30.

90. Leeman K. Transient tachypnea of the newborn. In: Eichenwald EC, Hansen AR, Martin CR, Stark AR, eds. *Cloherty and Stark's Manual of Neonatal Care*. 9th ed. Wolters Kluwer; 2023: 454-457.

91. Alhassen Z, Vali P, Guglani L, Lakshminrusimha S, Ryan RM. Recent advances in pathophysiology and management of transient tachypnea of newborn. *J Perinatol*. 2021;41(1):6-16.

92. Stoll BJ, Puopolo KM, Hansen NI, et al. Early-onset neonatal sepsis 2015 to 2017, the rise of escherichia coli, and the need for novel prevention strategies. *JAMA Pediatr*. 2020;174(7):e200593.

93. Hooven TA, Polin RA. Pneumonia. *Semin Fetal Neonatal Med*. 2017;22(4):206-213.

94. Hay S. Meconium aspiration. In: Eichenwald EC, Hansen AR, Martin CR, Stark AR, eds. *Cloherty and Stark's Manual of Neonatal Care*. 9th ed. Wolters Kluwer; 2023: 482-487.

95. Valentine GC, Wallen LD. Neonatal bacterial sepsis and meningitis. In: Gleason CA, Sawyer T, eds. *Avery's Diseases of the Newborn*. 11th ed. Elsevier; 2024: 439-449.

96. Ostrea E, Cortez J, Villanueva-Uy M, Gamiao J. The impact of prenatal exposure to nonnarcotic drugs: Maternal, fetal, neonatal, and long-term outcomes. In: Boardman J, Groves A, Ramasethu J, eds. *Avery & MacDonald's Neonatology: Pathophysiology and Management of the Newborn*. 8th ed. Wolters Kluwer; 2021: 164-184.

97. Grigoriadis S, Vonderporten EH, Mamisashvili L, et al. Prenatal exposure to antidepressants and persistent pulmonary hypertension of the newborn: Systematic review and meta-analysis. *BMJ*. 2014;(348):f6932.

98. Badillo A, Gingalewski C. Congenital diaphragmatic hernia: Treatment and outcomes. *Semin Perinatol*. 2014;38(2):92-6.

99. Lee SY, Jackson JE, Lakshiminrusimha S, Brown EG, Farmer DL. Anatomic disorders of the chest and airways. In: Gleason CA, Sawyer T, eds. *Avery's Diseases of the Newborn*. 11th ed. Elsevier; 2024: 626-658.

100. Wild KT, Rintoul NE, Puder M, Hansen AR. Surgical conditions in the newborn. In: Eichenwald EC, Hansen AR, Martin CR, Stark AR, eds. *Cloherty and Stark's Manual of Neonatal Care*. 9th ed. Wolters Kluwer; 2023: 982-1012.

101. Lakshminrusimha S, Keszler M, Yoder B. Care of the infant with congenital diaphragmatic hernia. In: Keszler M, Gautham KS, eds. *Goldsmith's Assisted Ventilation of the Neonate*. Elsevier; 2022: 444-455.

102. Dingeldein M. Selected gastrointestinal anomalies in the neonate. In: Martin RJ, Fanaroff AA, Walsh MC, eds. *Fanaroff and Martin's Neonatal-Perinatal Medicine: Diseases of the Fetus and Infant*. 12th ed. Elsevier; 2025: 1626-1652.

103. Taylor JA, Neu J. Disorders of the gastrointestinal tract. In: Boardman JP, Groves AM, Ramasethu J, eds. *Avery & MacDonald's Neonatology: Pathophysiolgy and Management of the Newborn*. 10th ed. Wolters Kluwer; 2021: 545-563.

104. Oermann CM. Congenital anomalies of the intrathoracic airways and tracheoesophageal fistula. In: Redding G, Hoppin AG, eds. *UpToDate*. Wolters Kluwer; Updated February 28, 2024. Accessed March 15, 2024. https://www.uptodate.com/contents/congenital-anomalies-of-the-intrathoracic-airways-and-tracheoesophageal-fistula

105. Koo N, Sims T, Arensman RM, et al. Medical and surgical interventions for respiratory distress and airway management. In: Keszler M, Gautham KS, eds. *Goldsmith's Assisted Ventilation of the Neonate*. 7th ed. Elsevier; 2022: 471-489.

106. Bluher AE, Darrow DH. Stridor in the newborn. *Pediatr Clin North Am*. 2019;66(2):475-488.

107. American Academy of Pediatrics and American Heart Association. Lesson 10: Special considerations. In: Weiner GM, Zaichkin J, eds. *Textbook of Neonatal Resuscitation*. 8th ed. AAP; 2021: 243-263.

108. Kumar S, Jain M, Sogi S, Thukral A. McGovern nipple: An alternative for nose breathing in newborn with CHARGE syndrome, having bilateral choanal atresia. *J Indian Soc Pedod Prev Dent*. 2020;38(2):204-207.

109. Martin DM, Oley CA, Van Ravenswaaij-Arts CM. Charge syndrome. In: Carey JC, Battaglia A, Viskochil D, Cassidy SB, eds. *Cassidy and Allanson's Management of Genetic Syndromes*. John Wiley & Sons; 2021: 157-170.

110. DiBlasi R. Respiratory care of the newborn. In: Keszler M, Gautham KS, eds. *Goldsmith's Assisted Ventilation of the Neonate.* 7th ed. Elsevier; 2022: 360-382.

111. Qureshi MJ, Kumar M. Laryngeal mask airway versus bag-mask ventilation or endotracheal intubation for neonatal resuscitation. *Cochrane Database Syst Rev.* 2018;3(3):CD003314.

112. Vali P, Laskminrusimha S. Laryngeal mask airway: An alternate option for all phases of neonatal resuscitation. *Pediatr Res.* 2022;92(3):626-628.

113. Moussa A, Sawyer T, Puia-Dumitrescu M, et al. Does videolaryngoscopy improve tracheal intubation first attempt success in the NICUs? A report from the NEAR4NEOS. *J Perinatol.* 2022;42(9):1210-1215.

Ⓑ Blood Pressure Module

1. Noori S, Seri I. Cardiovascular compromise in the newborn infant. In: Gleason CA, Sawyer T, eds. *Avery's Diseases of the Newborn.* 11th ed. Elsevier; 2024: 675-701.

2. Noori S, Seri I. Principles of developmental cardiovascular physiology and pathophysiology. In: Seri I, Kluckow M, Polin RA, eds. *Hemodynamics and Cardiology: Neonatology Questions and Controversies.* 3rd ed. Elsevier; 2019: 3-27.

3. Gupta S, Donn SM. Assessment of neonatal perfusion. *Semin Fetal Neonatal Med.* 2020;25(5):101144.

4. American Heart Association. Part 9: Recognizing shock. In: Kadlec KD, McBride ME, Meeks R, et al., eds. *Pediatric Advanced Life Support Provider Manual eBook.* American Heart Association; 2020: e12-e17.

5. Noori S, Friedlich PS, Seri I. Pathophysiology of shock in the fetus and neonate. In: Polin RA, Abman SH, Rowitch DH, Benitz WE, Fox WW, eds. *Fetal and Neonatal Physiology.* 6th ed. Elsevier; 2022: 1662-1671.

6. Fraga MV. Shock. In: Eichenwald EC, Hansen AR, Martin CR, Stark AR, eds. *Cloherty and Stark's Manual of Neonatal Care.* 9th ed. Wolters Kluwer; 2023: 525-533.

7. de Boode WP. Advanced hemodynamic monitoring in the neonatal intensive care unit. *Clin Perinatol.* 2020;47(3):423-434.

8. McNamara PJ, Weisz D, Jain A, Giesinger RE. Hemodynamics. In: Boardman J, Groves A, Ramasethu J, eds. *Avery & MacDonald's Neonatology: Pathophysiology and Management of the Newborn.* 8th ed. Wolters Kluwer; 2021: 418-458.

9. Park MK, Salamat M. Fetal and perinatal circulation. In: Park MK, Salamat M, eds. *Park's Pediatric Cardiology for Practitioners.* 7th ed. Elsevier; 2021: 92-95.

10. Park MK, Salamat M. Congestive heart failure. In: Park MK, Salamat M, eds. *Park's Pediatric Cardiology for Practitioners.* 7th ed. Elsevier; 2021: 346-356.

11. El-Khuffash A, McNamara P, Noori S. Diagnosis, evaluation, and monitoring of patent ductus arteriosus in the very preterm infant. In: Seri I, Kluckow M, Polin RA, eds. *Hemodynamics and Cardiology: Neonatology Questions and Controversies.* 3rd ed. Elsevier; 2019: 387-410.

12. American Heart Association. Part 11: Recognizing arrhythmias. In: Kadlec KD, McBride ME, Meeks R, et al., eds. *Pediatric Advanced Life Support Provider Manual eBook.* American Heart Association; 2020: e14-e17.

13. Karlsen KA, Cowley CG. *S.T.A.B.L.E. Cardiac Module: Recognition and Stabilization of Neonates with Severe CHD.* 2nd ed. S.T.A.B.L.E., Inc.; 2021.

14. American Heart Association. Part 4: Systematic approach to the seriously ill or injured child. In: Kadlec KD, McBride ME, Meeks R, et al., eds. *Pediatric Advanced Life Support Provider Manual eBook.* American Heart Association; 2020: e7-e17.

15. Park MK, Salamat M. Disturbances of atrioventricular conduction. In: Park MK, Salamat M, eds. *Park's Pediatric Cardiology for Practitioners.* 7th ed. Elsevier; 2021: 335-337.

16. Gehris RP. Dermatology. In: Zitelli BJ, McIntire SC, Nowalk AJ, eds. *Zitelli and Davis' Atlas of Pediatric Physical Diagnosis.* 7th ed. Elsevier; 2018: 275-340.

17. Kluckow M, Seri I. Cardiovascular compromise in the preterm infant during the first postnatal day. In: Seri I, Kluckow M, Polin RA, eds. *Hemodynamics and Cardiology: Neonatology Questions and Controversies.* 3rd ed. Elsevier; 2019: 471-488.

18. Raju NV, Maisels MJ, Kring E, Schwarz-Warner L. Capillary refill time in the hands and feet of normal newborn infants. *Clin Pediatr (Phila).* 1999;38(3):139-44.

19. Miletin J, Pichova K, Dempsey EM. Bedside detection of low systemic flow in the very low birth weight infant on day 1 of life. *Eur J Pediatr.* 2009;168(7):809-13.

20. Lobos AT, Lee S, Menon K. Capillary refill time and cardiac output in children undergoing cardiac catheterization. *Pediatr Crit Care Med.* 2012;13(2):136-40.

21. Batton B. Neonatal blood pressure standards: What is "normal"? *Clin Perinatol.* 2020;47(3):469-485.

22. Batton B. Neonatal shock: Etiology, clinical manifestations, and evaluation. In: Martin R, Tehrani N, eds. *UpToDate.* Wolters Kluwer; Updated December 02, 2022. Accessed November 23, 2023. https://www.uptodate.com/contents/neonatal-shock-etiology-clinical-manifestations-and-evaluation

23. Kharrat A, Rios DI, Weisz DE, et al. The relationship between blood pressure parameters and left ventricular output in neonates. *J Perinatol.* 2019;39(5):619-625.

24. Batton B. Assessment and management of low blood pressure in extremely preterm infants. In: Martin R, Tehrani N, eds. *UpToDate.* Wolters Kluwer; Updated May 22, 2023. Accessed November 23, 2023. https://www.uptodate.com/contents/assessment-and-management-of-low-blood-pressure-in-extremely-preterm-infants

25. Takci S, Yigit S, Korkmaz A, Yurdakok M. Comparison between oscillometric and invasive blood pressure measurements in critically ill premature infants. *Acta Paediatr.* 2012;101(2):132-5.

26. Zubrow AB, Hulman S, Kushner H, Falkner B. Determinants of blood pressure in infants admitted to neonatal intensive care units: A prospective multicenter study. *J Perinatol.* 1995;15(6):470-9.

27. Kent AL, Kecskes Z, Shadbolt B, Falk MC. Normative blood pressure data in the early neonatal period. *Pediatr Nephrol.* 2007;22(9):1335-41.

28. Kent AL, Meskell S, Falk MC, Shadbolt B. Normative blood pressure data in non-ventilated premature neonates from 28-36 weeks gestation. *Pediatr Nephrol.* 2009;24(1):141-6.

29. Elsayed Y, Ahmed F. Blood pressure normative values in preterm infants during postnatal transition. *Pediatr Res.* 2024;95(3):698-704.

30. Kiss JK, Gajda A, Mari J, Nemeth J, Bereczki C. Oscillometric arterial blood pressure in haemodynamically stable neonates in the first 2 weeks of life. *Pediatr Nephrol.* 2023;38(10):3369-3378.

B Blood Pressure Module

31. Dionne JM, Bremner SA, Baygani SK, et al. Method of blood pressure measurement in neonates and infants: A systematic review and analysis. *J Pediatr*. 2020;221:23-31.e5.

32. Dasnadi S, Aliaga S, Laughon M, Warner DD, Price WA. Factors influencing the accuracy of noninvasive blood pressure measurements in NICU infants. *Am J Perinatol*. 2015;32(7):639-44.

33. Di Fiore J, Raffay T. Neonatal cardiorespiratory monitoring. In: Martin RJ, Fanaroff AA, Walsh MC, eds. *Fanaroff and Martin's Neonatal-Perinatal Medicine: Diseases of the Fetus and Infant*. 12th ed. Elsevier; 2025: 622-633.

34. Devinck A, Keukelier H, De Savoye I, Desmet L, Smets K. Neonatal blood pressure monitoring: Visual assessment is an unreliable method for selecting cuff sizes. *Acta Paediatr*. 2013;102(10):961-4.

35. Kunk R, McCain GC. Comparison of upper arm and calf oscillometric blood pressure measurement in preterm infants. *J Perinatol*. 1996;16(2 Pt 1):89-92.

36. Park MK, Salamat M. Left-to-right shunt lesions. In: Park MK, Salamat M, eds. *Park's Pediatric Cardiology for Practitioners*. 7th ed. Elsevier; 2021: 120-142.

37. Park MK, Salamat M. Obstructive lesions. In: Park MK, Salamat M, eds. *Park's Pediatric Cardiology for Practitioners*. 7th ed. Elsevier; 2021: 143-159.

38. Park MK, Salamat M. Physical examination. In: Park MK, Salamat M, eds. *Park's Pediatric Cardiology for Practitioners*. 7th ed. Elsevier; 2021: 6-30.

39. Vargo L. Cardiovascular assessment. In: Tappero EP, Honeyfield ME, eds. *Physical Assessment of the Newborn*. 5th ed. NICU Ink; 2015: 93-110.

40. Driscoll D. History and physical evaluation. In: Shaddy RE, Penny DJ, Feltes TF, Cetta F, Mital S, eds. *Moss and Adams' Heart Disease in Infants, Children, and Adolescents*. 10th ed. Wolters Kluwer; 2022: 243-250.

41. Johnson G. Clinical examination. In: Long W, Tooley W, McNamara D, eds. *Fetal and Neonatal Cardiology*. W.B. Saunders Company; 1990: 223-235.

42. Keszler M, Abubakar K. Physiologic principles. In: Keszler M, Gautham KS, eds. *Goldsmith's Assisted Ventilation of the Neonate*. 7th ed. Elsevier; 2022: 10-32.

43. Andropoulos DB, Dunbar BS, Shekerdemian LS, Checchia PA, Chang AC. Cardiovascular intensive care. In: Shaddy RE, Penny DJ, Feltes TF, Cetta F, Mital S, eds. *Moss and Adams' Heart Disease in Infants, Children, and Adolescents*. 10th ed. Wolters Kluwer; 2022: 627-677.

44. Abrams SA, Tiosano D. Disorders of calcium, phosphorus, and magnesium metabolism in the neonate. In: Martin RJ, Fanaroff AA, Walsh MC, eds. *Fanaroff and Martin's Neonatal-Perinatal Medicine: Diseases of the Fetus and Infant*. 12th ed. Elsevier; 2025: 1697-1727.

45. Nicks BA. Acute lactic acidosis. Medscape. Updated September 26, 2022. Accessed January 11, 2024. https://emedicine.medscape.com/article/768159-overview

46. Gunnerson KJ. Lactic acidosis. Medscape. Updated September 11, 2020. Accessed January 11, 2024. https://emedicine.medscape.com/article/167027-overview

47. Owusu-Ansah A, Letterio J, Ahuja SP. Red blood cell disorders in the fetus and neonate. In: Martin RJ, Fanaroff AA, Walsh MC, eds. *Fanaroff and Martin's Neonatal-Perinatal Medicine: Diseases of the Fetus and Infant*. 12th ed. Elsevier; 2025: 1520-1552.

48. US National Library of Medicine. Partial thromboplastin time (PTT). MedlinePlus. Updated February 02, 2023. Accessed December 5, 2023. https://medlineplus.gov/ency/article/003653.htm#:~:text=Partial%20thromboplastin%20time%20(PTT)%20is,the%20coagulation%20(clotting)%20system

49. US National Library of Medicine. Prothrombin time test and INR (PT/INR). MedlinePlus. Updated September 21, 2022. Accessed December 5, 2023. https://medlineplus.gov/lab-tests/prothrombin-time-test-and-inr-ptinr/

50. Wright CJ, Posencheg MA, Seri I. Fluid, electrolyte, and acid-base balance. In: Gleason CA, Sawyer T, eds. *Avery's Diseases of the Newborn*. 11th ed. Elsevier; 2024: 231-252.

51. Wandrup J, Kroner J, Pryds O, Kastrup KW. Age-related reference values for ionized calcium in the first week of life in premature and full-term neonates. *Scand J Clin Lab Invest*. 1988;48(3):255-60.

52. Loughead JL, Mimouni F, Tsang RC. Serum ionized calcium concentrations in normal neonates. *Am J Dis Child*. 1988;142(5):516-8.

53. Zehnder JL. Clinical use of coagulation tests. In: Leung LLK, Tirnauer JS, eds. *UpToDate*. Wolters Kluwer; Updated December 29, 2023. Accessed January 11, 2024. https://www.uptodate.com/contents/clinical-use-of-coagulation-tests

54. Travers C, Ambalavanan N. Blood gases: Technical aspects and interpretation. In: Keszler M, Gautham KS, eds. *Goldsmith's Assisted Ventilation of the Neonate*. 7th ed. Elsevier; 2022: 93-110.

55. da Graca RL, Hassinger DC, Flynn PA, Sison CP, Nesin M, Auld PA. Longitudinal changes of brain-type natriuretic peptide in preterm neonates. *Pediatrics*. 2006;117(6):2183-9.

56. El-Khuffash A, Molloy EJ. Are B-type natriuretic peptide (BNP) and N-terminal-pro-BNP useful in neonates? *Arch Dis Child Fetal Neonatal Ed*. 2007;92(4):F320-4.

57. Davlouros PA, Karatza AA, Xanthopoulou I, et al. Diagnostic role of plasma BNP levels in neonates with signs of congenital heart disease. *Int J Cardiol*. 2011;147(1):42-6.

58. Cantinotti M, Passino C, Storti S, Ripoli A, Zyw L, Clerico A. Clinical relevance of time course of BNP levels in neonates with congenital heart diseases. *Clin Chim Acta*. 2011;412(23-24):2300-4.

59. Kulkarni M, Gokulakrishnan G, Price J, Fernandes CJ, Leeflang M, Pammi M. Diagnosing significant PDA using natriuretic peptides in preterm neonates: a systematic review. *Pediatrics*. 2015;135(2):e510-25.

60. Chong D, Chua YT, Chong SL, Ong GY. What raises troponins in the paediatric population? *Pediatr Cardiol*. 2018;39(8):1530-1534.

61. Zaidi AN, Daniels CJ. Myocardial Ischemia in the pediatric population. In: Allen HD, Shaddy RE, Penny DJ, Feltes TF, Cetta F, eds. *Moss and Adams' Heart Disease in Infants, Children, and Adolescents*. 9th ed. Wolters Kluwer; 2016: 1455-1463.

62. Shlomai NO, Friedman SE, Gielchinsky Y. Multiple gestation: Fetal and maternal considerations. In: Martin RJ, Fanaroff AA, Walsh MC, eds. *Fanaroff and Martin's Neonatal-Perinatal Medicine: Diseases of the Fetus and Infant*. 12th ed. Elsevier; 2025: 361-372.

63. Prazad PA, Rajpal MN, Mangurten HH. Birth injuries. In: Martin RJ, Fanaroff AA, Walsh MC, eds. *Fanaroff and Martin's Neonatal-Perinatal Medicine: Diseases of the Fetus and Infant*. 12th ed. Elsevier; 2025: 475-503.

64. Kapadia V, Wyckoff MH. Chest compressions, medications, and special problems in neonatal resuscitation. In: Martin RJ, Fanaroff AA, Walsh MC, eds. *Fanaroff and Martin's Neonatal-Perinatal Medicine: Diseases of the Fetus and Infant*. 12th ed. Elsevier; 2025: 569-581.

65. Chakravorty S, Roberts I. Red blood cells and their disorders. In: Boardman J, Groves A, Ramasethu J, eds. *Avery & MacDonald's Neonatology: Pathophysiology and Management of the Newborn*. 8th ed. Wolters Kluwer; 2021: 694-707.

66. American Heart Association. Part 10: Managing shock. In: Kadlec KD, McBride ME, Meeks R, et al., eds. *Pediatric Advanced Life Support Provider Manual eBook*. American Heart Association; 2020: e13-e17.

67. Apnea and bradycardia (A's and B's): On call. In: Gomella TL, Eyal FG, Bany-Mohammed F, eds. *Gomella's Neonatology: Management, Procedures, On-Call Problems, Diseases, and Drugs*. 8th ed. McGraw Hill Medical; 2020: 442-459.

68. Stayer K, Hutchins L. Emergency and critical care management. In: Kleinman K, Mcdaniel L, Molloy M, eds. *The Harriet Lane Handbook*. 22nd ed. Elsevier; 2021: 3-32.

69. Davis AL, Carcillo JA, Aneja RK, et al. American College of Critical Care Medicine Clinical Practice Parameters for Hemodynamic Support of Pediatric and Neonatal Septic Shock: Executive summary. *Pediatr Crit Care Med*. 2017;18(9):884-890.

70. Davis AL, Carcillo JA, Aneja RK, et al. American College of Critical Care Medicine Clinical Practice Parameters for Hemodynamic Support of Pediatric and Neonatal Septic Shock. *Crit Care Med*. 2017;45(6):1061-1093.

71. Batton B. Neonatal shock: Management. In: Martin R, Tehrani N, eds. *UpToDate*. Wolters Kluwer; Updated April 17, 2024. Accessed April 20, 2024. https://www.uptodate.com/contents/neonatal-shock-management

72. de Waal K, Seri I. Assessment and management of septic shock and hypovolemia. In: Seri I, Kluckow M, Polin RA, eds. *Hemodynamics and Cardiology: Neonatology Questions and Controversies*. 3rd ed. Elsevier; 2019: 489-501.

73. Andropoulos DB, Yuki K, Koutsogiannaki S. Physiology and cellular biology of the developing circulation. In: Andropoulos DB, Mossad EB, Gottlieb EA, eds. *Anesthesia for Congenital Heart Disease*. 4th ed. John Wiley & Sons Ltd; 2023: 166-189.

74. Sloan SR. Blood products used in the newborn. In: Eichenwald EC, Hansen AR, Martin CR, Stark AR, eds. *Cloherty and Stark's Manual of Neonatal Care*. 9th ed. Wolters Kluwer; 2023: 594-603.

75. Ohls R. Red blood cell (RBC) transfusions in the neonate. In: Garcia-Prats JA, Tobian A, Tehrani N, eds. *UpToDate*. Wolters Kluwer; Updated April 30, 2023. Accessed December 5, 2023. https://www.uptodate.com/contents/red-blood-cell-rbc-transfusions-in-the-neonate

76. Carlberg K. Neonatal erythrocyte disorders. In: Gleason CA, Sawyer T, eds. *Avery's Diseases of the Newborn*. 11th ed. Elsevier; 2024: 996-1024.

77. Goel R, Punzalan RC, Wong ECC. Neonatal and pediatric transfusion practice. In: Cohn C, Delaney M, Johnson ST, Katz LM, Schwartz J, eds. *Technical Manual*. 21st ed. American Association of Blood Banks; 2023: 729-761.

78. Mo YD, Jacquot C. Transfusion therapy: Evidence and recommendations for clinical practice. In: Cohn C, Delaney M, Johnson ST, Katz LM, Schwartz J, eds. *Technical Manual*. 21st ed. American Association of Blood Banks; 2023: 589-621.

79. Andrews J, Clarke G. Perinatal issues in transfusion practice. In: Cohn C, Delaney M, Johnson ST, Katz LM, Schwartz J, eds. *Technical Manual*. 21st ed. American Association of Blood Banks; 2023: 709-727.

80. Teruya J. Red blood cell transfusions in infants and children: Selection of blood products. In: Tobian A, Armsby C, eds. *UpToDate*. Wolters Kluwer; Updated August 30, 2023. Accessed December 5, 2023. https://www.uptodate.com/contents/red-blood-cell-transfusion-in-infants-and-children-selection-of-blood-products

81. Ipe TS, Alquist CR. Transfusion-service-related activities: Pretransfusion testing and storage, monitoring, processing, distribution, and inventory management of blood components. In: Cohn C, Delaney M, Johnson ST, Katz LM, Schwartz J, eds. *Technical Manual*. 21st ed. American Association of Blood Banks; 2023: 529-561.

82. Benheim A, North J. Pericardiocentesis. In: Ramasethu J, Seo S, eds. *MacDonald's Atlas of Procedures in Neonatology*. 6th ed. Wolters Kluwer; 2020: 321-326.

83. Gupta AO, Dirnberger DR. Thoracostomy. In: Ramasethu J, Seo S, eds. *MacDonald's Atlas of Procedures in Neonatology*. 6th ed. Wolters Kluwer; 2020: 307-320.

84. Benitz WE, Bhombal S. Patent ductus arteriosus. In: Martin RJ, Fanaroff AA, Walsh MC, eds. *Fanaroff and Martin's Neonatal-Perinatal Medicine: Diseases of the Fetus and Infant*. 12th ed. Elsevier; 2025: 1401-1409.

85. Krishnamurthy G, Ratner V, Levasseur S, Rubenstein SD. Congenital heart disease in the newborn period. In: Polin RA, Yoder MC, eds. *Workbook in Practical Neonatology*. 5th ed. Elsevier Saunders; 2015: 244-269.

86. Clyman RI. Mechanisms regulating closure of the ductus arteriosus. In: Polin RA, Abman SH, Rowitch DH, Benitz WE, eds. *Fetal and Neonatal Physiology*. 6th ed. Elsevier; 2022: 553-564.

87. American Pharmacists Association. *Lexicomp Pediatric & Neonatal Dosage Handbook with International Trade Names Index*. 24th ed. Wolters Kluwer; 2018.

88. Wagner JB, Artman M. Pharmacology. In: Shaddy RE, Penny DJ, Feltes TF, Cetta F, Mital S, eds. *Moss and Adams' Heart Disease in Infants, Children, and Adolescents*. 10th ed. Wolters Kluwer; 2022: 1800-1824.

89. Phad N, de Waal K. What inotrope and why? *Clin Perinatol*. 2020;47(3):529-547.

90. Evans N. Hemodynamically based pharmacologic management of circulatory compromise in the newborn. In: Seri I, Kluckow M, Polin RA, eds. *Hemodynamics and Cardiology: Neonatology Questions and Controversies*. 3rd ed. Elsevier; 2019: 521-534.

91. Manaker S. Use of vasopressors and inotropes. In: Gong M, Finlay G, eds. *UpToDate*. Wolters Kluwer; Updated December 8, 2023. Accessed December 14, 2023. https://www.uptodate.com/contents/use-of-vasopressors-and-inotropes

92. Cunningham FG, Leveno KJ, Dashe JS, Hoffman BL, Spong CY, Casey BM. Complications of the term newborn. In: Cunningham FG, Leveno KJ, Dashe JS, Hoffman BL, Spong CY, Casey BM, eds. *Williams Obstetrics*. 26th ed. McGraw Hill; 2022: 599-614.

93. Hoppe KK, Bosse B. Complicated deliveries. In: Gleason CA, Sawyer T, eds. *Avery's Diseases of the Newborn*. 11th ed. Elsevier; 2024: 135-146.

94. McQuivey RW. Vacuum-assisted delivery: A review. *J Matern Fetal Neonatal Med*. 2004;16(3):171-80.

95. Davis DJ. Neonatal subgaleal hemorrhage: Diagnosis and management. *CMAJ*. 2001;164(10):1452-3.

96. Doumouchtsis SK, Arulkumaran S. Head trauma after instrumental births. *Clin Perinatol*. 2008;35(1):69-83, viii.

97. El-Dib M, Parziale MP, Johnson L, et al. Encephalopathy in neonates with subgaleal hemorrhage is a key predictor of outcome. *Pediatr Res*. 2019;86(2):234-241.

98. Eseonu CI, Sacino AN, Ahn ES. Early surgical intervention for a large newborn cephalohematoma. *Pediatr Neurosurg*. 2016;51(4):210-3.

99. Christensen TR, Bahr TM, Henry E, et al. Neonatal subgaleal hemorrhage: Twenty years of trends in incidence, associations, and outcomes. *J Perinatol*. 2023;43(5):573-577.

100. Colditz MJ, Lai MM, Cartwright DW, Colditz PB. Subgaleal haemorrhage in the newborn: A call for early diagnosis and aggressive management. *J Paediatr Child Health*. 2015;51(2):140-6.

101. Demissie K, Rhoads GG, Smulian JC, et al. Operative vaginal delivery and neonatal and infant adverse outcomes: Population based retrospective analysis. *BMJ*. 2004;329(7456):24-9.

102. Towner D, Castro MA, Eby-Wilkens E, Gilbert WM. Effect of mode of delivery in nulliparous women on neonatal intracranial injury. *N Engl J Med*. 1999;341(23):1709-14.

103. Gardella C, Taylor M, Benedetti T, Hitti J, Critchlow C. The effect of sequential use of vacuum and forceps for assisted vaginal delivery on neonatal and maternal outcomes. *Am J Obstet Gynecol*. 2001;185(4):896-902.

Ⓛ Lab Work Module

1. Mukherjee D, Ryan RM. Postnatal bacterial infections. In: Martin RJ, Fanaroff AA, Walsh MC, eds. *Fanaroff and Martin's Neonatal-Perinatal Medicine: Diseases of the Fetus and Infant*. 12th ed. Elsevier; 2025: 857-880.

2. Koenig JM, Bliss JM, Sperandio M. Normal and abnormal neutrophil physiology in the newborn. In: Polin RA, Abman SH, Rowitch DH, Benitz WE, eds. *Fetal and Neonatal Physiology*. 6th ed. Philadelphia: Elsevier; 2022: 1215-1231.

3. Blackburn S. Immune system and host defense mechanisms. In: Blackburn ST, ed. *Maternal, Fetal, Neonatal Physiology: A Clinical Perspective*. 5th ed. St. Louis: Elsevier; 2018: 435-470.

4. Valentine GC, Wallen LD. Neonatal bacterial sepsis and meningitis. In: Gleason CA, Sawyer T, eds. *Avery's Diseases of the Newborn*. 11th ed. Elsevier; 2024: 439-449.

5. Wynn JI. Pathophysiology of neonatal sepsis. In: Polin RA, Abman SH, Rowitch DH, Benitz WE, eds. *Fetal and Neonatal Physiology*. 6th ed. Elsevier; 2022: 1606-1623.

6. Kollman T, Dauby N, Harbeson D, Fidanza M, Marchant A. Host defense mechanisms against bacteria. In: Polin RA, Abman SH, Rowitch DH, Benitz WE, eds. *Fetal and Neonatal Physiology*. 6th ed. Elsevier; 2022: 1158-1167.

7. Stoll BJ, Puopolo KM, Hansen NI, et al. Early-onset neonatal sepsis 2015 to 2017, the rise of Escherichia coli, and the need for novel prevention strategies. *JAMA Pediatr*. 2020;174(7):e200593.

8. Polin RA. Management of neonates with suspected or proven early-onset bacterial sepsis. *Pediatrics*. 2012;129(5):1006-1015.

9. Gardner S, Enzman-Hines M, Nyp M. Respiratory diseases. In: Gardner S, Carter BS, Enzman-Hines M, Niermeyer S, eds. *Merenstein & Gardner's Handbook of Neonatal Intensive Care*. 9th ed. Elsevier; 2021: 729-835.

10. Karlsen KA, Cowley CG. *S.T.A.B.L.E. Cardiac Module: Recognition and Stabilization of Neonates with Severe CHD*. 2nd ed. S.T.A.B.L.E., Inc.; 2021.

11. Gomella TL, Eyal FG, Bany-Mohammed F. Inborn errors of metabolism with acute neonatal onset. In: Gomella TL, Eyal FG, Bany-Mohammed F, eds. *Gomella's Neonatology: Management, Procedures, On-Call Problems, Diseases, and Drugs*. 8th ed. McGraw Hill; 2020: 915-937.

12. Cantey JB, Lee JH. Biomarkers for the diagnosis of neonatal sepsis. *Clin Perinatol*. 2021;48(2):215-227.

13. Pammi M, Brand C, Weisman LE. Infection in the neonate. In: Gardner S, Carter BS, Enzman-Hines M, Niermeyer S, eds. *Merenstein & Gardner's Handbook of Neonatal Intensive Care*. 9th ed. Elsevier; 2021: 692-727.

14. Perry MC, Yaeger SK, Noorbakhsh K, Cruz AT, Hickey RW. Hypothermia in young infants: Frequency and yield of sepsis workup. *Pediatr Emerg Care*. 2021;37(8):e449-e455.

15. Gomella T, Eyal FG, Bany-Mohammed F. Sepsis. In: Gomella TL, Eyal FG, Bany-Mohammed F, eds. *Gomella's Neonatology: Management, Procedures, On-Call Problems, Diseases, and Drugs*. 8th ed. McGraw Hill; 2020: 1175-1189.

16. Camacho-Gonzalez A, Spearman PW, Stoll BJ. Neonatal infectious diseases: Evaluation of neonatal sepsis. *Pediatr Clin North Am*. 2013;60(2):367-389.

17. Engelkirk PG, Duben-Engelkirk J, Fader R. *Burton's Microbiology for the Health Sciences*. 11th ed. Wolters Kluwer; 2019.

18. Desai AP, Lim PPC, Ogundare MO, Gonzalez BE. Viral infections in the neonate. In: Martin RJ, Fanaroff AA, Walsh MC, eds. *Fanaroff and Martin's Neonatal-Perinatal Medicine: Diseases of the Fetus and Infant*. Elsevier; 2025: 917-933.

19. Stokes C, Melvin AJ. Viral infections in the fetus and newborn. In: Gleason CA, Sawyer T, eds. *Avery's Diseases of the Newborn*. 11th ed. Elsevier; 2024: 450-486.

20. Pinninti SG, Kimberlin DW. Maternal and neonatal herpes simplex virus infections. *Am J Perinatol*. 2013;30(2):113-119.

21. Committee on Infectious Diseases, Academy of Pediatrics, Kimberlin DW, Barnett ED, Lynfield R, Sawyer MH. Herpes simplex. *Red Book: 2021–2024 Report of the Committee on Infectious Diseases*. American Academy of Pediatrics; 2021.

22. Pinninti SG, Kimberlin DW. Congenital infections. In: Boardman JP, Groves AM, Ramasethu J, eds. *Avery & MacDonald's Neonatology: Pathophysiology and Management of the Newborn*. 10th ed. Wolters Kluwer; 2021: 748-766.

23. Looker KJ, Magaret AS, May MT, et al. First estimates of the global and regional incidence of neonatal herpes infection. *Lancet Glob Health*. 2017;5(3):e300-e309.

24. James SH, Kimberlin DW. Neonatal herpes simplex virus infection: Epidemiology and treatment. *Clin Perinatol*. 2015;42(1):47-59, viii.

25. Polin RA, Hooven TA, Randis TM. Perinatal infections and chorioamnionitis. In: Martin RJ, Fanaroff AA, Walsh MC, eds. *Fanaroff and Martin's Neonatal-Perinatal Medicine: Diseases of the Fetus and Infant*. Elsevier; 2025: 414-424.

26. Dhudasia MB, Flannery DD, Puopolo KM. Evaluation and management of infection in the newborn. In: *Avery & MacDonald's Neonatology: Pathophysiology and Management of the Newborn*. 10th ed. Wolters Kluwer; 2021: 766-778.

27. Jung E, Romero R, Yeo L, Chaemsaithong P, Gomez-Lopez N. Intra-amniotic infection/inflammation and the fetal inflammatory response syndrome. In: Polin RA, Abman SH, Rowitch DH, Benitz WE, eds. *Fetal and Neonatal Physiology*. 6th ed. Elsevier; 2022: 111-129.

28. Tita AT, Andrews WW. Diagnosis and management of clinical chorioamnionitis. *Clin Perinatol.* 2010;37(2):339-354.

29. Ericson JE, Laughon MM. Chorioamnionitis: Implications for the neonate. *Clin Perinatol.* 2015;42(1):155-165, ix.

30. American College of Obstetricians and Gynecologists' Committee on Obstetric Practice, Heine RP, Puopolo KM, Beigi R, Silverman NS, El-Sayed YY. Committee opinion No. 712: Intrapartum management of intraamniotic infection. *Obstet Gynecol.* 2017;130(2):e95-e101.

31. Kallapur SG, Jobe AH. Antenatal factors that influence postnatal lung development and injury. In: Polin RA, Abman SH, Rowitch DH, Benitz WE, eds. *Fetal and Neonatal Physiology*. 6th ed. Elsevier; 2022: 748-756.

32. Schelonka RL, Chai MK, Yoder BA, Hensley D, Brockett RM, Ascher DP. Volume of blood required to detect common neonatal pathogens. *J Pediatr.* 1996;129(2):275-278.

33. Connell TG, Rele M, Cowley D, Buttery JP, Curtis N. How reliable is a negative blood culture result? Volume of blood submitted for culture in routine practice in a children's hospital. *Pediatrics.* 2007;119(5):891-896.

34. Benitz WE. Adjunct laboratory tests in the diagnosis of early-onset neonatal sepsis. *Clin Perinatol.* 2010;37(2):421-438.

35. Schibler KR, Christensen RD. Eosinophils and neutrophils. In: de Alarcon PA, Werner EJ, Christensen RD, Sola-Visner MC, eds. *Neonatal Hematology: Pathogenesis, Diagnosis, and Management of Hematologic Problems*. 3rd ed. Cambridge University Press; 2021: 261-278.

36. Burstein B, Beltempo M, Fontela PS. Role of c-reactive protein for late-onset neonatal sepsis. *JAMA Pediatr.* 2021;175(1):101-102.

37. Molloy EJ, Strunk T. Role of c-reactive protein for late-onset neonatal sepsis. *JAMA Pediatr.* 2021;175(1):100-101.

38. Cortes JS, Losada PX, Fernandez LX, et al. Interleukin-6 as a biomarker of early-onset neonatal sepsis. *Am J Perinatol.* 2021;38(S 01):e338-e346.

39. Jain VG, Willis KA, Jobe A, Ambalavanan N. Chorioamnionitis and neonatal outcomes. *Pediatr Res.* 2022;91(2):289-296.

40. Rouse DJ, Landon M, Leveno KJ, et al. The maternal-fetal medicine units cesarean registry: Chorioamnionitis at term and its duration-relationship to outcomes. *Am J Obstet Gynecol.* 2004;191(1):211-216.

41. Daifotis HA, Smith MM, Denoble AE, Dotters-Katz SK. Risk factors for postpartum maternal infection following spontaneous vaginal delivery complicated by chorioamnionitis. *AJP Rep.* 2020;10(2):e159-e164.

42. Higgins RD, Saade G, Polin RA, et al. Evaluation and management of women and newborns with a maternal diagnosis of chorioamnionitis: Summary of a workshop. *Obstet Gynecol.* 2016;127(3):426-436.

43. Ona S, Easter SR, Prabhu M, et al. Diagnostic validity of the proposed Eunice Kennedy Shriver National Institute of Child Health and Human Development criteria for intrauterine inflammation or infection. *Obstet Gynecol.* 2019;133(1):33-39.

44. Hornik CP, Benjamin DK, Becker KC, et al. Use of the complete blood cell count in early-onset neonatal sepsis. *Pediatr Infect Dis J.* 2012;31(8):799-802.

45. Celik IH, Hanna M, Canpolat FE, Mohan P. Diagnosis of neonatal sepsis: The past, present and future. *Pediatr Res.* 2022;91(2):337-350.

46. Christensen RD, Rothstein G, Hill HR, Hall RT. Fatal early onset group B streptococcal sepsis with normal leukocyte counts. *Pediatr Infect Dis.* 1985;4(3):242-245.

47. Puopolo KM, Benitz WE, Zaoutis TE, Committee on Fetus and Newborn, Committee on Infectious Diseases. Management of neonates born at ≥35 0/7 weeks' gestation with suspected or proven early-onset bacterial sepsis. *Pediatrics.* 2018;142(6):e20182894.

48. Schmutz N, Henry E, Jopling J, Christensen RD. Expected ranges for blood neutrophil concentrations of neonates: The Manroe and Mouzinho charts revisited. *J Perinatol.* 2008;28(4):275-281.

49. Wiedmeier SE, Henry E, Christensen RD. Hematological abnormalities during the first week of life among neonates with trisomy 18 and trisomy 13: Data from a multi-hospital healthcare system. *Am J Med Genet A.* 2008;146A(3):312-320.

50. Benjamin JT, Molloy EJ, Maheshwari A. Developmental immunology. In: Martin RJ, Fanaroff AA, Walsh MC, eds. *Fanaroff and Martin's Neonatal-Perinatal Medicine: Diseases of the Fetus and Infant*. 12th ed. Elsevier; 2025: 820-856.

51. Christensen RD, Rothstein G. Exhaustion of mature marrow neutrophils in neonates with sepsis. *J Pediatr.* 1980;96(2):316-318.

52. Lawrence S, Nizet V. Neutrophil granulopoiesis and hemostasis. In: Polin RA, Abman SH, Rowitch DH, Benitz WE, eds. *Fetal and Neonatal Physiology*. 6th ed. Elsevier; 2022: 1093-1104.

53. Hall JE, Hall ME. Resistance of the body to infection: I. Leukocytes, granulocytes, the monocyte-macrophage system, and inflammation. *Guyton and Hall Textbook of Medical Physiology*. 14th ed. Elsevier; 2021:449-458.

54. Hematological tests. In: Mastenbjörk M, Meloni S, eds. *Lab Values: Everything You Need to Know about Laboratory Medicine and its Importance in the Diagnosis of Diseases*. 2nd ed. Medical Creations; 2020: 11-30.

55. Min B, Brown MA, Legros G. Understanding the roles of basophils: Breaking dawn. *Immunology.* 2012;135(3):192-197.

56. Juul SE, Haynes JW, McPherson RJ. Evaluation of eosinophilia in hospitalized preterm infants. *J Perinatol.* 2005;25(3):182-188.

57. Khalili AS, Sferra TJ. Disorders of digestion in the neonate. In: Martin RJ, Fanaroff AA, Walsh MC, eds. *Fanaroff and Martin's Neonatal-Perinatal Medicine: Diseases of the Fetus and Infant*. Elsevier; 2025: 1615-1625.

58. Calihan J. Hematology. In: Kleinman K, McDaniel L, Molloy M, eds. *The Harriet Lane Handbook*. 22nd ed. Elsevier; 2021: 328-367.

59. Christensen RD. Reference intervals in neonatal hematology. In: De Alarcon PA, Werner EJ, Christensen RD, Sola-Visner MC, eds. *Neonatal Hematology: Pathogenesis, Diagnosis, and Management of Hematologic Problems*. 3rd ed. Cambridge University Press; 2021: 440-469.

References

L Lab Work Module

60. Hornik CP, Benjamin DK, Becker KC, et al. Use of the complete blood cell count in late-onset neonatal sepsis. *Pediatr Infect Dis J.* 2012;31(8):803-807.

61. Murphy K, Weiner J. Use of leukocyte counts in evaluation of early-onset neonatal sepsis. *Pediatr Infect Dis J.* 2012;31(1):16-19.

62. Christensen RD, Bradley PP, Rothstein G. The leukocyte left shift in clinical and experimental neonatal sepsis. *J Pediatr.* 1981;98(1):101-105.

63. Mouzinho A, Rosenfeld CR, Sanchez PJ, Risser R. Revised reference ranges for circulating neutrophils in very-low-birth-weight neonates. *Pediatrics.* 1994;94(1):76-82.

64. Koenig JM, Christensen RD. The mechanism responsible for diminished neutrophil production in neonates delivered of women with pregnancy-induced hypertension. *Am J Obstet Gynecol.* 1991;165(2):467-473.

65. Koenig JM, Yoder MC. Neonatal neutrophils: The good, the bad, and the ugly. *Clin Perinatol.* 2004;31(1):39-51.

66. Koenig JM, Christensen RD. Incidence, neutrophil kinetics, and natural history of neonatal neutropenia associated with maternal hypertension. *N Engl J Med.* 1989;321(9):557-562.

67. Manroe BL, Weinberg AG, Rosenfeld CR, Browne R. The neonatal blood count in health and disease. I. Reference values for neutrophilic cells. *J Pediatr.* 1979;95(1):89-98.

68. Sola MC. Evaluation and treatment of severe and prolonged thrombocytopenia in neonates. *Clin Perinatol.* 2004;31(1):1-14.

69. McPherson RJ, Juul S. Patterns of thrombocytosis and thrombocytopenia in hospitalized neonates. *J Perinatol.* 2005;25(3):166-172.

70. Sola-Visner M, Saxonhouse MA, Brown RE. Neonatal thrombocytopenia: What we do and don't know. *Early Hum Dev.* 2008;84(8):499-506.

71. Davenport P, Sola-Visner M. Acquired thrombocytopenias. In: De Alarcon PA, Werner EJ, Christensen RD, Sola-Visner MC, eds. *Neonatal Hematology: Pathogenesis, Diagnosis, and Management of Hematologic Problems.* 3rd ed. Cambridge University Press; 2021: 210-222.

72. Mitchell W, Bussel J. Fetal and neonatal alloimmune thrombocytopenias. In: De Alarcon PA, Werner EJ, Christensen RD, Sola-Visner MC, eds. *Neonatal Hematology: Pathogenesis, Diagnosis, and Management of Hematologic Problems.* 3rd ed. Cambridge University Press; 2021: 223-242.

73. Wiedmeier SE, Henry E, Sola-Visner MC, Christensen RD. Platelet reference ranges for neonates, defined using data from over 47,000 patients in a multihospital healthcare system. *J Perinatol.* 2009;29(2):130-136.

74. Henry E, Christensen RD. Reference intervals in neonatal hematology. *Clin Perinatol.* 2015;42(3):483-497.

75. Deschmann E, Sola-Visner M. Approach to the thrombocytopenic neonate. In: De Alarcon PA, Werner EJ, Christensen RD, Sola-Visner MC, eds. *Neonatal Hematology: Pathogenesis, Diagnosis, and Management of Hematologic Problems.* 3rd ed. Cambridge University Press; 2021: 201-209.

76. Kuzniewicz MW, Mukhopadhyay S, Li S, Walsh EM, Puopolo KM. Time to positivity of neonatal blood cultures for early-onset sepsis. *Pediatr Infect Dis J.* 2020;39(7):634-640.

77. Ur Rehman Durrani N, Rochow N, Alghamdi J, Pelc A, Fusch C, Dutta S. Minimum duration of antibiotic treatment based on blood culture in rule out neonatal sepsis. *Pediatr Infect Dis J.* 2019;38(5):528-532.

78. Achten NB, Klingenberg C, Benitz WE, et al. Association of use of the neonatal early-onset sepsis calculator with reduction in antibiotic therapy and safety: A systematic review and meta-analysis. *JAMA Pediatr.* 2019;173(11):1032-1040.

79. Snoek L, van Kassel MN, Krommenhoek JF, et al. Neonatal early-onset infections: Comparing the sensitivity of the neonatal early-onset sepsis calculator to the Dutch and the updated NICE guidelines in an observational cohort of culture-positive cases. *EClinicalMedicine.* 2022;44:101270.

80. Kuzniewicz MW, Puopolo KM, Fischer A, et al. A quantitative, risk-based approach to the management of neonatal early-onset sepsis. *JAMA Pediatr.* 2017;171(4):365-371.

81. Kuzniewicz MW, Walsh EM, Li S, Fischer A, Escobar GJ. Development and implementation of an early-onset sepsis calculator to guide antibiotic management in late preterm and term neonates. *Jt Comm J Qual Patient Saf.* 2016;42(5):232-239.

82. Puopolo KM, Draper D, Wi S, et al. Estimating the probability of neonatal early-onset infection on the basis of maternal risk factors. *Pediatrics.* 2011;128(5):e1155-1163.

83. Escobar GJ, Puopolo KM, Wi S, et al. Stratification of risk of early-onset sepsis in newborns ≥34 weeks' gestation. *Pediatrics.* 2014;133(1):30-36.

84. Ellington M, Kasat K, Williams K, et al. Improving antibiotic stewardship among asymptomatic newborns using the early-onset sepsis risk calculator. *Pediatr Qual Saf.* 2021;6(5):e459.

85. Dhudasia MB, Mukhopadhyay S, Puopolo KM. Implementation of the sepsis risk calculator at an academic birth hospital. *Hosp Pediatr.* 2018;8(5):243-250.

86. Flannery DD, Puopolo KM. Neonatal early-onset sepsis. *Neoreviews.* 2022;23(11):756-770.

87. Kuzniewicz MW, Puopolo KM. Antibiotic stewardship for early-onset sepsis. *Semin Perinatol.* 2020;44(8):151325.

88. Ampicillin (Pediatric and Neonatal Lexi-Drugs). *UpToDate-Lexidrug.* Wolters Kluwer; April 2, 2024. Accessed April 4, 2024. https://online-lexi-com.ezproxy.lib.utah.edu/lco/action/search?q=ampicillin&t=name&acs=true&acq=Ampicillin –

89. Percy A. Procedures. In: Kleinman K, Mcdaniel L, Molloy M, eds. *The Harriet Lane Handbook.* 22nd ed. Elsevier; 2021: 61-97.

90. Sheffield MJ, Lambert DK, Henry E, Christensen RD. Effect of ampicillin on the bleeding time of neonatal intensive care unit patients. *J Perinatol.* 2010;30(8):527-530.

91. Sheffield MJ, Lambert DK, Baer VL, et al. Effect of ampicillin on bleeding time in very low birth-weight neonates during the first week after birth. *J Perinatol.* 2011;31(7):477-480.

92. Gentamicin (Systemic) (Pediatric and Neonatal Lexi-Drugs). *UpToDate-Lexidrug.* Wolters Kluwer; April 2, 2024. Accessed April 4, 2024. https://online-lexi-com.ezproxy.lib.utah.edu/lco/action/search?q=gentamicin+systemic&t=name&acs=true&acq=gentamicin –

93. Dsouza V, Kothari N, Mishra U, et al. Reducing antibiotic use in asymptomatic term infants exposed to maternal chorioamnionitis: Predictive role of sepsis risk calculator. *J Paediatr Child Health.* 2022;58(11).

94. Kaplan M, Wong RJ, Bensen R, Sibley E, Stevenson DK. Neonatal jaundice and liver disease. In: Martin RJ, Fanaroff AA, Walsh MC, eds. *Fanaroff and Martin's Neonatal-Perinatal Medicine: Diseases of the Fetus and Infant.* 12th ed. Elsevier; 2025: 1874-1877.

95. Buendia M, Thoni N. Gastroenterology. In: Kleinman K, Mcdaniel L, Molloy M, eds. *The Harriet Lane Handbook.* 22nd ed. Elsevier; 2021: 283-299.

96. Wright CJ, Posencheg MA, Seri I. Fluid, electrolyte, and acid-base balance. In: Gleason CA, Sawyer T, eds. *Avery's Diseases of the Newborn*. 11th ed. Elsevier; 2024: 231-252.

97. Curtis SN. Fluid, electrolytes, and acid-base homeostasis. In: Martin RJ, Fanaroff AA, Walsh MC, eds. *Fanaroff and Martin's Neonatal-Perinatal Medicine: Diseases of the Fetus and Infant*. 12th ed. Elsevier; 2025: 1948-1965.

98. Vogt BA. The kidney and urinary tract of the neonate. In: Martin RJ, Fanaroff AA, Walsh MC, eds. *Fanaroff and Martin's Neonatal-Perinatal Medicine: Diseases of the Fetus and Infant*. 12th ed. Elsevier; 2025: 1966-1989.

99. Workeneh BT, Agraharkar M, Gupta R, Lederer E, Batuman V. Acute kidney injury (AKI). Medscape. Updated December 10, 2022. Accessed August 14, 2022. https://emedicine.medscape.com/article/243492-overview.

100. Wandrup J, Kroner J, Pryds O, Kastrup KW. Age-related reference values for ionized calcium in the first week of life in premature and full-term neonates. *Scand J Clin Lab Invest*. 1988;48(3):255-260.

101. Loughead JL, Mimouni F, Tsang RC. Serum ionized calcium concentrations in normal neonates. *Am J Dis Child*. 1988;142(5):516-518.

102. Andropoulos DB, Dunbar BS, Shekerdemian LS, Checchia PA, Chang AC. Cardiovascular intensive care. In: Shaddy RE, Penny DJ, Feltes TF, Cetta F, Mital S, eds. *Moss and Adams' Heart Disease in Infants, Children, and Adolescents*. 10th ed. Wolters Kluwer; 2022: 627-677.

103. Namgung R, Tsang RC. Neonatal calcium, phosphorus, and magnesium homeostasis. In: Polin RA, Fox WW, Abman SH, eds. *Fetal and Neonatal Physiology*. 4th ed. Elsevier Saunders; 2011: 384-402.

104. Abrams SA, Tiosano D. Disorders of calcium, phosphorus, and magnesium metabolism in the neonate. In: Martin RJ, Fanaroff AA, Walsh MC, eds. *Fanaroff and Martin's Neonatal-Perinatal Medicine: Diseases of the Fetus and Infant*. 12th ed. Elsevier; 2025: 1697-1727.

105. Cannon B, Snyder CS. Disorders of cardiac rhythm and conduction in newborns In: Martin RJ, Fanaroff AA, Walsh MC, eds. *Fanaroff and Martin's Neonatal-Perinatal Medicine: Diseases of the Fetus and Infant*. 12th ed. Elsevier; 2025: 1452-1469.

106. Bodamer OA. Neuromuscular junction disorders in newborns and infants. In: Patterson MC, Goddeau RP, eds. *UpToDate*. Wolters Kluwer; Updated August 10, 2023. Accessed December 5, 2023. https://www-uptodate: neuromuscular-junction-disorders-in-newborns-and-infants.

107. Owusu-Ansah A, Letterio J, Ahuja SP. Red blood cell disorders in the fetus and neonate. In: Martin RJ, Fanaroff AA, Walsh MC, eds. *Fanaroff and Martin's Neonatal-Perinatal Medicine: Diseases of the Fetus and Infant*. 12th ed. Elsevier; 2025: 1520-1552.

108. MedlinePlus. Partial thromboplastin time (PTT) test. Updated December 15, 2022. Accessed January 11, 2024. https://medlineplus.gov/lab-tests/partial-thromboplastin-time-ptt-test/

109. MedlinePlus. Prothrombin time test and INR (PT/INR). Updated September 21, 2022. December 5, 2023. https://medlineplus.gov/lab-tests/prothrombin-time-test-and-inr-ptinr/

110. Zehnder JL. Clinical use of coagulation tests. In: Leung LLK, Tirnauer JS, eds. *UpToDate*. Wolters Kluwer; Updated December 29, 2023. Accessed January 11, 2023. https://www-uptodate-com. clinical-use-of-coagulation-tests

111. Tripathi N, Jialal I. Conjugated hyperbilirubinemia. StatPearls [Internet]. Updated July 24, 2023. Accessed December 5, 2023. https://www.ncbi.nlm.nih.gov/books/NBK562172/

112. Puopolo KM, Mukhopadhay S, Frymoyer A, Benitz WE. The term newborn: Early-onset sepsis. *Clin Perinatol*. 2021;48(3):471-484.

113. Rabi Y, Kowal D, Ambalavanan N. Blood gases: Technical aspects and interpretation. In: Goldsmith JP, Karotkin EH, Keszler M, Suresh GK, eds. *Assisted Ventilation of the Neonate*. 6th ed. Elsevier; 2017: 80-96.

114. American Heart Association. Part 9: Management of shock. In: Samson RA, Schexnayder SM, Hazinski MF, Meeks R, Knight LJ, eds. *Pediatric Advanced Life Support Provider Manual*. American Heart Association; 2016: 197-238.

115. American Heart Association. Part 3: Systematic Approach to the Seriously Ill or Injured Child. In: Samson RA, Schexnayder SM, Hazinski MF, Meeks R, Knight LJ, eds. *Pediatric Advanced Life Support Provider Manual*. American Heart Association; 2016: 29-67.

116. Tung S. Pulmonology and sleep medicine. In: Kleinman K, Mcdaniel L, Molloy M, eds. *The Harriet Lane Handbook*. 22nd ed. Elsevier; 2021: 586-605.

117. Keszler M, Abubakar K. Physiologic principles. In: Goldsmith JP, Karotkin EH, Keszler M, Suresh GK, eds. *Assisted Ventilation of the Neonate*. 6th ed. Elsevier; 2017: 8-30.

118. Nicks BA. Acute lactic acidosis. Medscape. Updated September 26, 2022. Accessed December 5, 2023. https://emedicine.medscape.com/article/768159-overview

119. Gunnerson KJ. Lactic Acidosis. Medscape. September 11, 2020. Accessed August 14, 2022. https://emedicine.medscape.com/article/167027-overview.

120. Greenwood JC, Orloski CJ. End points of sepsis resuscitation. *Emerg Med Clin North Am*. 2017;35(1):93-107.

121. Strimbu K, Tavel JA. What are biomarkers? *Current Opinion in HIV and AIDS*. 2010;5(6):463-466.

122. Biomarkers Definitions Working Group. Biomarkers and surrogate endpoints: Preferred definitions and conceptual framework. *Clin Pharmacol Ther*. 2001;69(3):89-95.

123. Christensen RD, Bradley PP, Rothstein G. The leukocyte left shift in clinical and experimental neonatal sepsis. *J Pediatr*. 1981;98(1):101-105.

124. Franz AR, Steinbach G, Kron M, Pohlandt F. Interleukin-8: A valuable tool to restrict antibiotic therapy in newborn infants. *Acta Paediatr*. 2001;90(9):1025-1032.

125. Ebenebe CU, Hesse F, Blohm ME, Jung R, Kunzmann S, Singer D. Diagnostic accuracy of interleukin-6 for early-onset sepsis in preterm neonates. *J Matern Fetal Neonatal Med*. 2021;34(2):253-258.

126. Resch B, Gusenleitner W, Muller WD. Procalcitonin and interleukin-6 in the diagnosis of early-onset sepsis of the neonate. *Acta Paediatr*. 2003;92(2):243-245.

127. Schelonka RL, Maheshwari A, Carlo WA, et al. T cell cytokines and the risk of blood stream infection in extremely low birth weight infants. *Cytokine*. 2011;53(2):249-255.

128. Hedegaard SS, Wisborg K, Hvas AM. Diagnostic utility of biomarkers for neonatal sepsis—A systematic review. *Infect Dis (Lond)*. 2015;47(3):117-124.

L Lab Work Module

129. Bohnhorst B, Lange M, Bartels DB, Bejo L, Hoy L, Peter C. Procalcitonin and valuable clinical symptoms in the early detection of neonatal late-onset bacterial infection. *Acta Paediatr.* 2012;101(1):19-25.

130. Bengner J, Quttineh M, Gaddlin PO, Salomonsson K, Faresjo M. Serum amyloid A - A prime candidate for identification of neonatal sepsis. *Clin Immunol.* 2021;(229):108787.

131. Newman TB, Draper D, Puopolo KM, Wi S, Escobar GJ. Combining immature and total neutrophil counts to predict early onset sepsis in term and late preterm newborns: Use of the I/T2. *Pediatr Infect Dis J.* 2014;33(8):798-802.

132. Delanghe JR, Speeckaert MM. Translational research and biomarkers in neonatal sepsis. *Clin Chim Acta.* 2015;451(Pt A):46-64.

133. Steinberger E, Hofer N, Resch B. Cord blood procalcitonin and Interleukin-6 are highly sensitive and specific in the prediction of early-onset sepsis in preterm infants. *Scand J Clin Lab Invest.* 2014;74(5):432-436.

134. Cobo T, Kacerovsky M, Andrys C, et al. Umbilical cord blood IL-6 as predictor of early-onset neonatal sepsis in women with preterm prelabour rupture of membranes. *PLoS One.* 2013;8(7):e69341.

135. Howman RA, Charles AK, Jacques A, et al. Inflammatory and haematological markers in the maternal, umbilical cord and infant circulation in histological chorioamnionitis. *PLoS One.* 2012;7(12):e51836.

136. Chiesa C, Signore F, Assumma M, et al. Serial measurements of C-reactive protein and interleukin-6 in the immediate postnatal period: Reference intervals and analysis of maternal and perinatal confounders. *Clin Chem.* 2001;47(6):1016-1022.

137. Chiesa C, Pellegrini G, Panero A, et al. C-reactive protein, interleukin-6, and procalcitonin in the immediate postnatal period: Influence of illness severity, risk status, antenatal and perinatal complications, and infection. *Clin Chem.* 2003;49(1):60-68.

138. Buhimschi CS, Bhandari V, Dulay AT, et al. Proteomics mapping of cord blood identifies haptoglobin "switch-on" pattern as biomarker of early-onset neonatal sepsis in preterm newborns. *PLoS One.* 2011;6(10):e26111.

139. Fan Y, Yu JL. Umbilical blood biomarkers for predicting early-onset neonatal sepsis. *World J Pediatr.* 2012;8(2):101-108.

140. Kothari A, Morgan M, Haake DA. Emerging technologies for rapid identification of bloodstream pathogens. *Clin Infect Dis.* 2014;59(2):272-278.

141. Altunhan H, Annagur A, Ors R, Mehmetoglu I. Procalcitonin measurement at 24 hours of age may be helpful in the prompt diagnosis of early-onset neonatal sepsis. *Int J Infect Dis.* 2011;15(12):e854-858.

142. Mally P, Xu J, Hendricks-Munoz K. Biomarkers for neonatal sepsis: Recent developments. *Res Rep Neonatol.* 2014;2014(4):157-168.

143. Eschborn S, Weitkamp JH. Procalcitonin versus C-reactive protein: Review of kinetics and performance for diagnosis of neonatal sepsis. *J Perinatol.* 2019;39(7):893-903.

144. van der Hoeven A, van der Beek MT, Lopriore E, Steggerda SJ, Bekker V. Predicting neonatal early onset sepsis: A 14-year cohort study. *Pediatr Infect Dis J.* 2022;41(1):72-77.

145. Stocker M, van Herk W, El Helou S, et al. C-reactive protein, procalcitonin, and white blood count to rule out neonatal early-onset sepsis within 36 hours: A secondary analysis of the neonatal procalcitonin intervention study. *Clin Infect Dis.* 2021;73(2):e383-e390.

146. Stocker M, Hop WC, van Rossum AM. Neonatal Procalcitonin Intervention Study (NeoPInS): Effect of procalcitonin-guided decision making on duration of antibiotic therapy in suspected neonatal early-onset sepsis: A multi-centre randomized superiority and non-inferiority Intervention Study. *BMC Pediatr.* 2010;(10):89.

147. Kaapa P, Koistinen E. Maternal and neonatal C-reactive protein after interventions during delivery. *Acta Obstet Gynecol Scand.* 1993;72(7):543-546.

148. Kushner I, Antonelli M. Acute phase reactants. In: Furst DE, Seo P, eds. *UpToDate.* Wolters Kluwer; Updated March 13, 2023. Accessed December 5, 2023. https://pro.uptodatefree.ir/Show/7483

149. Celik IH, Demirel G, Canpolat FE, Erdeve O, Dilmen U. Inflammatory responses to hepatitis B virus vaccine in healthy term infants. *Eur J Pediatr.* 2013;172(6):839-842.

150. Chiesa C, Panero A, Rossi N, et al. Reliability of procalcitonin concentrations for the diagnosis of sepsis in critically ill neonates. *Clin Infect Dis.* 1998;26(3):664-672.

151. Arnon S, Litmanovitz I. Diagnostic tests in neonatal sepsis. *Curr Opin Infect Dis.* 2008;21(3):223-227.

152. Wang J, Wang Z, Zhang M, Lou Z, Deng J, Li Q. Diagnostic value of mean platelet volume for neonatal sepsis: A systematic review and meta-analysis. *Medicine (Baltimore).* 2020;99(32):e21649.

153. Christensen RD, Yoder BA, Baer VL, Snow GL, Butler A. Early-onset neutropenia in small-for-gestational-age infants. *Pediatrics.* 2015;136(5):e1259-1267.

154. Engle WA, McGuire WA, Schreiner RL, Yu PL. Neutrophil storage pool depletion in neonates with sepsis and neutropenia. *J Pediatr.* 1988;113(4):747-749.

155. Carballo C, Foucar K, Swanson P, Papile LA, Watterberg KL. Effect of high altitude on neutrophil counts in newborn infants. *J Pediatr.* 1991;119(3):464-466.

E Emotional Support Module

Als H, Duffy FH, McAnulty GB. Effectiveness of individualized neurodevelopmental care in the newborn intensive care unit (NICU). *Acta Paediatr Suppl.* 1996;(416):21-30.

Als H, Gilkerson L. The role of relationship-based developmentally supportive newborn intensive care in strengthening outcome of preterm infants. *Semin Perinatol.* 1997;21(3):178-89.

Billimoria ZC, Woodward GA. Neonatal transport. In: Gleason CA, Sawyer T, eds. *Avery's Diseases of the Newborn.* 11th ed. Elsevier; 2024: 217-229.

Boundy EO, Dastjerdi R, Spiegelman D, et al. Kangaroo mother care and neonatal outcomes: A meta-analysis. *Pediatrics.* 2016;137(1):1-16.

Brandon D, McGrath JM. Missed caregiving: A call to action for health system leadership. *Adv Neonatal Care.* 2022;22(5):379-380.

Caporali C, Pisoni C, Gasparini L, et al. A global perspective on parental stress in the neonatal intensive care unit: a meta-analytic study. *J Perinatol.* 2020;40(12):1739-1752.

ⓔ Emotional Support Module

Carty CL, Soghier LM, Kritikos KI, et al. The giving parents support study: A randomized clinical trial of a parent navigator intervention to improve outcomes after neonatal intensive care unit discharge. *Contemp Clin Trials*. 2018;70:117-134.

Chan GJ, Valsangkar B, Kajeepeta S, Boundy EO, Wall S. What is kangaroo mother care? Systematic review of the literature. *J Glob Health*. 2016;6(1):010701.

Dodge A, Gibson C, Williams M, Ross K. Exploring the needs and coping strategies of New Zealand parents in the neonatal environment. *J Paediatr Child Health*. 2022;58(6):1060-1065.

Fratantoni K, Soghier L, Kritikos K, et al. Giving parents support: A randomized trial of peer support for parents after NICU discharge. *J Perinatol*. 2022;42(6):730-737.

Friedman SH, Thomson-Salo F, Ballard AR. Support for the family. In: Martin RJ, Fanaroff AA, Walsh MC, eds. *Fanaroff and Martin's Neonatal-Perinatal Medicine: Diseases of the Fetus and Infant*. 12th ed. Elsevier; 2025: 739-751.

Gardner SL, Carter BS. Grief and perinatal loss. In: Gardner S, Carter BS, Enzman-Hines M, Niermeyer S, eds. *Merenstein & Gardner's Handbook of Neonatal Intensive Care*. 9th ed. Elsevier; 2021: 1096-1140.

Gardner SL, Voos K. Families in crisis: Theoretical and practical considerations. In: Gardner S, Carter, BS, Enzman-Hines M, Niermeyer S, eds. *Merenstein & Gardner's Handbook of Neonatal Intensive Care*. 9th ed. Elsevier; 2021: 1039-1095.

Holm KG, Aagaard H, Maastrup R, et al. How to support fathers of preterm infants in early parenthood - An integrative review. *J Pediatr Nurs*. 2022;(67):e38-e47.

Kim AR, Kim SY, Yun JE. Attachment and relationship-based interventions for families during neonatal intensive care hospitalization: A study protocol for a systematic review and meta-analysis. *Syst Rev*. 2020;9(1):61.

Kleinman ME. Neonatal transport. In: Eichenwald EC, Hansen AR, Martin CR, Stark AR, eds. *Cloherty and Stark's Manual of Neonatal Care*. 9th ed. Wolters Kluwer; 2023: 208-221.

Lefkowitz DS, Baxt C, Evans JR. Prevalence and correlates of posttraumatic stress and postpartum depression in parents of infants in the neonatal intensive care unit (NICU). *J Clin Psychol Med Settings*. 2010;17(3):230-7.

Macho P. Individualized developmental care in the NICU: A concept analysis. *Adv Neonatal Care*. 2017;17(3):162-174.

McCarty DB. Recognizing our biases, understanding the evidence, and responding equitably: Application of the socioecological model to reduce racial disparities in the NICU. *Adv Neonatal Care*. 2023;23(1):31-39.

Moore ER, Bergman N, Anderson GC, Medley N. Early skin-to-skin contact for mothers and their healthy newborn infants. *Cochrane Database Syst Rev*. 2016;11(11):CD003519.

National Perinatal Association. *Transcultural Aspects of Perinatal Care: A Resource Guide*. American Academy of Pediatrics; 2004.

Noergaard B, Ammentorp J, Garne E, Fenger-Gron J, Kofoed PE. Fathers' stress in a neonatal intensive care unit. *Adv Neonatal Care*. 2018;18(5):413-422.

Okito O, Yui Y, Wallace L, et al. Parental resilience and psychological distress in the neonatal intensive care unit. *J Perinatol*. 2022;42(11):1504-1511.

Ortiz R, Sibinga EM. The role of mindfulness in reducing the adverse effects of childhood stress and trauma. *Children (Basel)*. 2017;4(3):16.

Prouhet PM, Gregory MR, Russell CL, Yaeger LH. Fathers' stress in the neonatal intensive care unit: A systematic review. *Adv Neonatal Care*. 2018;18(2):105-120.

Ricciardi S, Blatz MA. Developmental care - Understanding and applying the science. In: Fanaroff AA, Fanaroff JM, eds. *Klaus and Fanaroff's Care of the High-Risk Neonate*. 7th ed. Elsevier; 2020: 171-189.

Rossen L, Hutchinson D, Wilson J, et al. Predictors of postnatal mother-infant bonding: The role of antenatal bonding, maternal substance use and mental health. *Arch Womens Ment Health*. 2016;19(4):609-22.

Sanders MR, Hall SL. Trauma-informed care in the newborn intensive care unit: Promoting safety, security and connectedness. *J Perinatol*. 2018;38(1):3-10.

Soghier LM, Kritikos KI, Carty CL, et al. Parental depression symptoms at neonatal intensive care unit discharge and associated risk factors. *J Pediatr*. 2020;(227):163-169.e1.

Torr C. Culturally competent care in the neonatal intensive care unit, strategies to address outcome disparities. *J Perinatol*. 2022;42(10):1424-1427.

Trombetta T, Giordano M, Santoniccolo F, Vismara L, Della Vedova AM, Rolle L. Pre-natal attachment and parent-to-infant attachment: A systematic review. *Front Psychol*. 2021;(12):620942.

Younge T, Jacobs M, Tuchman L, Streisand R, Soghier L, Fratantoni K. Sociodemographic risk factors, parental stress and social support in the neonatal intensive care unit. *Arch Dis Child Fetal Neonatal Ed*. 2023;108(2):165-169.

ⓠ Quality Improvement Module

1. Gupta M, Posencheg M. Patient safety and quality improvement. In: Eichenwald EC, Hansen AR, Martin CR, Stark AR, eds. *Cloherty and Stark's Manual of Neonatal Care*. 9th ed. Wolters Kluwer; 2023: 1104-1119.

2. Lapcharoensap W, Lee HC. Tackling quality improvement in the delivery room. *Clin Perinatol*. 2017;44(3):663-681.

3. James JT. A new, evidence-based estimate of patient harms associated with hospital care. *J Patient Saf*. 2013;9(3):122-8.

4. Kohn LT, Corrigan JM, Donaldson MS, Committee on Quality of Health Care in America. *To Err is Human: Building a Safer Health Care System*. National Academy Press; 2000.

5. Yamada NK, Yaeger KA, Halamek LP. Analysis and classification of errors made by teams during neonatal resuscitation. *Resuscitation*. 2015;96:109-13.

6. Weingart C, Herstich T, Baker P, et al. Making good better: Implementing a standardized handoff in pediatric transport. *Air Med J*. 2013;32(1):40-6.

7. Sawyer T, Lee HC, Aziz K. Anticipation and preparation for every delivery room resuscitation. *Semin Fetal Neonatal Med*. 2018;23(5):312-320.

8. Epps HR, Levin PE. The TeamSTEPPS approach to safety and quality. *J Pediatr Orthop*. 2015;35(5 Suppl 1):S30-3.

9. Natafgi N, Zhu X, Baloh J, Vellinga K, Vaughn T, Ward MM. Critical access hospital use of TeamSTEPPS to implement shift-change handoff communication. *J Nurs Care Qual*. 2017;32(1):77-86.

10. Reed T, Horsley TL, Muccino K, et al. Simulation using TeamSTEPPS to promote interprofessional education and collaborative practice. *Nurse Educ*. 2017;42(3):E1-E5.

Quality Improvement Module

11. Yamada NK, Fuerch JH, Halamek LP. Impact of standardized communication techniques on errors during simulated neonatal resuscitation. *Am J Perinatol*. 2016;33(4):385-92.

12. Litke-Wager C, Delaney H, Mu T, Sawyer T. Impact of task-oriented role assignment on neonatal resuscitation performance: A simulation-based randomized controlled trial. *Am J Perinatol*. 2021;38(9):914-921.

13. Halamek LP. Using simulation to support evidence-based design of safer health care environments. *Am J Perinatol*. November 11, 2022.

14. Katakam L, Suresh GK. Identifying a quality improvement project. *J Perinatol*. 2017;37(10):1161-1165.

15. Hollnagel E, Wears RL, Braithwaite J. *From Safety-I to Safety-II: A White Paper*. 2015:1-43.

16. The Joint Commission. Sentinel Event Alert 30: Preventing infant death and injury during delivery. July 21, 2004. Accessed January 11, 2024. https://www.jointcommission.org/resources/sentinel-event/sentinel-event-alert-newsletters/sentinel-event-alert-issue-30-preventing-infant-death-and-injury-during-delivery/

17. Sawyer T, Gray MM. Procedural training and assessment of competency utilizing simulation. *Semin Perinatol*. 2016;40(7):438-446.

18. Anderson JM, Warren JB. Using simulation to enhance the acquisition and retention of clinical skills in neonatology. *Semin Perinatol*. 2011;35(2):59-67.

19. Merien AE, van de Ven J, Mol BW, Houterman S, Oei SG. Multidisciplinary team training in a simulation setting for acute obstetric emergencies: A systematic review. *Obstet Gynecol*. 2010;115(5):1021 31.

20. Draycott TJ, Crofts JF, Ash JP, et al. Improving neonatal outcome through practical shoulder dystocia training. *Obstet Gynecol*. 2008;112(1):14-20.

21. Lindhard MS, Thim S, Laursen HS, Schram AW, Paltved C, Henriksen TB. Simulation-based neonatal resuscitation team training: A systematic review. *Pediatrics*. 2021;147(4):e2020042010.

22. Sawyer T, Stavroudis TA, Ades A, et al. Simulation in neonatal-perinatal medicine fellowship programs. *Am J Perinatol*. 2020;37(12):1258-1263.

23. Sawyer T, Eppich W, Brett-Fleegler M, Grant V, Cheng A. More than one way to debrief: A critical review of healthcare simulation debriefing methods. *Simul Healthc*. 2016;11(3):209-17.

24. Sawyer T, Umoren RA, Gray MM. Neonatal resuscitation: Advances in training and practice. *Adv Med Educ Pract*. 2017;(8):11-19.

25. Lapcharoensap W, Bennett MV, Powers RJ, et al. Effects of delivery room quality improvement on premature infant outcomes. *J Perinatol*. 2017;37(4):349-354.

26. Fioratou E, Flin R, Glavin R. No simple fix for fixation errors: Cognitive processes and their clinical applications. *Anaesthesia*. 2010;65(1):61-9.

27. Halamek LP, Weiner GM. State-of-the art training in neonatal resuscitation. *Semin Perinatol*. 2022;46(6):151628.

28. Yousef N, Moreau R, Soghier L. Simulation in neonatal care: Towards a change in traditional training? *Eur J Pediatr*. 2022;181(4):1429-1436.

29. Bhola M. Importance of simulation in neonatology. In: Martin RJ, Fanaroff AA, Walsh MC, eds. *Fanaroff and Martin's Neonatal-Perinatal Medicine: Diseases of the Fetus and Infant*. 12th ed. Elsevier; 2025: 100-107.

30. Kolbe M, Eppich W, Rudolph J, et al. Managing psychological safety in debriefings: A dynamic balancing act. *BMJ Simul Technol Enhanc Learn*. 2020;6(3):164-171.

31. Rudolph JW, Raemer DB, Simon R. Establishing a safe container for learning in simulation: The role of the presimulation briefing. *Simul Healthc*. 2014;9(6):339-49.

32. Gaba DM, Howard SK, Fish KJ, Smith BE, Sowb YA. Simulation-based training in anesthesia crisis resource management (ACRM): A decade of experience. *Simulation & Gaming*. 2001;32(2):175-193.

33. Rudolph JW, Simon R, Raemer DB, Eppich WJ. Debriefing as formative assessment: Closing performance gaps in medical education. *Acad Emerg Med*. 2008;15(11):1010-6.

34. Halamek LP, Cady RAH, Sterling MR. Using briefing, simulation and debriefing to improve human and system performance. *Semin Perinatol*. 2019;43(8):151178.

35. Hughes KM, Benenson RS, Krichten AE, Clancy KD, Ryan JP, Hammond C. A crew resource management program tailored to trauma resuscitation improves team behavior and communication. *J Am Coll Surg*. 2014;219(3):545-51.

36. Berwick DM, Leape LL. Reducing errors in medicine. *Qual Health Care*. 1999;8(3):145-6.

37. Reason J. Human error: Models and management. *BMJ*. 2000;320(7237):768-70.

38. Shepherd M. Improving health care systems following an incident investigation. *Conf Proc IEEE Eng Med Biol Soc*. 2004;(5):3500-2.

39. Yamada NK, Kamlin COF, Halamek LP. Optimal human and system performance during neonatal resuscitation. *Semin Fetal Neonatal Med*. 2018;23(5):306-311.

40. Yamada NK, Catchpole K, Salas E. The role of human factors in neonatal patient safety. *Semin Perinatol*. 2019;43(8):151174.

41. Bell T, Sprajcer M, Flenady T, Sahay A. Fatigue in nurses and medication administration errors: A scoping review. *J Clin Nurs*. 2023;32(17-18):5445-5460.

42. Liu KW, Shih YF, Chiang YJ, et al. Reducing medication errors in children's hospitals. *J Patient Saf*. 2023; 19(3):151-157.

43. Culbreth RE, Spratling R, Scates L, Frederick L, Kenney J, Gardenhire DS. Associations between safety perceptions and medical error reporting among neonatal intensive care unit staff. *J Clin Nurs*. 2021;30(21-22):3230-3237.

44. Wolfe AHJ, Hinds PS, du Plessis AJ, Gordish-Dressman H, Arnold RM, Soghier L. Defining objective measures of physician stress in simulated critical communication encounters. *Crit Care Explor*. 2022;4(7):e0721.

45. Eppich W. "Speaking Up" for patient safety in the pediatric emergency department. *Clinical Pediatric Emergency Medicine*. 2015;16(2):83-89.

46. Riskin A, Erez A, Foulk TA, et al. The impact of rudeness on medical team performance: A randomized trial. *Pediatrics*. 2015;136(3):487-95.

47. Gougoulis A, Trawber R, Hird K, Sweetman G. 'Take 10 to talk about it': Use of a scripted, post-event debriefing tool in a neonatal intensive care unit. *J Paediatr Child Health*. 2020;56(7):1134-1139.

48. Coggins A, Hong SS, Baliga K, Halamek LP. Immediate faculty feedback using debriefing timing data and conversational diagrams. *Adv Simul (Lond)*. 2022;7(1):7.

49. Rudolph JW, Simon R, Dufresne RL, Raemer DB. There's no such thing as "nonjudgmental" debriefing: A theory and method for debriefing with good judgment. *Simul Healthc*. 2006;1(1):49-55.

50. Ahmad FB, Anderson RN. The leading causes of death in the US for 2020. *Jama*. 2021;325(18):1829-1830.

51. Gupta M, Kaplan HC. Measurement for quality improvement: Using data to drive change. *J Perinatol*. 2020;40(6):962-971.

52. Howell EA, Zeitlin J. Quality of care and disparities in obstetrics. *Obstet Gynecol Clin North Am*. 2017;44(1):13-25.

53. Schwartz HP, Bigham MT, Schoettker PJ, Meyer K, Trautman MS, Insoft RM, American Academy of Pediatrics Section on Transport M. Quality metrics in neonatal and pediatric critical care transport: A national delphi project. *Pediatr Crit Care Med*. 2015;16(8):711-7.

54. Crane S, Sloane PD, Elder NC, Cohen LW, Laughtenschlager N, Zimmrman S. Advances in patient safety and medical liability. Implementing near-miss reporting and improvement tracking in primary care practices: Lessons learned. Agency for Healthcare Research and Quality. August, 2017. Accessed April 12, 2024. https://www.ahrq.gov/patient-safety/reports/liability/crane.html#:~:text=Near%2Dmiss%20events%20are%20errors,before%20a%20patient%20is%20harmed

The letter f after a page number indicates a figure and the letter t indicates a table.